Communicating Rare Diseases and Disorders in the Digital Age

Liliana Vale Costa
University of Aveiro, Portugal

Sónia Oliveira
University of Aveiro, Portugal

A volume in the Advances in Medical Technologies and Clinical Practice (AMTCP) Book Series

IGI Global
DISSEMINATOR OF KNOWLEDGE

Published in the United States of America by
IGI Global
Medical Information Science Reference (an imprint of IGI Global)
701 E. Chocolate Avenue
Hershey PA, USA 17033
Tel: 717-533-8845
Fax: 717-533-8661
E-mail: cust@igi-global.com
Web site: http://www.igi-global.com

Library of Congress Cataloging-in-Publication Data

Names: Costa, Liliana Vale, editor. | Oliveira, Sónia, 1986- editor.
Title: Communicating rare diseases and disorders in the digital age / Liliana Vale Costa, Sónia Oliveira, editors.
Description: Hershey, PA : Medical Information Science Reference, [2020] | Includes bibliographical references and index. | Summary: "This book explores the use of computer-mediated communication in rare diseases and disorders"-- Provided by publisher.
Identifiers: LCCN 2019036436 (print) | LCCN 2019036437 (ebook) | ISBN 9781799820888 (hardcover) | ISBN 9781799820895 (ebook)
Subjects: MESH: Rare Diseases | Health Communication | Social Media
Classification: LCC RA971.6 (print) | LCC RA971.6 (ebook) | NLM QZ 140 | DDC 362.10285--dc23
LC record available at https://lccn.loc.gov/2019036436
LC ebook record available at https://lccn.loc.gov/2019036437

This book is published in the IGI Global book series Advances in Medical Technologies and Clinical Practice (AMTCP) (ISSN: 2327-9354; eISSN: 2327-9370)

British Cataloguing in Publication Data
A Cataloguing in Publication record for this book is available from the British Library.

Advances in Medical Technologies and Clinical Practice (AMTCP) Book Series

ISSN:2327-9354
EISSN:2327-9370

MISSION

Medical technological innovation continues to provide avenues of research for faster and safer diagnosis and treatments for patients. Practitioners must stay up to date with these latest advancements to provide the best care for nursing and clinical practices.

The **Advances in Medical Technologies and Clinical Practice (AMTCP) Book Series** brings together the most recent research on the latest technology used in areas of nursing informatics, clinical technology, biomedicine, diagnostic technologies, and more. Researchers, students, and practitioners in this field will benefit from this fundamental coverage on the use of technology in clinical practices.

COVERAGE

- Medical Imaging
- Diagnostic Technologies
- Clinical High-Performance Computing
- Telemedicine
- Clinical Studies
- Clinical Data Mining
- Neural Engineering
- Biometrics
- E-Health
- Nutrition

Titles in this Series

For a list of additional titles in this series, please visit:
https://www.igi-global.com/book-series/advances-medical-technologies-clinical-practice/73682

Exploring the Role of ICTs in Healthy Aging
David Mendes (Universidade de Évora, Portugal) César Fonseca (Universidade de Évora, Portugal) Manuel José Lopes (Universidade de Évora, Portugal) José García-Alonso (University of Coimbra, Spain) and Juan Manuel Murillo (University of Coimbra, Spain)
Medical Information Science Reference • © 2020 • 300pp • H/C (ISBN: 9781799819370) • US $285.00

Artificial Intelligence Paradigms in Smart Health Informatics Systems
Abdel-Badeeh M. Salem (Ain Shams University, Egypt) and Senthil Kumar A V (Hindusthan College of Arts and Science, India)
Medical Information Science Reference • © 2020 • 300pp • H/C (ISBN: 9781799811015) • US $265.00

Incorporating the Internet of Things in Healthcare Applications and Wearable Devices
P. B. Pankajavalli (Bharathiar University, India) and G. S. Karthick (Bharathiar University, India)
Medical Information Science Reference • © 2020 • 288pp • H/C (ISBN: 9781799810902) • US $285.00

Impacts of Information Technology on Patient Care and Empowerment
Roger W. McHaney (Kansas State University, USA) Iris Reychev (Ariel University, Israel) Joseph Azuri (Maccabi Healthcare Services, Israel) Mark E. McHaney (U.S. Air Force, USA) and Rami Moshonov (Assuta Medical Centers, Israel)
Medical Information Science Reference • © 2020 • 452pp • H/C (ISBN: 9781799800477) • US $295.00

Handbook of Research on Clinical Applications of Computerized Occlusal Analysis in Dental Medicine
Robert B. Kerstein, DMD (Tufts University School of Dental Medicine, USA & Private Dental Practice Limited to Prosthodontics and Computerized Occlusal Analysis, USA)

For an entire list of titles in this series, please visit:
https://www.igi-global.com/book-series/advances-medical-technologies-clinical-practice/73682

IGI Global
DISSEMINATOR OF KNOWLEDGE

701 East Chocolate Avenue, Hershey, PA 17033, USA
Tel: 717-533-8845 x100 • Fax: 717-533-8661
E-Mail: cust@igi-global.com • www.igi-global.com

Editorial Advisory Board

Table of Contents

Detailed Table of Contents

access to healthcare, and their quality of life may be affected. A key challenge is also the physician-patient interaction that differs from traditional medical care settings by demanding physicians' experience in dealing, for example, with psychological problems associated with the diagnosis process. Information and Communication Technologies can facilitate the interaction between the sources of information and patients, overcoming geographical distances. This chapter discusses the role of Information and Communication to extract health data in rare diseases and reinforce physician-patient interactions. It argues that Information and Communication are crucial to meet patients' needs, drivers, and decision-making that tend to occur during the patient's journey (pre-diagnosis, diagnosis, and post-diagnosis).

Chapter 3
Designing Sustainable Social Media Health Communication Campaigns for Promoting Rare Diseases 113
Isabell Koinig, University of Klagenfurt, Austria
Sandra Diehl, University of Klagenfurt, Austria

The third goal of the United Nations Sustainable Development Agenda aims to ensure individual's wellbeing and a long and healthy life. As such, health is perceived as an essential part of sustainable development. While progress has been made over the past decades, far too little attention has been paid to misdiagnosed and rare diseases. In the context of promoting "health for all", communication is of uttermost importance. By means of a content analysis for selected rare disease campaigns, the present contribution seeks to highlight the way the UN's health goal is communicated as part of health campaigns for rare diseases. Amongst others, this chapter sets out to understand how the goal is communicated, which aspects are stressed, and whether there are differences in message strategies across different platforms relative to rare diseases. Ultimately, the potential of social media for communicating rare diseases is carved out. Research limitations and directions for future research are also addressed.

Chapter 4
Digital Media in Rare Diseases or "Knowledge Is Power": The Role of EURORDIS in Creating Awareness and Diagnosing Rare Diseases 154
Célia Felícia Belim Rodrigues, Instituto Superior de Ciências Sociais e Políticas, Universidade de Lisboa, Portugal

This chapter focuses on the use of digital media by EURORDIS-Rare Diseases Europe and is specifically committed to understand its contribution to the awareness and diagnosis of rare diseases. To perceive the use of digital media and role in creating awareness of rare diseases, the contents of its website and Facebook page were analyzed. In specific, a promotional video of EURORDIS and a collection of 12 videographically documented stories from 2018 and 2019. The results show

the use of various types of content and inherently practices, such as information, clarification, personalization, support, appeal, and empowerment, and of several rhetorical resources. In the dimension of pathos, the author finds elements that motivate awareness and inspire the receiver. Some elements of the logos used are credibility of sender(ethos), testimony (ethos), description of disease and identification of symptoms, exemplification and personalization, factual data, statistic data, and the use of metaphors and repetition.

Rare diseases and disorders are, as the names suggest, a strange or unusual health condition, and so the coverage given by the media is not as extensive as it could be. However, researchers point out that this situation is changing little by little, and there is now more information about those who suffer from these conditions, and their experience. It is quite interesting to see how the public media, especially in the case of Spain, are making a great effort to give a voice and space to people affected by such diseases. In the case of public media, there are many other aspects to be considered. Firstly, the Spanish Broadcasting Corporation, Radio Televisión Española (RTVE) is not tied to private finance. Secondly, these channels are expected to be more independent and, subsequently, there may be no additional pressure to reach high audience share or obtain external funding from private media companies. This is especially interesting in the case of radio broadcasting, as it tends to be a medium with a high level of credibility, and closeness to the audience.

There are more than 360 associations of patients with rare diseases in Spain that strive for visibility to obtain funding and encourage clinical pathologies. The Spanish Year of Rare Diseases has been a considerable effort to be part of media agenda since 2013 and a "collective voice" throughout the media has been encouraged with the international initiatives devoted to the cause. Over the past years, representation of patients with rare diseases in Spanish media has been very superficial, despite the renewed interest during the Spanish Year of Rare Diseases. Certain cases as "Paco Sanz" or "Los Padres de la Pequeña Nadia" have negatively affected this representation by using the disease to pursue economic benefit. This chapter reports on the representation of rare diseases through Spanish media and the way it evolved

The neuropsychiatric adult onset Tay-Sachs disease is relatively unknown. Although clinical features and mode of presentation are variable, there are common symptoms and signs of, for example, spinocerebellar atrophy, motor neuron disease, psychiatric disorder, and neuroimaging features of cerebellar atrophy. This chapter reviews the neuropsychiatric features of Late Onset Tay-Sachs disease, discussing possible interconnections between psychosis and the cerebellum in this disease. Understanding this interlink offers some important insights into the rarity of the disease that together with the diverse clinical onset and manifestations are responsible for a marked delay in diagnosis and even misdiagnosis. Genetic testing for the activity of Hexosaminidase A, prompted by the presence of cerebellar atrophy will establish the diagnosis. In all, the combination of cerebellar degeneration together with atypical psychiatric features is in line with the ongoing assumption that the cerebellum and its thalamo-cortical outflow are responsible for psychosis, and in particular, schizophrenia.

This chapter examines the portrayal of rare and misdiagnosed diseases in 9 movies from 1980 to 2018. The analysis embodies the representation of rare diseases and the suggested audiovisual strategies to comprehend the message conveyed. Most of the movies introduced the disease by highlighting its symptoms. The binomial culture of cure and care often emerges, as well as the patient's desire for the mundane pleasures in life and over dependence in a health system. The high hopes in research advances and lack of information are majorly covered in the caregivers' attempts to seek tests and drug trials and their mediator's role in patient-physician interactions. The audiovisual strategies adopted vary between the accelerated montage to communicate the contrast between the frenetic side of everyday life and the patient's process of coping with the disease, deep focus from patients to parents, and close-ups to show the individual's reactions and perspectives.

This decade, patients with chronic conditions take advantage of technological resources to share experiences, look for help, and get together in groups. Social media has become a productive spot of health information for users. This chapter clarifies the administrators' user experience of social media health groups within the context of the Inflammatory Bowel Disease (IBD). Semi-structured interviews with 7 Portuguese and Brazilian managers of Facebook groups were carried out. The authors propose a model of participation in online communities that take into account the variables of Presence–Interconnection between users in daily lives; Relationship–Aspects of experience where users meet; Reputation–Positioning of users related to the status; Groups–Relationship issues between members; Conversations – Extension of the user interaction; Sharing–Represents the exchange, distribution, and reception and Education–The information transmitted. Findings reinforced that administrators' groups use social media to lead patients´ empowerment.

Preface

INTRODUCTION

During the process of writing this preface, some headlines draw the attention in the media, such as "This Mom Is Buying Mutant Mice From China To Find A Cure For Her Son's Rare Genetic Disease."[1] This piece of news written by Dan Vergano to BuzzFeed News Reporter registers the story of a strong mother moving mountains in an attempt to find a cure for her son's rare genetic disease. SLC6A1 disease is so rare that the name simply consists of the designation of the affected gene, SLC6A1. Only about a hundred people in the world seems to have been diagnosed with this disease. Indeed, these parents often face many challenges shared by other parents of children with a rare disease: lack of sensitivity and awareness from clinicians, late diagnosis and late appropriate testing, emotional and psychological burdens from having to deal with a rare disease, stigma, lack of therapeutic solutions, and lack of peer-support groups as of parents with children with similar (or not) rare diseases; plus the financial burden. The readers would not possibly have access to this story without the use of digital media, a family willing to share it and a science reporter from an online media willing to listen and publish the content.[1]

Alongside this scenario, a major problem with rare diseases diagnosis is the lack of accurate information that, consequently, may lead to successive delays. Rare diseases patients often have to manage inaccurate treatments or rehabilitation interventions and, social and emotional consequences. Although attention has been increasingly drawn to rare diseases since the US Orphan Drug Act of 1983, there is still a long way to go. There are still enormous problems with studies design and the amount of conditions studied. The lack of patients' tracking and information about the diseases' causes and incidence add to this problem, as well as the "rarity" factor, i.e. the small pool of subjects to work with.

Health communication rely heavily on the expertise from the health professional/practitioners and, in such a broad spectrum of rare diseases, patients may find it hard to obtain timely information, accurate diagnosis, appropriate treatments and surgeries, medication or/and psychological counseling in their own countries. In fact, most health professionals probably will never encounter a rare disease patient throughout their careers. However, all clinicians should be informed and sensitive to the existence of rare conditions.

The use of Information and Communication Technologies (ICT) open up avenues for future research and development on health communication, pathophysiology, epidemiology, innovative provider-patient mediated interactions, rare diseases initiatives, media and health campaigns, biostatistics and public health monitoring. Indeed, ICT potential to facilitate interaction and overcome geographic distances is enormous when it comes to information seeking and sharing and disease coping and management. Thus, the potential to raise awareness and change the current paradigm is significant.

Rare diseases are often characterized by a low prevalence in general population. They can have a genetic origin or be environment-generated and are often debilitating and even life-threatening. An orphan disease, however, is not necessarily a rare disease. Orphan diseases may not fit into the rare disease definition, representing health conditions that are somewhat common but that lack effective treatments. Orphan diseases usually affect people in underdeveloped countries, and owing to economic and profit restrictions, there is a lack of investment on drugs and treatments. Whereas a rare disease affects a low proportion of patients in comparison with the total population of a country; considering that this is a small market, governments, physicians, patients, media and general community need to ensure patients' equitable access to the necessary therapies, treatments and drugs. Therefore, legislation and policies claiming such as a basic Human Right that is access to healthcare must be established and enforced worldwide.

The number of associations and institutions related to rare diseases has increased drastically in the last years. These new stakeholders are committed to improving rare disease patients' access to health care and support. Several initiatives are being undertaken throughout the year to raise awareness and funding for research and development. Moreover, besides the pathophysiology and etiology of rare diseases, investments have been made to improve the emotional and psychological burden of rare disease patients and caregivers. Information and Communication Technologies (ICT) have also been playing a key role in these interactions.

Such initiatives as the Rare Diseases Day (Feb 28th) rely significantly on ICT to spread a message and to raise awareness towards rare diseases. By using different media, this initiative highlights the need for better coordination of medical, social, and support services to decrease the burden that rare diseases – often complex, chronic, and disabling - have on the everyday lives of patients, their families, and caregivers. The interest in this topic by some scientific journals is also important in order promote investment into rare diseases research.

Indeed, rare diseases conditions often progress fast and are unmanageable, with very diverse causes – e.g. genetic, hereditary, infectious agents and other environmental factors. Furthermore, they involve different areas of expertise/ specialty - e.g. neurology, mental and behavioral disorders, endocrinology, among others - that only combined may decipher the epigenetic causes and find treatments to fight the disease.

Although there are thousands of rare diseases, only very few have designated treatments. The policies and investment on these diseases also vary from country to country. For example, a rare disease in the European Union and Australia is defined as affecting 1 in 2,000 people while in the USA to be considered rare it must affect 1 in 200,000 people, and 1 in 50,000 in Japan.

Given that we are living in a global society and the use of Information Communication Technologies have potential to empower rare disease patients and patients' organizations, there is hope that a shift in healthcare towards cures instead of treatments may occur. That way, gene therapies and epigenetics are likely to be key to improve healthcare systems and overpass the health burden.

A good sign is that despite the challenges in diagnosing, managing and treating rare diseases, progress is being made, and not only societies are more sensitive to the topic but pharmaceutical companies are also increasingly interested in these diseases. These latter may be owing to the financial and tax breaks incentives that orphan drug status offers. The number of requests for orphan designation and drugs granted for market authorization is on the rise, and that is a good indication of interest and progress. Progress has been made, particularly, for cancer and hematological disorders, but many stumbling blocks were turned into steppingstones in the management and treatment of other rare conditions, namely rare endocrine diseases.

Recently, U.S. Food and Drug Administration (FDA) issued their approval of a new drug against a rare disease, the second-ever drug based on RNAi (RNA interference) that can mute defective genes. The medicine approved is intended to treat a rare genetic condition entitled Acute Hepatic Porphyria that can cause attacks of severe abdominal pain. The drug givosiran, branded as Givlaari, will market at the 'reasonable' sum of $575,000 *per* year. The drug is intended to benefit just a small number of acute hepatic porphyria patients, who suffer from frequent attacks. Thus, the market pool is rather small. But the drug's approval is a good sign for other companies to develop drugs based on the RNAi technique and invest in rare disease problematics (FDA news release of 11/20/2019 "FDA approves first treatment for inherited rare disease"[2]). Rather than knowing these advances in the field from such direct information sources as FDA, most of the health stakeholders may have heard about this approval in different forums, as mentioned in Kate Sheridan's article in StatNews ("FDA approves Alnylam's Givlaari, second-ever drug based on RNAi, November 20th 2019[3]), or in rare diseases social media (e.g. Facebook) groups.

Therefore, the aim of this book is to provide theoretical and empirical research about the use of computer-mediated communication in rare diseases and disorders. It differs from other published books as it is transdisciplinary, bringing to the fore current advances in health communication, computer science and epidemiology. In addition, the book covers the following important issues in health-related communication and disease management: the use of social media and awareness to rare diseases, media coverage and the use of social networks to health support and care.

TARGET AUDIENCE

The target audience of this book are students, researchers, and practitioners with interests in health communication, rare diseases, technology-enabled health, epidemiology, information, social media, genetics, computer-mediated communication and marketing. As the book addresses health computer-mediated communication aspects and disease management, it will be beneficial to such stakeholders as physicians, patients, researchers, health professionals and practitioners, caregivers and decision-makers.

INSIDE THIS BOOK

The book 'Communicating Rare Diseases and Disorders in the Digital Age' combine different knowledge bases – *i.e.* a triadic interrelationship between the concepts of Health-related Communication, Rare Diseases and Information and Communication Technologies. This book is divided into 11 chapters, being structured as follows:

The book begins with the chapter "Talking about Rare Diseases: A Compendium on Rare Diseases and Online News." In this chapter, the difference between orphan and rare diseases is clarified and the common characteristics of rare diseases and coverage in online news are presented. In addition, the author provides an overview of the following rare diseases categories: Rare Diseases in Neurology, Rare Mental and Behavioral Disorders, Rare Diseases of the Endocrine System, Rare Diseases of the Immune System, Rare Eye and Ear Diseases, Rare Pulmonary Diseases, Rare Cardiac Diseases, Rare Vascular Diseases, Rare Hepatic Diseases, Rare Gastrointestinal Diseases, Rare Diseases of Genitourinary (or Urogenital) System, Rare Bacterial, Viral and Fungal Infections, Rare Allergic Diseases, Rare Skin Diseases, Rare Musculoskeletal Diseases, Rare Congenital and Genetic Diseases, Rare Diseases in Anesthesiology, Rare Diseases in Hematology, Rare Diseases of the Lymphatic System, Rare Nutritional and Metabolic Diseases, Rare Multisystemic Diseases,

Rare Gynecological and Obstetrical Diseases, Rare Tumors, Rare Diseases due to Plastic Surgery, Rare Diseases due to External Causes like Poisoning, General Surgery or Injury, Abnormal Clinical and Laboratory Findings, and Others. Some of the challenges in researching rare cancers and rare diseases diagnosis and treatment options are also summarized.

Chapter 2 entitled "Health-Related Communication and Rare Diseases: A Passport for the Patient Journey", the author discusses the role of Information and Communication Technologies to inform about rare diseases and strengthen the interactions between physicians, patients and caregivers. The author presents the patients' journey and the patients' needs, drivers, decision-making process and subsequent challenges that are posed during pre-diagnosis, diagnosis and post-diagnosis. Indeed, the different stages of the patient's journey involve such important variables as family communication, psychology, emotions and physician-patient social interactions, and communities in order obtain to health-related information and to cope with a rare disease.

In Chapter 3, the strategies for "Designing 'Sustainable' Social Media Health Communication Campaigns for Rare Diseases" are unraveled. Specifically, the communication goals, message strategies across different platforms and the role of social media are addressed in three different campaigns: Rare Disease Day, Ataxia and Epidermolysis Bullosa (EB) Campaigns. For each campaign, the authors analyze the informative appeals, visual appeals, cues to action, different types of social support (i.e. emotional, instrumental, informational and appraisal), and the channels and advertisements used in raising awareness for rare diseases. This Chapter proposes a set of recommendations for Health Care Marketers to design effective cross-media (health) campaigns within the socio-cultural context associated to rare diseases.

Chapter 4, "Digital Media in Rare Diseases or 'Knowledge is Power': The Role of EURORDIS in Creating Awareness and Diagnosing Rare Diseases," covers the use of digital media by the organization EURORDIS – Rare Diseases Europe. The content shared and practices of digital communication undertaken by this organization are analyzed, aiming at creating awareness and facilitating the process of diagnosis of rare diseases. Specifically, the content was analyzed in terms of persuasion – *ethos* (credibility of the sender of the message – *e.g.* medical/health professional), *pathos* (emotion aroused in the public that may encourage awareness, inspiration, empathy or curiosity) and *logos* (reasoning and arguments used).

Chapter 5 entitled "Public Media Coverage of Rare Diseases and Disorders: The Case of Spanish Public Broadcasting Corporation" highlights the duty of Public Broadcasting Corporations to inform and serve the audience. Focusing on the case of the Radio Televisión Española (RTVE), the study reports on the way health-related information about rare diseases are covered and the interconnection established with their audience in terms of visibility, credibility and intimacy.

Chapter 6, "Representation of Patients With Rare Diseases in Spanish Media," covers the use of social media in Spain to ensure association's visibility in order to obtain funding and be involved in both cure and treatment research. The author also reports the challenges that these patients' organizations face in terms of their reputation, given the very recent Spanish cases that negatively affected their representation – e.g. 'Paco Sanz' and 'Los Padres de La Pequeña Nadia.'

Chapter 7 entitled "Networks in Rare Diseases: Identities, Partnership, and Advocacy in Brazil" provides background on the status of Rare Diseases in Brazil. The authors draw attention to the fact that patient organizations are crucial actors in social movements, using social media to convey ideas and discourses that encourage lay expertise on rare diseases and shape patients' self-identity and triadic relationships involving patients-family and society.

Chapter 8 encompasses a discussion about the experience of parents with children afflicted by a rare disease. The chapter is entitled "Challenges of Parents With Children with Rare Diseases in Portugal: A Relational Perspective". This novel study in the Portuguese context describes the challenges experienced by the parental figures of children with rare diseases in Portugal. Parents of children with different rare disorders, including spina bifida, Angelman syndrome, Prader-Willi syndrome, Peters anomaly and osteogenesis imperfecta, were followed up. The authors discuss the differences in the perception and care of the children among the parental figures, as well as the influence of factors such as age and health of the relationship into the coping strategies adopted by the parents. This research identified several key factors into the coping strategies of parents at hands with a diagnose of a rare disease in a child. Additionally, the chapter contributes to a more complete and practical knowledge of the reality that rare diseases patients' caregivers may face. It draws attention to the family nucleus of a rare disease patient, highlighting the importance of the family and of a differentiated support plan for both parents. The authors stress the importance of an intervention plan for these families, which underline important changes in the current country's laws and guidelines to improve the health status and proper support of these patients, as well as of their carers.

In Chapter 9, "Neuropsychiatry in Late Onset Tay-Sachs Disease: Key Features and Possible Etiology of Psychosis," a case of late onset of the rare Tay-Sachs disease is reported. The author discusses a specific group of rare inherited diseases termed GM2 gangliosidoses. Within this group of three related genetic disorders, the author focuses in the most common Tay-Sachs disease. Tay-Sachs disease was one of the first rare diseases to benefit from a mass screening tool test in medical genetics, developed in the 1960s-1970s. Tay-Sachs causes the progressive degeneration of nerve cells resulting in compromised mental and physical abilities. The continuous progress in biological tools allowed to identify several late-onset variants of this disease that cause various neuropsychiatric conditions. Although anyone can be a carrier of Tay-Sachs disease, it is more prevalent among people of Ashkenazi (Eastern Europe) Jewish descendance. Early diagnosis stands as highly important to delay the worsen of the condition. In the chapter, the author discusses the interconnections between psychosis and the cerebellum of patients with this disease, based on a case of a patient with Late Onset Tay-Sachs (LOTS).

Chapter 10, "Portraying Rare and Misdiagnosed Diseases in Movies: A Content Analysis, 1980-2018," addresses the portrayal of rare and misdiagnosed diseases in movies, suggesting the audiovisual strategies that are possibly used to comprehend the message conveyed. Concerning the topics that are often covered, these vary between the overly dependence in a health system, high hopes in research and attempts to seek for drug trials and patients-physicians' interactions.

Chapter 11, "How Is the Administrator's Experience in Managing Health Facebook Groups? The Impact of Social Media on Patients With IBD," covers the online groups' administrators role in social media to help with Inflammatory Bowel Disease (IBD) information gathering, communication and management. The authors analyze IBD Facebook groups in Portugal and Brazil accordingly with a model of participation in online communities and taking into account the variables of Presence (The interconnection with patient's daily lives), Relationship (Credibility of the contents) and Groups.

The content of each chapter included in this book is the sole responsibility of the respective authors.

FINAL REMARKS

This book expands the knowledge that results from the combination of health communication, rare diseases and digital technology. A myriad of movies, radio, TV-shows and social networks depict a number of rare diseases and its portrayal tend to affect the socio-cultural aspects inherent to the disease and patients' empowerment. Alongside the advances on Information and Communication Technologies, the knowledge on the pathogenesis, diagnosis and therapies has grown significantly but further work needs to be carried out relative to rare and misdiagnosed diseases.

The lack of information and experience in dealing with such diseases and disorders seem to lead to decentralized and multiple sources of information that patients often have to decipher by themselves. Cooperation within different knowledge bases and strengthening global communities of patients, caregivers and health professionals seem, therefore, essential to create some 'cross-borders' pressure within health policies, represent these diseases in public genomic databases, and to ensure the circulation of information and investment in orphan drugs and treatments.

The chapter contributions for this book suggest several courses of action for advances in epigenetic and genomic information projects, bioethics and policymaking combined with biomedical and clinical research, as well as emotional and psychological management of disease for both patients and caregivers. Associations and international entities and events, such as NORD, EURORDIS, Rare Voices Australia (RVA) and International Rare Disease Day also play an important role in informing and safeguarding patients and caregivers affected by rare diseases and in pressuring for the improving of legislation and policymaking, ensuring research investment and the development of treatments and cures for orphan and rare conditions.

Liliana Vale Costa
University of Aveiro, Portugal

Sónia Oliveira
University of Aveiro, Portugal

ENDNOTES

1 The story can be read at https://www.buzzfeednews.com/article/danvergano/this-mom-is-buying-mutant-mice-from-china-to-find-a-cure (access date: 20-Nov-2019)

2 FDA approves first treatment for inherited rare disease, https://www.fda.gov/news-events/press-announcements/fda-approves-first-treatment-inherited-rare-disease (access date: 20-Nov-2019)

3 FDA approves Alnylam's Givlaari second- ever drug based on RNAi, shorturl.at/gBEGV (access date: 20-Nov-2019)

Acknowledgment

The editors appreciate the assistance of all reviewers and editorial members, who revised and improved the quality of each chapter. A special thanks to all the authors who contributed with their chapters. The work here, passionately, shared has been carried out over the past few years and represents a statement of the many challenges one can encounter when intertwining the topics of health-related communication and rare diseases.

Last but not least, the editors would like to dedicate this book to their students in order to inspire them to these topics of research.

To all the patients and caregivers being challenged by a rare or misdiagnosed disease, we wish lots of strength and optimism in the face of challenges. We will continue to study the way media can facilitate health-related information about rare and misdiagnosed diseases.

Liliana Vale Costa
University of Aveiro, Portugal

Sónia Oliveira
University of Aveiro, Portugal

Chapter 1
Talking About Rare Diseases: A Compendium on Rare Diseases and Online News

Sonia M. Rodrigues Oliveira
https://orcid.org/0000-0002-0707-5203
Hunter Medical Research Institute, Australia & University of Aveiro, Portugal

ABSTRACT

Originally, rare diseases and orphan diseases were not synonyms. Rare diseases became known as orphan diseases because pharmaceutical companies were not interested in developing treatments for them. The Orphan Drug Act (USA) used financial incentives for orphan drug development. Herewith, a definition for rare disease was also established. This differs slightly across countries. Some rare diseases respond to drugs that are not orphan drugs. Orphan diseases refer to neglected diseases and even common disorders as endometrial cancer and infantile diabetes. Nonetheless, nowadays very often rare and orphan are used as synonyms. The causes for rare diseases are very diverse. The majority are thought to be genetic. Most lack proper diagnosis, treatment, or known therapeutic targets. However, rare disease patients account for a huge proportion of the health burden. This chapter discusses rare (and orphan) diseases, what has been reported about them, and how they appear to the general public. The different categories of rare diseases are introduced.

DOI: 10.4018/978-1-7998-2088-8.ch001

INTRODUCTION

CHARGE and HUNTER may seem like random names of a fictional superhero, but they are in fact rare inherited genetic disorders. Charge and Hunter syndromes belong to a group of diseases loosely called rare diseases. The group designation comes from the rarity of the disease among the population. Together with low prevalence in the population, these diseases are often associated with problems in diagnosis and treatment.

Financial incentive programs were created to encourage companies to develop new drugs for rare diseases. In this sense, a rare disease definition was needed to establish which conditions would qualify for new incentive programs. Countries have their own official definitions of a rare disease. [1] In the European Union and in Australia, a rare disease is a specific, clinically serious disorder affecting fewer than 1 in 2,000 people, i.e. less than 0.05% of the population (EC Regulation on Orphan Medicinal Products) (EURORDIS, 2005), while the USA Congress defined in the Orphan Drug Act of 1983 a rare disease as a condition that affects fewer than 200,000 people.

The market size for rare diseases is much smaller in comparison with other common diseases. Thus, these incentive programs and acts, which include tax breaks, lower fees, research support and exclusivity periods for emerging therapies were essential to create economic motivation for the pharmaceutical industry to invest into research and development of drugs for rare diseases. The lack of interest by the industry in to develop these drugs has also led them to be named as "orphan drugs". In fact, there are thousands of known rare diseases yet only a few hundred of them have treatment. Before these incentive programs and legal acts, only a handful of rare diseases had designated therapies.

Nonetheless, the accessibility to patients of these emergent therapies remains challenging. A good example is the recent Food and Drug Administration – FDA's approval of a vaccine against pediatric spinal muscular atrophy, Zolgensma (AVXS-101)[2] with a price tag of over 2 million dollars[3]. Many government healthcare funds cannot assure these high prices. Thus, many rare disease patients are left untreated despite the existence of treatment in the market. An example is Malaysian patients of Hunter disease. Less than half of these patients receive treatment. However, a recent effort is being made to inform and sensitize health care professionals to these disorders for example, through ministries publishing and release of rare diseases guidelines for diagnosis and treatments (Teik, Keong, Hock, Latif, & Rawi, 2012). It may be that without social and mediatic pressure, governments simply do not recognize the urgency of making available emerging therapies to these patients.

For potential cures, patients alone often cannot gather these values but even tougher for payers is to disburse the full cost upfront. Additionally, health care billing and insurance systems are not set up to pay for cures. Thus, politicians need to be creative and proactive to assure the equity of rare disease patients. They need to study options as, for example, special allocation funds or special fiscal treatment for companies working to help these patients. In order to understand the challenges of rare disease patients, pharmaceutical companies' stakeholders, patients, industry, clinicians and researchers need to establish proactive dialogues and engage in collaborative projects. Special days and dedicated symposiums can help to raise awareness and interest. These initiatives should invite and be attended by leading figures and policy makers in the management of rare diseases.

Zolgensma maker Novartis Pharmaceuticals, may just have set the pace into bridging the gap between expensive gene therapies and people who would greatly benefit from them. This could shift healthcare paradigms towards cures instead of treatments, opening the door to future gene therapies that are not solely focused on rare diseases and whereas governments are pushed to act and give better health care systems to their people.

BACKGROUND

Diseases usually belong to one of four main types of disease: infectious, deficiency, hereditary (genetic and non-genetic), and physiological. Rare diseases often comprehend more than one category if they affect multiple tissues or organs and not all diseases fall into a category.

ORPHANET (EU) and NIH-GARD (U.S.A. National Institutes of Health - Genetic and Rare Diseases Information Center) maintain the same nomenclature of rare diseases, but the US Orphan drug Act (1983) and the European Union Regulation on Orphan Medicinal Products (1999) have different definitions of rare disease. In the United States of America, a rare disease is defined as a condition that affects fewer than 200,000 people, and not more than 1 person per 2,000 in the European population. However, the use of identical nomenclature is essential for improving visibility of rare diseases in health and research information. Both Orphanet and NIH-NORD (National Organization for Rare Disorders) also attribute unique and stable identifier numbers, the ORPHA and GARD numbers (sometimes indicated here for some rare diseases). In these databases, a disorder can be a disease, a malformation syndrome, a clinical syndrome, a morphological or a biological anomaly or a specific clinical situation (in the course of a disorder or disease).[1] There are over 2190 rare diseases listed in Orphanet and many more are described by GARD.

In general, a rare disease is defined as a disease rarely found in the general population and this makes it seems like very few people in the world are affected. But in a population of billions of people, several hundred thousand of people suffer of some sort of rare ailment. Moreover, it is important to highlight that the number of rare disease patients varies considerably from disease to disease. Some of these people, suffer from an even rarer disease, affecting only a few thousand or less to even a dozen or so, worldwide. Most rare diseases are this "rarer."

Usually, rare diseases are misdiagnosed and mistaken for a common disease or for some other rare disorder. Nonetheless, it is comprehended that due to their rareness, a physician attains clinical experience in rare diseases with a very small fraction of the total number of rare diseases (Berman, 2014). Every doctor should consider oneself as amateurish when it comes to rare diseases.

Most genetic and metabolic diseases are foreign to both the public and clinicians. However, it is estimated that 6 to 10% of the total population are rare disease patients (EURORDIS, 2005; Knight & Senior, 2006).

Most health professionals struggle to recall many of them and their symptoms. Genetics is at the basis of ~80% of rare diseases, which are often chronic and life-threatening (The Lancet & Endocrinology, 2019). Many of these diseases have no cure and the treatment involves managing symptoms and complications. The onset of symptoms can range from early childhood to adulthood. The diagnosis lingers due to the complex nature and small numbers of known cases. Rare diseases also include rare childhood cancers and other better-known conditions both present from birth, such as Cystic Fibrosis, Amyotrophic Lateral Sclerosis (ALS) and Phenylketonuria or, as with Huntington's disease, with symptoms arising in adulthood. One rare disease may affect only a handful of patients worldwide while another can affect several thousands of people. There are over 6000 rare diseases recognized. Altogether, they may affect 1.2 million people in Australia, somewhere between 25 and 30 million people in the US, and 30 million people in Europe hence, being a major health burden to societies (EURORDIS, 2019; Knight & Senior, 2006). Although many nations as the United States of America, the EU and Australia have enacted orphan drug legislation, they lack coordinated approaches from governments, physicians and patient groups.

Research around rare genetic diseases is particularly challenging because of small patient cohorts and commercial viability, hindering the interest into the development of therapies. Collaborations, research fields crosstalk and incentives for breakthrough technologies are needed to overcome these health challenges. Moreover, clinicians are particularly well placed to help patients of rare diseases and their families but a general strategy needs to be put in place in order to improve their overall care (Knight & Senior, 2006).

The present chapter proposes to summarize the current, general knowledge about rare and / or orphan diseases. It includes the current numbers on prevalence and / or incidence. Challenges in research and development and, media and public awareness are also acknowledged. The different categories of rare diseases are also introduced. A glossary of 'key terms' with small descriptions of the diseases and disorders mentioned throughout this chapter is also provided. This chapter should to be useful to a number of rare disease related stakeholders including, but not limited to, patients, caregivers, health professionals, researchers and students.

COMMON CHARACTERISTICS OF RARE DISEASES

Rare diseases are a group that includes over 6000 diseases that are often degenerative to life-threatening. In common, they share some traits (EURORDIS, 2005; "Rare Disease Day," 2019; WHO, 2013):

- Many onsets during childhood (as many as 50%);
- Patients often lose autonomy;
- The issue is aggravated by psychological and emotional burden due to lack of therapeutic assistance and hope and, lack of practical daily support with routines;
- Incurable and mostly without any effective treatment or form of mitigate the suffering and improve quality of life and life expectancy;
- Difficulty in managing mixed information and the general lack of information prevent patients from accessing adequate treatments;
- Most of the patients have a genetic basis (roughly, it can be estimated that one out of 15 people worldwide have a rare ("orphan") disease of most likely genetic origin).

RARE DISEASES CATEGORIES

Rare Diseases in Neurology

Neurological disorders are not to be confused with mental disorders. Mental disorders are "psychiatric illnesses" or diseases, which appear primarily as abnormalities of thought, feeling or behavior, producing either distress or impairment of function. Neurological diseases are a large group of over 600 diseases that affect the brain, spine and nerves. These include degenerative diseases as Alzheimer's disease, Parkinson's disease, Huntington's disease and dementia but, also, brain tumors, epilepsy, stroke, and ALS (Amyotrophic Lateral Sclerosis) and the rarest Creutzfeldt-Jakob disease (CJD); CJD affects 1 to 1.5 person per 1 million per year, worldwide and is a fatal brain disorder. [4]

Diseases as Tay-Sachs (rare inherited disorder that progressively destroys nerve cells in the brain and spinal cord) are also part of this group. As Tay-Sachs, many neurological rare diseases arise from specific inheritance patterns and may be more prevalent in particular ethnic groups – *e.g.* people of Ashkenazi (eastern and central European) Jewish heritage and in certain French-Canadian communities of Quebec, the Old Order Amish community in Pennsylvania, and the Cajun population of Louisiana are the most likely carriers of the mutations that cause Tay-Sachs disease.[5]

Common to most rare diseases, neurological rare diseases have ineffective diagnoses and treatments. There are many recognized neurological disorders, some relatively common, but many rare. Recognizing the clinical features of rare neurological diseases (RNDs) is immensely challenging. The Rare Neurological Disease Special Report[6], a collaboration of NORD (National Organization for Rare Disorders, USA) and Neurology Reviews, is published annually in the Rare Diseases Day (28th February or 29th February in leap years). This publication is a valuable reference to health care professionals providing an easily accessible and a reliable resource of information. The European Academy of Neurology (EAN) is also at the forefront in Europe to help raise awareness and improve knowledge aiming early diagnosis and research to identify disease mechanisms and potential therapies. [7]

Rare Mental and Behavioral Disorders

Psychological or mental disorders refer to patterns of behavioral or psychological symptoms that can impact multiple areas of life. Over 450 definitions of mental disorders are published in the 'Diagnostic and Statistical Manual of Mental Disorders (DSM)' [8] by the American Psychiatric Associations, the standard reference for psychiatry. Concomitantly, the World Health Organization (WHO) also includes a section on mental and behavioral disorders in its 'International Classification of Diseases (ICD)'[9], the international standard system for medical diseases classification.

Some of the main groups of mental disorders are:

- Mood disorders (such as depression or bipolar disorder);
- Anxiety disorders;
- Personality disorders;
- Psychotic disorders (such as schizophrenia);
- Eating disorders;
- Trauma-related disorders (such as post-traumatic stress disorder);
- Substance abuse disorders.

Such mental disorders as anxiety, schizophrenia and bipolar disorder are relatively common and well-understood. Thus, health professionals are well prepared to use a set of common diagnoses to come up with a differential diagnosis and treatment plan. Other disorders, however, are so rare that mental health clinicians may never encounter them in their careers. These include: the Stendhal Syndrome, Apotemnophilia or body integrity identity disorder, Alien Hand syndrome, Foreign Accent Syndrome (FAS), Capgras Syndrome, and Alice in Wonderland Syndrome and Clinical Lycanthropy.

Many movies like 'Confessions of a shopaholic' (directed by P.J. Hogan) brought back into 'popular' spotlight more common conditions like Oniomania (the technical name for being a shopaholic), but also rare ones like in 'Split' (from the director and writer: M. Night Shyamalanwith), the story of a Dissociative Identity Disorder (DID) patient. A myriad of movies and TV-shows depict terrible mental illness as the above mention DID or the Diogenes syndrome ('hoarding') however, they remain extremely misunderstood.

Mental health disorders have gotten a bad reputation in the past but as new information is gathered, people are able to learn more and not fear people afflicted by these conditions. With somewhere between 11% and 18% of the world population suffering from some sort of mental illness (Ritchie & Roser, 2019) it is hard to understand why rare mental disorders are still overlooked and under-studied.

The latest estimates of mental health disorder prevalence, disease burden rates, and mortality impacts across a number of prevalent mental disorders can be found at OurWorldInData.org database. NAMI, the National Alliance on Mental Illness10, also provides good data and information, and support, about mental diseases in the USA, including the rare ones. Nonetheless, official sources as NIH – GARD (National Centre for Advancing Translational Sciences – Genetic and Rare Diseases Information Centre) still are not publishing proper lists of rare behavioral and mental disorders, reducing it to just a few syndromes.[11]

Different countries may have different strategies and institutions offering support for mental health patients and families, as for example, SANE in Australia (SANE, 2019). However, countries generally fail in making its existence thoroughly known amongst the general public. As the public start to value mental and physical health equity, the stigma surrounding mental illness lessens and people are able to access better health care. This may lead up to a clearer grasp of rare mental disorders as more cases are being recognized and followed-up.

Rare Diseases of the Endocrine System

Rare diseases of the endocrine system have been listed by official agencies (NIH & GARD, 2019) and even have their own online platforms as, for example, '*Rare Endocrine Genetic Diseases | Hormone Health Network.*" at Hormone.org and provided by the Endocrine Society (Network, 2019).

According to these, there are over 175 different rare diseases that affect the endocrine system. In common with other rare diseases, the symptoms are often vague and confusing leaving physicians puzzled and patients without diagnosis for long periods of time. Hypoparathyroidism and Hypopituitarism are part of these diseases.

'Orphan' is a 2009 American-Canadian-German-French psychological horror film directed by Jaume Collet-Serra and written by David Leslie Johnson from a story by Alex Mace that depicts a case of hypopituitarism, a condition that stunted a character's physical growth and caused proportional dwarfism, thus having her spent most of her life posing as a little girl. Nonetheless, most of these rare endocrine conditions are not 'movie material', even though they affect immensely the patients' lives.

The rare endocrine-metabolic diseases are a recognized important area of medicine and pharmacology that include mechanisms and treatments largely misunderstood. These disorders hold also the complexity of involving different fields of physiology, endocrinology and pharmacology, and include rare diseases of the pituitary, thyroid and adrenal glands, paraganglia, ovary and testis but also bone and mineral metabolism disorders, energy and lipid metabolism, water metabolism and syndromes that involve different glands and neuroendocrine tumors (Marcucci et al., 2015). Therefore, type 1 Diabetes, type 2 Diabetes, osteoporosis, and thyroid cancer are common endocrine diseases.

General public websites[12] offer some information for patients. Rare endocrine diseases include several tumors and neoplasia, namely pheochromocytomas which, are catecholamine-secreting tumors that may arise from chromaffin cells of the adrenal medulla and the sympathetic ganglia (pheochromocytomas) or in extra-adrenal chromaffin cells (secreting paragangliomas) (Neumann, Young, & Eng, 2019). Recently, the current landscape for European registries of Rare Endocrine diseases was also analyzed, and similarly to other rare conditions, the need to improve awareness and participation in existing registered rare diseases was emphasized (Ali et al., 2019). Orphanet[13] and RD-connect[14] remain the most reliable sources of information also for endocrine rare diseases.

Rare Diseases of the Immune System

Rare diseases of the immune system often touch young and very young people having considerable social and economic impact. Rare immune system diseases make up a long and growing list of over 300 conditions often of deficiency of a cell or protein due to genetic mutation(s).[15]

Many rare diseases are Primary Immunodeficiencies (PIDs). This encompasses a large, growing group of over 300 diseases caused by the failure of some components of the immune system. PIDs are recognized as rare conditions whilst some are more common than others. They are generally caused by genetic defects of the immune system that are hereditary. Similarly, to other rare diseases, non-profit organizations also work in the International set to raise awareness and inform (for example, IPOPI -International Patient Organization for Primary Immunodeficiencies).[16] In recent years, the knowledge on pathogenesis, diagnosis and therapies has grown significantly. Nonetheless, much is yet to be done in order to motivate and attract the general public.

Asherson's Syndrome or Catastrophic Antiphospholipid Syndrome is one of the rarest autoimmune disorders registered and it is characterized by the development of rapidly progressive blood clots, over hours, days or weeks, potentially causing multiple organ systems failure. Specific symptoms vary as different organs are affected, complicating the diagnosis. The exact origin of the disease is unknown, but researchers believe that epigenetic factors (genetic-environmental interactions) play a role in the etiology of autoimmune diseases.[17]

Autoimmune diseases may range from relatively common to very rare. Common autoimmune diseases include thyroiditis, rheumatoid arthritis and diabetes, alopecia areata and multiple sclerosis and less common conditions, as lupus (Systemic Lupus Erythematosus (SLE)). Autoimmune diseases as lupus, however, may not be considered rare. Lupus is registered as a rare disorder in Europe[18], but not in the USA.[19] This is due to different definitions to orphan or rare diseases established by the parliaments.

Rare Eye and Ear Diseases

Rare eye and ear diseases have been linked to autoimmune diseases. This is the case of autoimmune inner ear disease which, is a rare disease that is triggered by the body's immune system mistakenly attacking the own inner ear. Symptoms include dizziness, ringing in the ears, and bilateral sensorineural hearing loss. The estimated prevalence is of about 15/100,000 (in the United States) and more common in middle-aged women than in men (Ciorba et al., 2018).

A search for rare eye and ear diseases, rapidly, returns results about the Cogan and the Susac syndromes, other two autoimmune disorders. Cogan's syndrome symptoms include pain and irritation in the eyes, decreases vision, hearing loss and vertigo. It also may provoke muscle and joint pain or inflammation of blood vessels (Berrocal, Vargas, Vaquero, y Cajal, & Ramírez-Camacho, 1999). Susac syndrome provokes three main problems: impaired brain function (encephalopathy), partial or complete blockage of blood vessels that supply blood to the retina), and inner ear disease (mainly, hearing loss). Usually, the disease show in MRI scans as 'snowball' lesions in the corpus callosum in the brain (Said, Lee, Sabat, & Zacharia, 2015; Vishnevskia-Dai et al., 2016).

At least 400 rare diseases include hearing loss as a symptom.[20] This can be of different types but mainly is sensorineural or conductive hearing loss. Some rare diseases can cause anatomical and functional changes in the ears as for example, the Turner syndrome or the Mondini dysplasia. Other rare diseases that include hearing loss as a symptom are KID syndrome, Donnai-Barrow syndrome, Wildervanck syndrome, and Krabbe disease. In the latter, symptoms can develop in the first six months of age and include muscle weakness, fever and vision and hearing loss. Ménière's disease and Alport syndrome are other rare disorders affecting hearing and the eyes.

In many other rare syndromes, hearing loss can start as early as at birth or soon after. Because of this, hearing screening tests are taken by babies in the first days of life in many countries including in the United States of America and in European countries, as Portugal. About 2 to 3 out of every 1,000 newborns in the United States are born with a detectable level of hearing loss in one or both ears (CDC, 2019; NIH, 2016). In Europe, the prevalence of hearing loss also sits at 0.1% of children (CDC, 2019). Hearing loss and/or vision is often a manifestation of rare syndromes.

Rare Pulmonary Diseases

Rare pulmonary diseases are a group of over 190 diseases affecting the lung. Rare lung diseases have had some attention from the scientific community and benefit from some 'easy-to-read' literature compilations about them. This is the case of the chapters published by the American Thoracic Society[21] (ATS, 2019) and by the European Respiratory Society - the European Lung White Book (ERS, 2019).

Rare pulmonary diseases also include autoimmune disorders (e.g. Anti-basement Membrane Syndrome, or Goodpasture syndrome, and Takayasy's Arteritis), and some neoplastic disorders (Benign or Malignant tumors). Amongst the neoplastic disorders is the adenosquamous carcinoma of the lung, a subtype of rare non-small cell lung cancer of difficult diagnosis and limited treatment options that makes up 0.4-4% of all lung cancer cases (C. Li & Lu, 2018).

Pulmonary fibrosis is probably one of the best-known orphan lung diseases. Several lung association's worldwide offer support and resources for patients of this life-threating disease (e.g. American lung association[22]). Pulmonary fibrosis causes irreversible lung scaring thus, breathing becomes increasingly difficult. The causes are not clear, and treatments include self-care measures, oxygen therapies and even lung transplant (Baddini-Martinez et al., 2015; NHS, 2019; N. H. NIH, Lung, and Blood Institute, 2019).

Other rare pulmonary disease also benefit from some support provided by the Rare Lung Diseases Consortium[23], which is registered in the Rare Diseases Clinical Research Network (RDCRN).[24] RDCRN provides funding to over 20 research groups across over 20 countries, and a data management and coordinating center bringing the gap between research, clinicians and patients by improving the availability of rare diseases information, treatment, clinical studies and awareness. This groundbreaking collaborative network of researchers and patients' organizations improved significantly the support to rare diseases research and general public awareness.

The investment in awareness and research of rare pulmonary disorders and in particular rare lung cancers has been great. Health professionals and patients are increasingly better informed. Both Europe and USA National Institutes of Health (NIH) even suggest patients diagnosed with a rare lung disease to be referred to specialist centers and to register to have access to clinical trials (EU Clinical Trials Register[25]; USA NIH[26]) (ERS, 2015). This is slowly allowing to find better diagnosis techniques and treatments for lung orphan diseases overcoming the general obstacle of rare diseases of lack of properly designed big clinical studies.

Rare Cardiac Diseases

Rare cardiac diseases have low incidence but a huge effect on the affected patients and their families. There are as many as 30 million people in Europe with some sort of rare heart condition. This adds up, with other rare diseases, to an enormous socio-economic burden in societies. Efficient diagnostic and therapeutic opportunities for patients are a major problem. Again, developing national and international collaboration networks, disseminating knowledge, targeting both physicians and patients, and promoting research and development should be top priority for countries' leaders and societies (Podolec, 2017).

Rare cardiac diseases can been divided into eight main classes as: of the heart (cardiomyopathies), congenital cardiovascular diseases, rare arrhythmias, cardiac tumors, cardiovascular diseases during pregnancy, of systemic circulation and of pulmonary circulation, and other unclassified types (Podolec, 2017). [27]

Restrictive cardiomyopathy is a rare type of cardiomyopathy (and one of the rarest heart diseases) that causes the heart muscle to become very rigid or stiff. An array of exams allow to diagnose specific subtypes of this disease allowing better follow-up and medical counselling (Rammos, Meladinis, Vovas, & Patsouras, 2017). Nonetheless, the etiology, incidence and diagnostic criteria of this cardiomyopathy remains controversial (Albakri, 2018).

Other rare cardiac disorders are less 'petrifying'. Brugada syndrome is one of them. This rare cardiac disease is characterized by problems with the electrical system of the heart causing arrythmias that left without treatment can be fatal. This syndrome can be responsible for some 'sudden deaths' registered worldwide by as much as 20%. The symptoms show up in adulthood and it is more frequent in males. It is due to genetic mutations and is registered to have a prevalence of about 5 in 10,000 people but, there is no incidence data as it is a recently identified syndrome.[28]

Similar to rare lung disorders, rare cardiac diseases also attract higher attention from drug companies, health professionals and societies. Higher investment results in more and faster results. Thanks to this today we have a pioneer treatment to improve survival in a progressive and fatal rare heart condition called transthyretin amyloid cardiomyopathy: the drug Tafamidis (Maurer et al., 2018a). International Societies as The European Society of Cardiology welcome and inform about these innovations.[29, 30]

Although independent evaluations are lacking, this outcome is a sign that incentives to drug companies to develop orphan drugs is bringing positive changes and results. To note that it took six years since the drug company got the authorization and started to recruit participants up to the final phase and results of the clinical trial. Before that, there were many years of research to identify therapeutic targets and hundreds of in vitro and in vivo tests. This is a long and costly process.

Rare Vascular Diseases

Often in association or part of cardiac rare diseases are also vascular rare diseases. Common vascular diseases include stroke, deep vein thrombosis and pulmonary embolism (blood clots). But rare diseases also affect blood's vascular system. These diseases are often found in association with other rare syndromes as Wegener's granulomatosis, Kawasaki syndrome or Churg-Strauss syndrome. Other rare vascular diseases include:

- Cystic adventitial disease (CAD) - The disease is registered in NIH-GARD, but nothing was input about it, and does not appear in the orphanet database. It is a rare vascular disorder that involves the arteries and rarely the veins, most commonly found in the popliteal artery (branches off from the femoral artery and is localized in the knee and back of the leg) of male patients; it is curable but represents a diagnostic challenge and unknown etiology (Li, King, Velasco, Kumar, & Gupta, 2017).
- Endofibrosis of the iliac artery – This rare condition is not registered in orphanet or NIH-GARD; it affects young endurance athletes and is characterized by focal intimal thickening of the artery made of loose connective tissue without atherosclerotic changes. The main symptom is unilateral leg claudication triggered by a near-maximal effort in a young athlete, thus the condition is often confused with other musculoskeletal or neurological condition. Prevalence is unknown (Brunelle, Baradaran, & Keeler, 2016).
- Polyarteritis nodosa – Multi-system disease characterized by widespread inflammation, weakening, and damage to small and medium-sized arteries; affects about 1 in 100,000 people.[31]
- Lymphomatoid granulomatosis - Infiltration and destruction of the veins and arteries by lesions caused by the overproduction (proliferation) of white blood cells called lymphocytes (lymphoproliferative disorder); It affects mostly men and is of unknown prevalence. [32]
- Hereditary lymphedema (there are two types called type I or Milroy's disease, and type II or Meige syndrome) – swelling (edema) that is present at or shortly after birth (congenital); type I prevalence is unknown and type II prevalence is of 1 in 6,000 people. [33]

Vascular rare diseases represent a particular health care challenge and for this, specific work groups were created as VASCERN, a European Reference Network (ERN). [34] VASCERN can support and inform clinicians and patients about rare vascular diseases and make healthcare assistance accessible cross-border. Similarly, to other ERNs, this platform aims to reduce the delay in diagnosis – one of the main issues with rare diseases - as well as improve awareness, reduce care gaps and redundant test and improve counselling, diagnosis tools and medical knowledge.

Rare Hepatic Diseases

Most people have been in contact with patients of liver disease. Governments have in place national plans to fight the rates of common liver diseases, such as hepatitis. However, there are over a hundred different types of liver diseases and many of them most people have not ever heard of, such as the Alagille syndrome or Primary

Sclerosing Cholangitis (PSC). Congenital liver diseases and polycystic liver disease are rare. Rare liver diseases can be divided into four groups: Autoimmune disorders (as autoimmune hepatitis or PSC, mentioned above and summarized in the glossary of this chapter), Biliary atresia and related diseases (e.g. Wilson disease or Biliary Atresia), Structural liver disease (cystic liver and vascular liver disease), and Liver disease in pregnancy.[35]

A common trace of many of liver diseases is that they have high incidence in, usually, young people and result in high morbidity and mortality. Advances in knowledge of these diseases is hindered by the small number of cases (rarity) and the limit number of studies on the etiology, pathophysiology and therapies for these conditions. Conversely, in recent years there has been an increase in rare liver disorders. In line with has been done to support rare heart and lung disease patients, centers of excellence in the clinical management of rare liver disease in adults and children were created. This is the case of the European ERN RARE-LIVER[35] or EASL.[36] These networks highlight an effort to inform clinicians and patients into the best clinical practice options, innovative solutions and standardized care, in order to provide high-quality care and information.

RARE-LIVER website is not as 'user-friendly' or complete as other IT solutions for other rare diseases, but it is a start to mend the gap between rare liver disease patients and health support. Additionally, EASL and AASL (American Association for the Study of the Liver) encourage further investment into research rare liver diseases by sponsoring conferences and support initiatives as #RareDiseaseDay (last day of February each year). EASL is a contributor of the general EU efforts to develop and adopt a comprehensive strategy on rare diseases. It is important to recall that rare liver conditions represent a huge health burden worldwide.

Rare Gastrointestinal Diseases

Digestive and/or gastrointestinal (GI) rare diseases account for over a hundred registries in NIH-GARD listing (https://rarediseases.info.nih.gov/diseases/diseases-by-category/6/digestive-diseases accessed 13-10-2019). Orphanet Journal of Rare Diseases also publishes a section dedicated to rare gastrointestinal diseases.[38] This group of diseases is characterized by sharing common clinical features with other conditions but with a special pathogenesis profile.

Probably the best-known example of rare GI diseases is inflammatory bowel disease which, is more common in children. Many GI disorders are inherited or have a genetic predisposition. This include inflammatory bowel disease but also pancreatitis, celiac sprue, Peutz-Jeghers syndrome, Neuroendocrine tumors, Hereditary Telangiectasia, and Menetrier's disease also known as hypertrophic gastritis. Other rare GI disorders are Hirschsprung's disease, chronic intestinal pseudo-obstruction (CIP), achalasia and short bowel syndrome (SBS), among others.[39] Many patients of these rare diseases still face stigma and embarrassment in to seeking help and diseases management.

Rare Diseases of Genitourinary (or Urogenital) System

The genitourinary system includes the entire urinary tract and the male genital tract. Problems can occur at any part of the system, from the production of urine by the nephrons to the eventual elimination of urine via the external urethral meatus or orifice. The male genital tract includes organs responsible for the production and transport of spermatozoa, the secretion of sex hormones, and erections. Most patients present for evaluation of the male genital tract because of inflammatory processes and tumors of these organs. The interaction between the urinary tract and male genital organs, such as the prostate, often creates diagnostic challenges (White, 1990).

There are many rare diseases affecting the kidneys and the urinary system. The list released by NIH-GARD is thus long.[40] Many of these diseases are either part of a problem in the urinary system itself (affecting kidneys cells or the urinary tract) or are part of a condition that causes additional symptoms in other organs (caused by inflammation or autoimmune disease). Of the later are example the Alport syndrome – mentioned in the 'rare eye and ear diseases' – and, the Goodpasture syndrome (mentioned in rare pulmonary diseases).

The Alport syndrome is a rare genetic defect in the type IV collagen chain that, because it is a structural component of ears, eyes, and kidneys, it causes glomerulonephritis (damage of the glomeruli, the filter units of the kidneys), end-stage kidney disease, and hearing loss (Genetics Home Reference, 2019a; McAdoo & Pusey, 2017). In the Goodpasture syndrome, a rare autoimmune disorder, antibodies attack the basement membrane in lungs and kidneys – at a subunit of type IV collagen, presumably -, leading to bleeding from the lungs and kidney failure (DeVrieze & Hurley, 2019).

Due to the importance of blood supply to and from the kidney, many rare diseases of the genitourinary system are vasculitis (group of disorders that damage the blood vessels by inflammation). Henoch-Schonlein purpura nephritis is one of this rare vasculitis of childhood that cause major kidney problems. This disease is characterized by abnormal deposits of immunoglobulin A (IgA, an antibody) in small blood vessels, leading to their inflammation. This causes purple-colored spots on the skin (purpura), joint pain, and gastrointestinal problems such as abdominal pain, nausea, bloody stools.[41]

Clinical Practice Guidelines have been shared for this disorder in countries like Australia[42] (Watson, Richardson, Holt, Jones, & Beresford, 2012) or the United Kingdom.[43]

Probably one of the rarest conditions of the genitourinary system is Emphysematous cystitis (EC). This is a gas-forming bacterial or fungal infection of the bladder wall. It is more prevalent in female patients with diabetes and it can be associated with more serious complications (e.g. pyelonephritis, a potentially organ- and/or life-threatening bacterial infection that characteristically causes scarring of the kidney) (Amano & Shimizu, 2014; Fumeo, Manfredi, & Volta, 2019).

Prevalence values are unknown and there is a probable underestimation of this disease. Genitourinary rare diseases can be congenital, functional or neoplastic/tumors. For instance, congenital scrotal agenesis is an extremely rare disorder characterized by the absence of scrotal rugae in the perineum between the penis and anus (Yılmaz et al., 2013).

Another group of conditions to these rare diseases are disorders of sex development (DSD) which include multiple congenital conditions where chromosomal, gonadal, and/or anatomical sex do not match. It can happen in about 1 in 5000 newborns and the treatments have improved and often fix the anomalies. The number of conditions under this umbrella is enormous but usually fall into the following categories: metabolic disorders (e.g. steroid synthesis disorder), androgen receptor disorder (Androgen Insensitivity Syndrome (complete (CAIS) and partial (PAIS)), gonadal development disorder (e.g. ovotesticular DSD), chromosomal aberrations (Turner syndrome and Charge syndrome).

These disorders (ORPHA:101433) are highly under-investigated and patients tend to develop stigmatizing attitudes and/or high personal stigma. However, sometimes rare and unusual urogenital disorders attract public attention, especially if occurring in famous people. Plus, publicity is given when these abnormalities are described by eminent physicians, some of them as hosts in TV-shows and so on. The European Reference Network (ERN) for rare and complex urogenital diseases and conditions – eUROGEN (http://eurogen-ern.eu) - is trying to overcome these obstacles in order for patients to access equitable, 'easily-approachable' health care, without fear or stigma. Unlike in previous categories, clinical practice guidelines for urogenital or genitourinary rare diseases were not found. In fact, Clinical practice guidelines for rare diseases are scarce and sometimes hard to identify while also varying in quality depending on the source (Pavan et al., 2017).

Rare Bacterial, Viral and Fungal Infections

A broad variety of microorganisms, fungus and parasites can cause infectious diseases. Many of which uncommon, as the sexually transmitted diseases lymphogranuloma venereum (LGV), chancroid and donovanosis for which there are cures and, the cytomegalovirus that is without a cure. Parasitic infections (e.g. Trichomoniasis) may be more or less common, as well.

Most people know what arthritis is, however, most will not know that there is a form called infectious arthritis. This is a rare occurring inflammation of one or more joints caused by infection by bacteria, viruses or, less frequently, fungi or parasites. Infectious arthritis can affect people of all ages and both sexes. It has a reported incidence of 2 to 10 cases per 100,000 individuals, and about half of all cases involve adults over the age of 60. For patients with immunologic disorders, the incidence increases to about 30-70 cases per 100,000 people. [44]

Infectious myositis is another rare disease given the relative resistance of the musculature to infection. Myositis too may be caused by numerous bacterial, fungal, parasitic, and viral agents, and is characterized by the inflammation of a muscle especially a voluntary muscle, characterized by pain, tenderness, swelling, and/or weakness (Crum-Cianflone, 2008).

Fungi can also in rare cases originate eye infections (rare infections that can develop after eye surgery), and rare infections as sporotrichosis and mycetoma. [45] These are more common in equatorial regions of Africa, Latin America, and Asia. Fungal eye infections, as keratitis, can have different causing fungi (e.g. *Gjaerumia minor*, a rare yeast) and are recognized as a major global public health problem, especially in developing countries, representing from 6 to 50% of all cases of culture proven infectious keratitis (Al-Falki, Alshehri, Joseph, & Hamid, 2018).

Sporotrichosis or "rosebush mycosis" is a subacute or chronic infection, caused by thermodimorphic (switch to yeast or mold form depending on the prevailing temperature) fungi of the genus Sporothrix. It is a cosmopolitan disease mainly of tropical and subtropical areas. Although registered worldwide, some species are more ubiquitous than others, thus there is a divergence in the geographic distribution and incidence of the etiological agents contributing to undetermined prevalence values (Orofino-Costa, Macedo, Rodrigues, & Bernardes-Engemann, 2017). The number of cases can vary from 48 to 98 cases per 100,000 individuals, and the double in children as in Peru, to 155 cases in 36 years in Japan and decreasing (Chakrabarti, Bonifaz, Gutierrez-Galhardo, Mochizuki, & Li, 2014). On another hand, mycetoma, also more common in tropical regions, is a neglected disease lacking accurate data on its incidence and prevalence. Mycetoma is a chronic disease, usually of the foot, where subcutaneous tissues of skin, muscle and bone are progressively destroyed by the infection. The global burden caused by this infection is unknown (Chakrabarti et al., 2014).

Rare infections can also be caused by prions, a protein that contains no genetic information. Prions are usually harmless, but if they fold into an abnormal shape, they can cause diseases in the brain and other parts of the nervous system. This is the case of the well-known bovine spongiform encephalopathy (BSE) or mad cow disease, and the Creutzfeldt-Jakob disease (CJD). Prion infection have also been implicated in Alzheimer's disease. Prion diseases are rare, but usually progress rapidly and are fatal. Because they affect mainly the nervous system, diseases caused by this agent are often considered rare diseases of the nervous system.

Rare infections have been registered and described by NIH:

- Bacterial, including Brucellosis, Bubonic plague, Chancroid, Cholera, Legionnaires' disease, Mycetoma, Necrotizing fasciitis, Tetanus, Typhus and Whooping cough;[46]
- Viral, including Rubella, Zika syndrome, Dengue Fever, Measles, Poliomyelitis, Rabies and Yellow Fever; [47]
- Fungal, including Aspergillosis, Candida glabrata, Mycetoma and Pneumocystosis[48], and in Orphanet as: infectious embryofetopathy, bacterial, parasitic and viral [49].

Rare Allergic Diseases

Allergies as hay fever, allergic rhinitis and asthma are among the commonest causes of chronic illness. But there are some allergies which are far more unusual. This is the case of:

- Aquagenic urticaria (skin rushes from contact with water); [50]
- Exercise-induced anaphylaxis and urticaria (severe allergic reaction to exercise, with symptoms as breakout of hives, gastrointestinal problems and even anaphylactic shock); [51]
- Dermographism (a form of urticaria where writing on the skin with touch causes a physical allergic reaction); [52]
- Solar urticaria or polymorphic light eruption, PLE (outbreak of hives when exposed to the sun) or heat urticaria (allergic reaction to when temperatures are above 43ºC or to sweat);
- Vibratory urticaria (physical urticaria with hives and rashes caused by vibrations); or
- Seminal plasma hypersensitivity (reaction to proteins in male sperm that may cause redness, swelling, itching and pain namely in the vagina; symptoms can be confused with vaginitis and fungal infections thus it is often misdiagnosed).

Allergic or eosinophilic gastroenteropathy (disorder of the stomach and small intestine; rarely the colon) is even rarer. It is a rare benign disease characterized by eosinophils (type of 'disease-fighting' white blood cell) infiltration that may involve several digestive tract layers. Its incidence and prevalence are incomplete as the disease is often undiagnosed or patients unregistered (Méndez-Sánchez, Chavez-Tapia, Vazquez-Elizondo, & Uribe, 2007). The symptoms may mimic other common illness or be more complex, and its pathogenesis is still not clear. It is, however, often associated with reactions associated with the ingestion of food antigens in infancy and childhood (Moon & Kleinman, 1995).

Food allergies are, however, very frequent but its clinical spectrum is vast. Some food allergies are also common as to milk, eggs, shellfish, fish, tree nuts, peanuts, wheat and soybeans. But others are rare, as to red meat, sesame seeds, avocados, gelatin, corn, mango or dried fruits (in the later, the allergy is more to sulfites, such as sulfur dioxide, used to preserve the fruits). Unlike asthma or allergic rhinitis there is no official definition of severe food allergy. Despite this, the prevalence thresholds are used to define rare allergic diseases among different organizations and/or countries, namely of allergies causing anaphylaxis or anaphylactic shock. However, in many cases of rare diseases the prevalence and incidence data are scarce.

Angioedema is another rare disease, hereditary and that can affect 1 in 10,000 to 1 in 150,000 individuals. It is characterized by unpredictable swelling that can affect any part of the body or multiple sites at once. Commonly affected areas include the extremities, genitalia, trunk, gastrointestinal tract, face, and larynx. Hereditary angioedema often occurs as part of an allergic response to exogenous substances and conditions. Such substances can be dietary in origin, e.g., shellfish and other seafood, or may be environmental, as is the case with temperature-related angioedema (Nzeako, Frigas, & Tremaine, 2001). Clinical practice guidelines have been published by organizations, namely the World Allergy Organization (M. Maurer et al., 2018b).

Rare Skin Diseases

Skin diseases differ significantly in severity and symptoms. They can appear and disappear or be chronic, painless or painful, they can be caused by the environment or be hereditary / genetic. Some are minor while others can be life-threating and while some are onset since birth, others only appear suddenly later in life. In common, they often have unidentified causes. Common skin disorders include eczema, seborrheic dermatitis, chickenpox, measles, warts, acne. Most people will have at least one of these skin conditions in their life. But others are rarer and little known. These include, just to name a few:

- Hidradenitis suppurativa (HS), a chronic inflammatory condition with no cure and unknown causes where lesions form on parts of the body where skin touches skin (e.g. underarms, groin, buttocks, upper thighs, and breasts) (Goldburg, Strober, & Payette, 2019).
- Harlequin ichthyosis, a rare genetic disorder (mutation in gene ABCA12) of unknown prevalence that causes children to be born with hard, thick skin that forms diamond-shaped scales across their bodies. This can affect movement

of limbs and chest and the shape of eyelids, mouth and nose, for example (Layton, 2005) (ORPHA:457);

- Morgellons disease, a rare condition in which small fibers and particles emerge from skin sores, creating the sensation that something is crawling on the skin. Patients complain of itchy skin rashes or sores, black fibrous material in and on the skin, anxiety, fatigue, and depression (Middelveen, Fesler, & Stricker, 2018). There is some debate if it is a physical disorder due to similarities to a mental illness called delusional infestation (Lai, Xu, Xu, & Hu, 2018);
- Elastoderma, a rare acquired condition of unknown cause and with a prevalence of less than 1 in a million individuals and, that is characterized by increased laxity of the skin on specific areas of the body, causing the skin to sag or hang down in loose folds [53] (ORPHA:228240).

Disorders as vitiligo (patches of skin become lighter or white because pigment-producing cells (melanocytes) die or stop producing melanin) are not considered rare as they are relatively common. However, they are of unknown cause and lack therapeutic targets, are thus orphan diseases. [54]

Rare Musculoskeletal Diseases

Many rare disorders derive from injuries or pain in the human musculoskeletal system which, include the joints, ligaments, muscles, nerves, tendons, and structures that support limbs, neck and back. These rare diseases have various symptoms. Some cause weakness of muscles and pain affecting some specific muscles, others affect the whole body. The list of musculoskeletal rare diseases is long [55] and include genetic disorders (e.g. osteogenesis imperfecta, progeria) and tumors of the bone (e.g. osteosarcoma) and soft tissues (e.g. synovial sarcoma). Hereditary disorders are associated with genes regulating the skeletal development, growth and homeostasis, and remains a diagnostic challenge. It is now patent that disease phenotypes caused by mutations in one gene, depend on the mutation type and location within the gene.

The amount in knowledge and treatment solutions achieved in the last 20 years sparked by the Orphan Drug Act is immense and continued research is extremely important. Many musculoskeletal rare diseases are also pediatric. Thus, bone health research is of extreme importance. Task forces on skeletal rare diseases were than created in order to spread knowledge on these rare diseases, as for example, the one created by the International Osteoporosis Foundation.[56] Working groups like this help to generate comprehensive information as well as to develop standardize classifications of rare skeletal diseases – ‘classification will help in the development of common and shared diagnostic and treatments for these patients and also in the creation of international registries of rare skeletal diseases' (Masi et al., 2015) -, and eventually produce guidelines for clinical practice.

Rare Congenital and Genetic Diseases

Rare congenital (from birth) or genetic diseases are probably the ones getting most attention nowadays. In fact, many diseases have a genetic component. The list is very long as one can see at NIH-GARD database[57]; and include diseases from categories above mentioned as of the nervous system, lung, cardiovascular, musculoskeletal, eyes and ears, among others.

Neurofibromatosis (NF) is one of these genetic disorders with huge impact in patients' life. This disease causes tumors to form on nerve tissues, including the brain and spinal cord. Often onset since childhood it takes a toll in the development and social integration. The tumors are usually benign and symptoms often mild, but they tend to cause complications including hearing loss, vision impairment, cardiovascular problems, learning difficulties and severe pain. Surgery can reduce the symptoms, but the disease has no cure. There are three types of neurofibromatosis, each with different signs and symptoms; being NF1 the most common. NF1 prevalence is of 1 in 2,500 to 3,000 births while NF2 occurs in 1 in 33,000 births.[58]

Schwannomatosis is another neurofibromatosis but due to a mutation in different genes and with onset in adulthood. It is rarer as it occurs in 1 in 40,000 to 1 in 1.7 million newborns[59] (ORPHA:93921). Neurofibromatosis are part of different categories of rare diseases due to its characteristics: Congenital and Genetic Diseases; Nervous System Diseases; Rare Cancers; and Skin Diseases. Treatments are currently being investigated, thanks to the continuous investment and governmental incentives as through the orphan drugs act.[60]

Concomitantly, patients are getting some mediatic attention often associated with acts of kindness as per the story shared by SBS in Australia of a West Papuan woman getting surgery in Sydney to mitigate NF symptoms; the story was shared on TV, online news and social media as in Facebook (Bhole, 2019). [61] This may represent a social pressure for politicians and scientists to keep on investing and developing new technology and therapeutics for rare disorders and infections.

Other rare congenital or genetic diseases brim the spotlight through mediatic attention. This is the case of the only known diagnosis of chromosome 6 deletion where the child, Olivia Farnsworth, feels no hunger, pain or need to sleep (Chauhan, 2018; Pickles, 2016; SWNS, 2016). Another case is of the unique triplication in chromosome 15 of Dylan Torrances making him completely disabled (Rose, 2016), or of Bertrand Mights whom suffers from a new glycosylation disorder caused by NGLY1 gene mutations - so new that only got found and diagnosed recently, after years of search (Mnookin, 2014).

Genetic diseases can secure significant funding and interest representing a different biomedical and health research challenge. Genetic diseases encompass single gene disorders, chromosome imbalances, epigenetics, complex disorders and even cancer. Thus, understanding how medical and technological advances can be used for proper diagnosis, disease management and treatment is crucial for patients' survival and quality of life.

Precision medicine is based on vast troves of genomic information, but diverse populations are still underrepresented in public genomic databases. Europe, however, is just starting to take big steps in this front. Thirteen European counties signed in 2018 a protocol so that genomic and genetic information can 'cross-borders' and improve European health research and clinical practice.[61] Genomic databases are weakened by lack of representation of diverse populations. For example, African, Latin American and Asian ancestral populations are underrepresented compared to European populations in two public databases, the Genome-Wide Association Study Catalog (GWAS) and the database of Genotypes and Phenotypes (dbGaP) (Landry, Ali, Williams, Rehm, & Bonham, 2018). Moreover, most studies on the genetics of diseases were performed in European populations.

This lack of diversity in genomic studies has implications for the risk prediction of diseases across global populations and harms the scientific understanding of the genetic mechanisms of a disease in all populations increasing health care inequities (Sirugo, Williams, & Tishkoff, 2019). It can be compared to the gender bias in research with studies on female-specific health and pain performed in male subjects. This situation has been too repeatedly approached in the media (Billock, 2018; Dusenbery, 2018; Glezerman, 2016; Westervelt, 2015). Thus, this agreement is particularly significant for rare diseases and cancer patients[62]; and represents the first step for equity in the access to personalized treatments and target drug therapies.

Governments promote some strategies for research, clinicians, and public health care in general. Newborn screenings help to detect registries of congenital and development (rare or not) diseases that can be addressed immediately and improve prognosis and outcomes[63] (Tridello, Castellani, Meneghelli, Tamanini, & Assael, 2018). USA through NIH - National Human Genome Research Institute (NHGRI) incentives investigators and health professionals to collaborate, promote funding opportunities while also providing information for health professionals, patients and people interested, as well as raising awareness in communities.[64] The combination of social media usage and awareness together with information dissemination and social media streaming is slowly but steadily improving rare diseases patients' outcomes by winning attention and investment.

Rare Diseases in Anesthesiology

Patients with a rare disease present unique challenges for primary care and anesthesiologists in specific. Because anesthesia does not follow the known mechanisms in rare disease patients as in normal individuals, recommendations on anesthesia clinical practice are made available in databases. [65] Literature has also been published addressing the issue and practice and management guidelines, as in "Anesthesia and Uncommon Diseases" (Fleisher, 2012).

Putting under anesthesia, a rare disease patient is however always a challenge and can lead to complications. Clinicians awareness of rare and uncommon diseases and possible complications is essential for proper anesthetic patient management.

Rare Diseases in Hematology

Blood cell formation, growth and development also can be disrupted, with cell types being produced abnormally and/or in large quantities. This can lead to blood cancers or other blood disorders. For example, myelodysplastic syndrome is a rare group of blood disorders that result from the improper development of blood cells within the bone marrow. It includes white blood cell dysfunctions that may be related to different diseases and, platelet and red blood cells abnormalities (e.g. Familial platelet disorder with associated myeloid malignancy (FPD/ AML), sickle cell thalassemia, Diamond-Blackfan anemia). Therefore, rare hematological or blood diseases include plasma-based disorders, anemia-type red blood cells, immune disorders, and while blood cell overproduction.

Some blood diseases are Aagenaes syndrome, Abetalipoproteinemia, Acquired hemophilia, Acute Erythroid leukemia, Fabry disease, Fanconi anemia, Yellow nail syndrome, Williams syndrome and Tufted Angloma, or rare blood cancers as myeloproliferative neoplasms (rare blood cancers are characterized by the overproduction of cells in the bone marrow, affecting less than six in 100,000 people) which include Polycythemia Vera, myelofibrosis, and essential thrombocythemia (Coles, Chan, Palczewski, Lewis, & Ho, 2019). Some of these blood diseases may be caused by low intake of iron or excessive blood loss due to menstruation, resulting in iron-deficiency anemia. Additionally, ulcers or cancer can cause blood loss in the gastrointestinal tract.

It has been a slow move into developing and certifying new therapies for these rare blood diseases. The first treatment was only approved in 2017 - vemurafenib, a drug for adults diagnosed with Erdheim-Chester disease (ECD), a rare blood cancer that originates in the bone marrow. This drug was approved in 2011 for treatment of melanoma with mutations in the BRAF gene (Voelker, 2017). Countries have created National Blood Cancer Networks; however, much is yet to be done to promote clinical research and international collaborations (e.g. Blood Cancer Network Ireland (BCNI). [66]

To support health professionals and patients of these rare diseases, Europe created a network of expert centers: EuroBloodNet - European Reference Network on Rare Hematological Diseases[67] and Enerca - European Network for Rare and Congenital Anemias.[68] The exchange of knowledge is the main objective in this context. Recently, new communication technologies have been pinpointed as key tools for the European Reference Networks (ERN), and thus institutions have increasingly adopted digitized and networked information in medical practice (Héon-Klin, 2017).

Rare Diseases of the Lymphatic System

Some diseases under the umbrella of the term 'blood cancers' affect the lymphatic system too, namely lymphomas, cancers that start in white blood cells (lymphocytes) and then accumulate in lymph nodes impairing the immune system. However, other diseases even more rarely affect the fluid-filled channels that are part of the lymphatic system.

They are non-malignant masses or spaces that are thought to be caused by development problems of the lymphatic system. These formations are often congenital, detected at birth or up to two years of age, and can affect any part of the body, except the brain. They are more prevalent in head and neck and tend to consist of soft, spongy, non-tender masses. The symptoms are diverse and depend upon the size and location of the malformation. Some can be huge, while others can potentially cause problems in the nearby structures or organs and disfigurement irrespective of its size.

Primary lymphedema (i.e., not caused by other health conditions as for example, from surgery to treat breast cancer) is one of these rare inherited conditions caused by abnormal development of lymph vessels. It is estimated to occur in 1 in every 100,000 individuals younger than 20 years old. [69] Meige disease, for example, is the most common type of primary lymphedema; it is congenital but with swelling only showing during or after puberty, it has unknown causes and prevalence.[70] It is characterized by the abnormal buildup of fluid in soft tissue due to a blockage in the lymphatic system.

Another is Castleman Disease, which encompasses a group of disorders with variable symptoms that include enlarged lymph nodes that share similar morphology when reviewed under the microscope. It is estimated that there are about 5,000 cases diagnosed each year and 30,000 individuals in the United States suffering with one of the forms of Castleman disease. [71] With similar symptoms, there is also Hodgkin lymphoma, a cancer of the lymphatic systems where tumors form in lymph nodes and/or the areas around these nodes. These tumors are more common in the spleen, stomach and chest, and it is a progressive and generally fatal cancer. The cause is unclear and accounts for less than 1% of all cases of cancer in the USA.[72]

The lymphatic system has a fundamental role in cardiovascular diseases, infection, immunity and cancer, and probably obesity. These are the major global health challenges of today. Rare diseases of the lymphatic system are complex in nature and can be localized, affect multiple sites, or be congenital. They can cause symptoms that range from mild to severe to life-threating and even be fatal. And, they can affect a small portion of the population but have devastating effects and are a health burden worldwide. Thus, focus in increasing current knowledge, promote research and develop therapeutic targets is essential.

Rare Nutritional and Metabolic Diseases

Metabolism is the chemical process by which the body transforms the food we eat into the 'fuel' that keeps us alive. Sometimes, this process fails. Metabolic disorders have variable causes that include a missing enzyme or vitamin, abnormal chemical reactions, disease of the liver, pancreas, endocrine glands or other organ involved in the metabolism, or nutritional deficiencies. These can result from genetics, a deficiency in a certain hormone or enzyme, consuming too much or too little or certain foods, amongst other factors. There are hundreds of metabolic rare diseases caused by gene mutations. Others can be linked to a nutritional deficiency and are visible in the skin (e.g. deficiency of vitamin C (scurvy) and of niacin or vitamin B3 (pellagra)) or in the body appearance (kwashiorkor disease or edematous malnutrition which, occurs due to chronic zinc deficiency and cause patients to suffer from edema (fluid retention) and an enlarged liver with fatty infiltrates) (Sarkany, Breathnach, Morris, Weismann, & Flynn, 2010).

Nutritional diseases not often are considered rare, but this may the case of Scurvy (vitamin C deficiency), Rickets (vitamin D deficiency), and Keshan disease (selenium deficiency) in the United States and in most of the Western countries.[73] Malabsorption can, sometimes, be behind these deficiencies as a consequence from genetic abnormalities.[74]

Hundreds of errors in metabolism have been registered with most being very rare. However, collectively these diseases may affect up to 1 in every 1,000 children. Many of these can only be treated by limiting the intake of the substance that the body cannot process. A listing of metabolic diseases registered in a US rare diseases database can be consulted at https://rarediseases.info.nih.gov/diseases/diseases-by-category/14 (accessed 17-10-2019) which, include the more common diseases:

- Gaucher's disease (inability to process fat, which accumulates in the liver, spleen and bone marrow. Enzyme replacement treatment is used to treat it.);
- Glucose galactose malabsorption (abnormal transport of glucose and galactose across the stomach lining, causing severe diarrhea and dehydration. The disease is often controlled by removing lactose, sucrose, and glucose from the diet.);
- Gestational *diabetes insipidus* (occurs only during pregnancy when an enzyme made by the placenta destroys anti-diuretic hormone (ADH) in the mother. This rare endocrine complication is associated with vasopressinase overproduction. It causes an imbalance of fluids in the body. This causes severe thirst. There is no cure, but treatments can decrease the thirst and urine output);
- Hepatoerythropoietic porphyria (inherited cutaneous porphyria caused by a deficiency of the enzyme uroporphyrinogen decarboxylase. Porphyrins are essential for the function of hemoglobin, a protein in red blood cells that links to porphyrin, binds iron, and carries oxygen to the organs and tissues. High levels of porphyrins can cause severe conditions.);
- Hereditary hemochromatosis (excess iron deposited in several organs. It is treated by removing blood from the body regularly (phlebotomy));
- Lesch-Nyhan syndrome (overproduction of uric acid resulting in neurological and behavioral problems. It may cause inflammation and kidney diseases too. It is a congenital genetic disease.);
- Maple syrup urine disease (the metabolism of some aminoacids is disturbed leading to neuronal degeneration. If not treated, it is fatal within months after birth. Treatment requires limiting the intake of branched chain aminoacids, leucine, isoleucine and valine. Human dietary sources of these aminoacids are foods that contain protein, such as meats and dairy products);
- Phenylketonuria (decreased metabolism of the amino acid phenylalanine due to failure to produce phenylalanine hydroxylase. This can lead to organ failure, seizures and intellectual disability. It is a genetic disease. Treatment requires limiting foods that contain phenylalanine and special supplements).

Another rare heritable metabolic disease is Tay-Sachs disease. This usually fatal genetic disease causes progressive damage to the nerve cells in the brain and spinal cord. As many other metabolic rare diseases, it is mostly commonly associated to a particular racial/ethnic group. In this case, Tay-Sachs diseases is more common among Ashkenazi Jews (Eastern and Central European) but has also been found in the French Canadians of South- eastern Quebec, the Cajuns of Southwest Louisiana, and other populations throughout the world. The severity of expression and the age at onset of Tay-Sachs varies. It can then be subdivided into infantile Tay-Sachs disease, Juvenile (subacute) Tay-Sachs Disease and Late-Onset Tay-Sachs disease.[75]

Symptoms associated with this disease include psychomotor regression, paralysis, dementia and blindness. They are the result of the excessive accumulation of some fats (lipids), known as gangliosides, in the central nervous system. Mutations in the HEXA gene result in deficiency of hexosaminidase A enzyme, responsible for breaking down these fatty substances called GM2 gangliosides. Thus, this substance accumulates to toxic levels mainly in the neurons, which causes the symptoms of Tay-Sachs Disease. [76]

Metabolic diseases are complex and rare. Most are misidentified and under-diagnosed. However, the public can be increasingly aware of their existence through media coverage or the share of personal stories in social media. For example, in Portugal very few will know what the CDG syndrome is - congenital disorder of glycosylation (ORPHA: 137). [77]

The first case seems to have been only registered in 1997 to a, then, 16-year-old adolescent.[78] Patients may initially be diagnosed with cerebral palsy or a different genetic disorder. CGD syndrome is extremely rare affecting about 1 in 50,000 to 100,000 children. Patients can now find some support among patients' associations. But before the 21st century, it was mostly unheard of. The strength of these children's parents together with the new IT and communication tools is changing the paradigm and raising awareness for this syndrome.[79] Thanks to this, CDG syndrome cases are appearing in the news and TV-shows, further raising awareness and potentially incentivizing biomedical research of orphan diseases like these.

Rare Multisystemic Diseases

Multisystemic diseases, as the designation suggests, refers to diseases that affect more than one system of bodily organs. These include many rare diseases aforementioned. One of them is autosomal systemic lupus erythematosus, mentioned in rare immune diseases. Lupus can have many clinical manifestations. It can affect the skin, eye, gastrointestinal tract, heart, lungs, muscles, kidneys and even the central nervous system. Moreover, lupus may have obstetrical implications by passing to the fetus – neonatal lupus - and inducing spontaneous abortions (ORPHA: 300345). [80] HERNS syndrome (Hereditary endotheliopathy with retinopathy, nephropathy, and stroke disease)[81] is now called Retinal vasculopathy with cerebral leukoencephalopathy and systemic manifestations (ORPHA: 247691). [82] This is a very rare genetic disease of unknown prevalence and treatment that affects the inner lining of the blood vessels, and whose name highlights the various bodily systems affected (Seifried, Sitzer, Jen, & Auburger, 2005).

Sarcoidosis is a non-rare example. This inflammatory condition mainly affects the lungs and immune system but can also cause cardiac, ocular, hepatic, neuronal, and nose and skin complications. Sarcoidosis occurs worldwide, with a prevalence of about 5-64 in 100,000 individuals and an incidence of 1.0-36 in 100,000 individuals per year (Valeyre et al., 2014).

Rare Gynecological and Obstetrical Diseases

Some rare diseases present particular pathophysiology and etiology when associated with pregnancy; some occur just during pregnancy and then they may disappear, or not. This is the case of the aforementioned gestational diabetes.

Gestational diseases may be considered a group of rare diseases that develop within the womb throughout an abnormal physiological condition. In some diseases, tumors or abnormal cells grow inside the tissues that form following conception and that may surround the embryo and transform the placenta. Infections may too become chronic. Many adrenal disorders and gynecological cancers are also rare.

The most widely recognized obstetrical disorder is probably gestational trophoblastic disease (GTD), a group of diseases that occur in the uterus during an abnormal pregnancy. It develops when abnormal cells or tumors propagate in the tissues after conception. These tumors are called 'moles' and are usually noncancerous.

Reproductive health is today a huge and increasing health burden worldwide of which our future depends on. Thus, rare female reproductive diseases cannot be overlooked. It is urgent to understand and to find treatments for diseases that include CHARGE syndrome (mentioned in genitourinary diseases) and HELLP syndrome (mentioned in hepatic diseases), and many others as BRCA hereditary breast and ovarian cancer syndrome. The current term of hereditary breast and ovarian (HBOC) syndrome is generally used for individuals with BRCA1 and BRCA2 genetic mutations. Arguably, it should be renamed because mutations in the BRCA genes can also be involved in tumors in men as in breast, prostate and pancreatic cancers and in melanomas. HBOC has been proposed to be renamed 'King syndrome' (Marabelli, Calvello, & Bonanni, 2019; Pritchard, 2019). BRCA syndrome got attention when celebrities patients announced their health issue (e.g. actress Angelina Jolie double Mastectomy and Oophorectomy).

The mediatization captured much general interest but if this has been reflected in medical research and findings is unknown. Nonetheless, many other disorders also require attention.[83] There are over a hundred ongoing research projects to understand and treat rare genetic gynecological and obstetrical diseases. [84] However, if any of them will be successful in finding a therapeutic target or treatment is yet an open question.

Figure 1. (A) Proportion of common, less common, rare and very rare cancers. (B) Parts of the body that are affected by rare cancers, Source: https://www.macmillan.org.uk (Access Date: September 10, 2019)

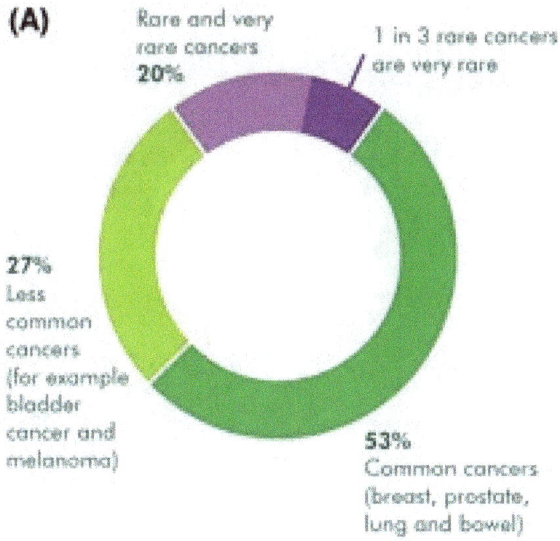

Rare Tumors

Cancer is a leading cause of death worldwide, accounting for an estimated 9.6 million deaths in 2018. [85] There is no correct definition for a rare cancer. Traditionally, a rare cancer is defined as a type of cancer that occurs in less than 6 people per year per 100,000 population. A less common cancer is one that affects between 6 and 12 people per year per 100,000 population (e.g. brain tumors, thyroid cancers, pancreatic cancers, testicular cancers, etc.). A very rare cancer affects fewer than 1 people per year per 100,000 population. According to this, most cancers except for breast, prostate, bowel, lung and melanoma, can be classified as rare or less common. In Europe, 1 in 5 people is diagnosed with a rare cancer annually (Pillai & Jayasree, 2017). The diagram (A) in Figure 1 shows the percentage of patients affected by a form or type of rare cancer. The diagram (B) in Figure 1 shows where in the body rare cancers may occur with, one in every 5 rare cancers affecting the blood or lymphatic system (e.g. leukemias and lymphomas).

There are many different rare tumors. They can be a subtype of a more common cancer or start in different types of cells, sometimes not related to the body part where it starts. It can affect anyone, child or young adult, and the personal, psychological and economic impact is enormous. It can occur in virtually any cell in the body and eventually spread to any tissue. Societies have invested greatly in trying to

Figure 2. From DeSantis et al. (2017), Distribution of Rare and Common Cancers, 2009 Through 2013, United States. NH indicates non-Hispanic. Source: North American Association of Central Cancer Registries, 2016

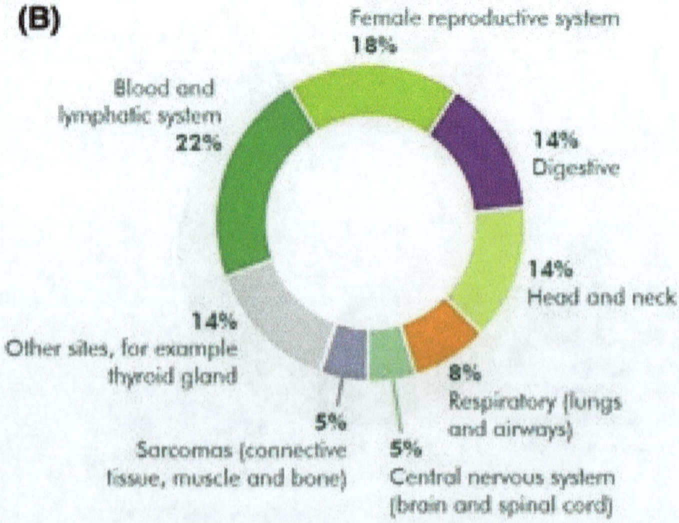

control, research and reduce cancer incidence and mortality. However, the progress has been very slow and hard to come by. Rare cancers need to be urgently put on nations' policy agenda. Recently created, rare cancers Europe, RCE (https://www.rarecancerseurope.org), is a multi-stakeholder initiative taking on its hands this goal.

Rare cancers can be grouped in several categories based in the RARECARE framework [86] and the International Classification of Diseases for Oncology (ICD-O 3rd edition, by WHO 2015), and as per listed by RCE [87]:

- Rare SKIN cancers and NON-CUTANEOUS MELANOMA;
- Rare THORACIC cancers (mesothelioma, thymoma, rare lung cancers, rare breast cancers);
- Rare UROGENITAL cancers (kidney cancers, bladder cancers, urinary tract cancers);
- Rare FEMALE GENITAL cancers (cervical and ovarian cancers);
- Rare MALE GENITAL cancers (prostate and testicular cancers);
- NEUROENDOCRINE cancers;
- ENDOCRINE ORGAN cancers (adrenal cancer, thyroid and parathyroid cancer);
- Rare CNS cancers (brain cancer);
- SARCOMAS;

- Rare DIGESTIVE cancers (esophageal cancers, stomach and small intestine cancer, colorectal and anal cancers, liver cancers, gallbladder cancers and cancers of the Intrahepatic/Extrahepatic Bile Tract (IBT/EBT), pancreatic cancers);
- Rare cancers of HEAD & NECK;
- Rare HAEMATOLOGIC cancers (lymphomas, leukemias, myelodysplastic and myeloproliferative disorders/neoplasms);
- PAEDIATRIC solid cancers.

Rare tumors patients often face lack of approved treatments and clinical trials access. However, even though a rare tumor is uncommon, together, rare tumors sum up to about 25% of all cancers being diagnosed (Gatta et al., 2011; Kato, Kurasaki, Ikeda, & Kurzrock, 2018). Just in the United States of America, rare cancers account for one fifth of the new annual diagnoses and more than two-thirds of children and adolescents affected (~70%, Figure 2) have a rare cancer type (DeSantis, Kramer, & Jemal, 2017).Variations in the percentages of rare cancers by sex, race/ethnicity, and age at diagnosis, and the distribution of rare and common cancers by cancer site are shown in Figure 2.

Rare cancers are unique and represent a challenge for health professionals and patients. Research to identify their causes and mechanisms is lacking and so is the development of strategies for prevention or early detection. Several factors limit the analysis, diagnosis and registration of rare cancers. Unspecified morphology contributes to difficulties in to make a precise diagnosis and correct documentation of cases. As biomolecular techniques continue to develop, and molecular markers are being identified, it is likely that the number of rare tumors identified will continue to raise. Collectively, rare cancers burden will contribute substantially to the health burden on societies and countries. At the same time, patients face great inequalities in the access to new treatments and medical expertise across the countries, and that is noticeable in the cancer-survival rates.

Additionally, rare cancers in adults are more ‘deadly’ than common cancers, killing more rare cancer patients within 5 years after diagnosis (American Cancer Society Inc, 2017; Gatta, Trama, & Capocaccia, 2019). Therefore, rare diseases patients, and rare cancer patients in particular, face multiple setbacks: incorrect or late diagnosis, lack of access to proper treatments and medical assistance, very limited number of clinical studies associated with few available registries and tissue banks and, as in all rare diseases, the lack of interest from pharmaceutical industry and biotechnology in to developing new medications due to the ‘assumed’ small sized market. Furthermore, there are evidences that rare cancer survivors face increased risk of a subsequent cancer (Finkelstein et al., 2019).

Research and development have focused historically in the most common cancers / diseases; thus, orphan drugs development have 'fallen' behind. But it is now accepted that research for rare cancers can further knowledge for all cancers, thus leading to increased investment. Rare cancer patients elevated risks of re-incidence also make them subjects of particular interest to better understand cancer causes and mechanisms. Additionally, understanding a rare tumor or cancer can also create insight into other cancers and diseases, rare or not.

The investment in managing and raising awareness about rare cancers has increased dramatically in the last few years. Networking and reference centers were created worldwide. Expertise and information diffusion have been improving the standards of care.

The European Medical Society for Medical Oncology (ESMO) released clinical practice guidelines for rare cancers.[88] ESMO also organizes congresses, workshops and shares news about the latest medications and findings in cancer biology.

Other international initiatives as the International Rare Cancer Initiative EORTC-US-UK global collaboration have taken on similar mission.[89] This later network initiative counts with over 5300 scientists, from over 37 countries and with over 50 studies ongoing in 2019. The main objective of these initiatives is to boost the development of orphan drugs to treat patients with rare tumors or cancers.

Rare Diseases Due to Plastic Surgery

Several body deformities or anomalies can be caused by rare diseases (e.g. Bosma Arhinia Microphthalmia Syndrome (BAM), which is characterized by three major features: 1) complete absence of the nose, 2) eye defects, and 3) absent sexual maturation; and it is extremely rare having registered less than 100 people affected worldwide in the last century [90]). These malformations are often treated or corrected by plastic surgery procedures. However, the opposite may occur, and plastic surgery can lead to rare diseases upsurge, namely to the development of rare types of cancer.

One of these cases was reported just this year, 2019, in July, with a massive global recall for textured breast implants made by Allergan. The implants were linked to over 30 cancer-related deaths, and to over 570 cases of an unusual cancer - anaplastic large-cell lymphoma, a rare cancer of the immune system (Grady, 2019). However, textured breast implants have been associated to rare lymphomas before. Another case earned mediatic attention in 2018 with a major worldwide recall for implants produced by the French manufacturer PIP, but the first alert for women whom receiving these implants about the risks of developing cancer came out in 2011 (Devlin & Osborne, 2018; Perrone & Neergaard, 2011).

Right in 2011, when the first cancer-related dead was reported, UK NHS (National Health Service in the United Kingdom) issued a concern, but at the time the regulatory agency (MHRA, medicines and healthcare products regulatory agency) argued insufficient evidences linking the implants to the cancer.[91] But reports from the scientific community suggesting that breast implants could be associated with anaplastic large cell lymphoma (ALCL) can be traced back as far as 1997 (Peters, 2014). However, more recent media coverage and public pressure together with increasing number of registered cancer patients and cancer-related deaths prompted improving of the studies design and continued reviews on the cases, hence allowing causation links to be objectively established. Silicone implants have also been suggested to be associated with other diseases, including autoimmune diseases as scleroderma, rheumatoid arthritis, and lupus, or cancers of the brain, respiratory tract, cervix, and vulva (Brown, Langone, & Brinton, 1998; Hirmand, Latrenta, & Hoffman, 1993).[92]

Recently, silicone implants in a large cohort of patients were associated with some rare diseases, autoimmune disorders and other conditions (Coroneos, Selber, Offodile, Butler, & Clemens, 2019). Although a causation relationship was not clearly established by some studies, they analyzed implants recently applied thus, the long-term consequences of having an implant were not considered.

Plastic surgeons are urged to monitor long-term safety of the implants that they apply and, to inform people seeking these surgeries about the risks and to make sure that the patients understand these risks. U.S.A. Food and Drug Administration (FDA) released guidelines designated 'Breast Implants - Certain Labeling Recommendations to Improve Patient Communication Draft Guidance' as early as in 2006.[93, 94] U.S. health officials and FDA continue now tracking reports of side-effects from implants. However, it took about two decades for breast implant-associated anaplastic large cell lymphoma (BIA-ALCL) to be accepted and registered as a clinical issue (Clemens, DeCoster, Fairchild, Bessonov, & Santanelli di Pompeo, 2019; Wohlgemuth, Brasil, & d'Acampora, 2019). The US National Comprehensive Cancer Network guidelines now include this problem in updated versions. Medicolegal considerations and bioethics are currently a very important discussion for health professionals and stakeholders engaged in policy-making efforts (Clemens et al., 2019).

The popularity of breast augmentation has more than doubled since 1997. Concerns about their safety remain despite the increasing number of people with breast implants. Furthermore, silicone implants are also increasingly sought by men. Bottom and pectoral implants are increasingly popular. Additionally, men pressure for certain body standards also lead them to take illegal substances and injections of silicone. Despite the scarce literature, there has been reports of silicone-related health issues namely, silicone-induced granulomatous hypercalcemia (a rare disease) (Hamadeh & Fares, 2018; Hamadeh, Fares, Maatouk, & Darwish, 2018).

Research shows that implants can be associated with health, cosmetic and economic risks, particularly over time, when the risk increases greatly. But long-term risks are unknown as properly designed and comprehensive studies remain to be done. FDA and European institutions require implant manufactures to conduct additional research to assess implants toxicology, breakage and durability. However, these studies are confidential and often suspected of bias. Cases of rare diseases caused by cosmetic surgery often are only revealed when affecting public figures or by patients and families mediatic pressure. Plastic surgeons need to be sensible to follow the side-effects of the procedures they perform in the long-term, particularly, when using implants. This may allow timely screening and diagnosis, and potentially better outcome for patients.

Rare Diseases Due to External Causes like Poisoning, General Surgery or Injury

Exposure to poisons such as industrial chemicals and heavy metals (e.g. arsenic, lead, mercury, etc.) can damage the nerves outside of the brain and spinal cord (peripheral nerves), causing weakness, numbness, and pain usually in the hands and feet. This condition is designated by peripheral neuropathy. Peripheral neuropathy can also be caused by injuries, infections, metabolic problems and inherited causes, besides exposure to toxins.

Over a hundred rare diseases are characterized by neuropathies. These include: systemic inflammatory disease associated with an acquired peripheral neuropathy (e.g. Crohn's disease), malignant lymphoma with peripheral neuropathy (e.g. non-Hodgkin's lymphoma), infectious disease with peripheral neuropathy (e.g. reactive arthrosis, or actinomycosis, i.e. when Actinomyces species of bacteria spread through the body because of tissue damage), systemic amyloidosis (ORPHA:85448 ; GARD: 2339), amyotrophic lateral sclerosis (ORPHA:803; GARD: 5786), acute motor and sensory axonal neuropathy (ORPHA:98917), neuralgic amyotrophy (ORPHA: 2901; GARD: 4228), Lewis-Sumner syndrome (ORPHA: 48162), amongst many others. Heavy metal poising is listed in rare diseases databases as NORD and Orphanet.[95,96]

Rare conditions can also arise from traumas or injuries. Examples include the Asherson's syndrome (mentioned in the subtopic 'Rare diseases of the immune system'), Gerstmann syndrome and the now named Central Pain syndrome. Ashersons's syndrome is an extremely rare disease where blood clots affect the several organs of the body. Infections, immunizations but also wounds caused by physical trauma or injury can lead to failures in the anticoagulation mechanisms of the body and be a 'trigger' for this condition. [97]

Related to this, women during pregnancy or after birth can also express the same symptoms, which can follow to HELLP syndrome (discussed in 'Rare hepatic diseases' and in 'Rare gynecological and obstetrical diseases') or other disorders. Gerstmann syndrome, on the other hand, is a rare neurological disorder that can occur due to a brain injury or a developmental problem. Cognitive impairment caused by this syndrome can arise in adults as a result of impaired blood flow to the brain (cerebrovascular disease) such as a stroke or other damage to the brain. But in rare cases, traumatic brain injury or a brain tumor in the parietal region of the brain (involved in sensation and perception) can cause the symptoms associated with Gerstmann syndrome.[98] The last example provided, the central pain syndromes, previously known as thalamic syndrome, Dejerine Roussy syndrome, Posterior thalamic syndrome, amongst others, is a rare neurological disorder resulting from damage of the pain-conducting pathways of the central nervous system. The current name recognizes that damage to the central nervous system can cause central pain, and stroke is not necessarily the cause. In fact, central pain syndromes have been associated with stroke, multiple sclerosis, tumors, epilepsy, Parkinson's disease, and trauma to the brain or spinal cord, being often associated with peripheral neuropathies (Nicholson, 2004; Siddall & Loeser, 2001).[99]

Abnormal Clinical and Laboratory Findings

Abnormalities of heart beat (e.g. palpitations or cardiac murmurs), abnormalities of breathing (mouth breathing, hiccup, etc.), stomach and pelvic pains, but also skin swellings and rashes, abnormal nervous and musculoskeletal movements, amongst many other disturbances of the systems of the body can be included in abnormal clinical and laboratory findings (International Statistical Classification of Diseases and Related Health Problems ICD-10 Chapter XVIII by WHO, 2016). Diseases as sudden infant death syndrome, hyperglycemia (high glucose levels in the blood) and dysuria (painful urination) follow under this category. While hyperglycemia and dysuria are relatively common, sudden infant death syndrome is relatively uncommon affecting 1 in 1,000 to 10,000 newborns.

The newborns die before the 12 months of age, suddenly and unexpectedly, without obvious cause. Even though emergency guidelines for the reporting and evaluation of sudden infant death syndrome have been developed, the causes and prevention remain elusive (Hunt & Hauck, 2006). Recent guidelines suggest cares during sleep and benefits with breastfeeding (Pathologists, 2016; Task Force on Sudden Infant Death, 2016).[100] But a strong correlation is yet to be demonstrated.

Even rarer, is sudden infant death-dysgenesis of the testes syndrome (ORPHA: 168593; GARD: 12382), which affects less than 1 in 1,000,000 newborns, having been described in particular in sibships of the Old Order Amish. A genetic mutation in the chromosome 6, in a testis-specific gene, cause these infants to die of sudden cardiorespiratory arrest before they reach the first year of life. The newborns are apparently normal at birth, but within the first months of life they develop signs of nerve dysfunction in the viscera that include bradycardia, hypothermia, severe gastroesophageal reflux, and abnormal cardiorespiratory patterns during sleep. Female sexual development is normal, but male babies may present ambiguous genitalia and testicular impairment due to abnormal fetal testes development (Puffenberger et al., 2004). [101]

Abnormal findings in medical and laboratorial testes are diverse and relatively common. Nonetheless, clinicians should be aware and sensitized to any rare conditions underlying these unusual findings. Current challenges include raised awareness and wider dissemination of guidelines and information.

Other Rare Diseases

There are emerging diseases being identified and described for which there are no assigned classification or code yet. This is particularly common with diseases arising from antibiotic resistance (e.g. resistance to beta-lactam antibiotics as penicillin) and resistance to antineoplastic drugs. Others include infections by virus at a scale never seen before.

This is the case of the Zika virus and its correlation to newborn malformations and abortions, that gave name to the rare disease / viral infection 'congenital Zika syndrome'.[102] Zika virus disease results from an emerging *Aedes* mosquito-borne virus and the disease is characterized, mostly, by absent to mild fever, conjunctivitis, muscle and joint pain and headaches, but also with serious neurological and autoimmune problems and, birth defects (microcephaly) if a woman gets infected while pregnant. [103] It was reported in South America (namely, in Brazil) in 2014, and in 2016 the causation relationship between Zika infection and microcephaly in newborns was established (Van der Linden, 2016). This led the World Health Organization (WHO) to declare Zika infection to be a Public Health Emergency of International Concern, and since then great efforts to understand the syndrome have been made (Van der Linden, 2016). [104] But other problems and disorders can also be related with exposure to risk-factors, traumas, social environment, physical environment, lifestyle, family history of neoplasms / cancer, presence of implants and postsurgical states, amongst others.

In a rapidly changing world, the global health spectrum is also changing. Common diseases are no longer common and new infections and problems are being identified. Furthermore, the development of improved and new cellular and molecular biology techniques is allowing to identify subtypes of diseases or even new malignancies never before pinpointed. For example, particular clinical features but also genetic testing allowed to identify the new Au-Kline syndrome, which is caused by mutations in a nuclear regulatory protein. The lack of this protein results in intellectual disability, development delays and other neurological problems.[105] This syndrome was only described in 2015 and only about 25 cases are known so far (Au, Innes, & Kline, 1993).

Some syndromes still own their designation to the genetic defect that causes it. This is the case of 10q26 deletion syndrome that is caused by the loss (deletion) of a small piece on the long (q) arm of chromosome 10 at position designated 10q26, in each cell. This small deletion is behind symptoms that include distinctive facial features, mild to moderate intellectual disability, growth problems, and developmental delay. This syndrome is inherited and there are about 100 cases reported, however the prevalence is unknown (Lin et al., 2016). [106, 107] Despite its rarity, there are some rare chromosome disorder support groups offering information and raising awareness (Lin et al., 2016; Rare chromosome disorder support group).

Ribose-5-phosphate isomerase (RPI) deficiency is probably the rarest human disease in the world with only three known patients in a 27-yearlong period. It is caused by mutations in the enzyme ribose-5-phosphate isomerase that lead to peripheral neuropathy and leukoencephalopathy (all of the brain white matter diseases). Inborn defects in pentose and polyol metabolism constitute a new area of inborn metabolic disorders (Huck et al., 2004; Wamelink et al., 2010). Leukoencephalopathy with evanescent white matter is on itself a rare genetic disease. This hereditary brain disease occurs primarily in children. The disease is chronic and progressive (Porciuncula, Spada, & Goulart, 2018).

CHALLENGES FACING RESEARCH INTO RARE CANCERS

Innovation and implementation into practice of novel findings (i.e. with translational results) are key for better health and patient care. Biomedical and health research are central and are under pressure by a changing society that demands new research, innovation and efficient strategies.

Knowledge about cancer biology remains sparse and full of gaps that interest multiple research groups worldwide. This also constitute an obstacle for patients and physicians. Only a few researchers in the world are able to study each rare cancer. Furthermore, a clear diagnosis for rare cancers is hampered by the lack of specialized tests, biomarkers and more important specialist referrals that often are required. The lack of evidence and experience with most of these cancers often make treatment a trial-error exercise.

Parallelly to the difficulties of diagnosis, the patients also struggle to find proper information and guidance about their disease. This puts a huge psychological, emotional and financial impact on the family and caregivers. The rarity of these tumors may single people out even more by not finding "disease-peers" for support and to share experiences. However, collectively, these rare tumors stand out and are a number too big to ignore.

DIAGNOSIS AND TREATMENT OPTIONS FOR RARE DISEASES

Accessibility of Drugs for Patients

Patients journey does not end with the diagnosis, as treatment is rarer than knowledge about the condition. Many associations and international entities were created in recent years to inform and safeguard patients and families affected by rare diseases. They help raise awareness and pressure stakeholders to improve legislation and research investment and to develop treatments and therapies for these patients. Thus, the interest and awareness of rare diseases has risen adamantly across the many disciplines of medical and life sciences. However, some rare diseases patients face particular challenges. For example, rare gastrointestinal (GI) tract disease patients face particular difficulties as these conditions are often not easily discussed due to stigma.

For children, these problems are enhanced affecting their physical, emotional and psychological wellbeing and development. Patient advocacy organizations for gastrointestinal rare diseases play a leading role in reducing this burden by offering information, support and raising awareness. They also encourage and sponsor collaborative relationships between patients and their families and health professionals, researchers, manufactures and other involved in the research and development of new drugs and treatments, as well as pressing policymakers and regulators.

At the same time, being part of initiatives like the International Rare Diseases Day further raise awareness for the trials that rare diseases patients live with, including rare cancers.

Health technologies and health communication also require scientific research to take steps forward. Researchers have made progress in learning how to identify, diagnose, treat and sometimes even prevent several rare diseases. However, the majority lacks approved or known treatments or therapies. Governmental institutions have been pivotal in to support research to improve the health of people with rare diseases.

Collaborative projects to study common themes and causes of related diseases are also sought out. Collaborations are intended to speed the development of treatments that will eventually be useful for both rare and common diseases. Just the U.S.A. have several institutes, centers, and programs dedicated to study rare diseases (e.g. National Center for Advancing Translational Sciences (NCATS) supports the following programs: Rare Diseases Clinical Research Network (RDCRN), Therapeutics for Rare and Neglected Diseases (TRND), Rare Diseases Registry Program (RaDaR) and, Genetic and Rare Diseases Information Center (GARD)). Thanks to the multiple administrative practices installed since the Orphan Act was approved in 1983, over 400 drugs and biological products for rare diseases were developed and approved to market in the U.S.A.

In an attempt to gather and promote international cooperation as well as to speed up the research and development of treatments for rare disease, the European Union created E-Rare or ERA – Net for research programs on rare diseases (http://www.erare.eu). Starting in 2006, with partners from European and non-European countries, they aim to maximize the resources and, to coordinate and to promote efforts for funding research in rare diseases.

To sum to all this, media coverage play an important role in increasing public awareness and formation of their views and attitudes toward certain issues. Thus, institutions should 'recruit' media support and engage with them to increase peoples interest and levels of information.

CLINICAL RESEARCH ON ORPHAN DRUGS

Small patient cohorts constitute one of the main challenges for rare disease clinical trials. Therefore, trials follow great planning and concern on how to conduct them with a small number of subjects, yet still gathering significative evidence regarding safety and effectiveness in order to obtain approval of the rare disease medicine or drug product. However, entities as FDA do not distinguish between orphan drugs or drugs for common maladies in the requirements for approval. In consequence, researchers should consider novel approaches to trial designs such as a complete single-patient trial design (or n-of-1 trial). Moreover, statistical methods for data analysis also require discussion (Chow & Chang, 2019).

A presentation from Anne Mathieu-Boué, MD from Novartis, in 2014, already identified some key points about the development of orphan drugs for rare cancers, in particular (Mathieu-Boué, 2014). Namely, legislation and norms, as the ones coming after the Orphan Act, are partially to turn research in rare diseases attractive; and studies in pediatric diseases and tumors are rare and raise long term safety issues. Companies and pharma sponsors face budget and production constraints, along with recruitment issues due to low prevalence of the tumors or diseases (i.e. small sample size) (Mathieu-Boué, 2014; Miller, 2010). But also, long and numerous regulated protocols, difficulty in assessing long-term safety, commercial and authorization challenges and lack of specialized staff, along with many other issues. Thus, collaborations that include data base sharing and tissue banks need to be promoted so that pharma companies are incentivized to overcome the focus in the cost issues (Miller, 2010).

Currently, research teams are taking a chance at advancing targeted therapies for better management of some rare diseases. Nonetheless, some challenges remain as, for example, to properly conduct clinical trials with few patients or taking an innovative clinical trial approach and getting approval or prevailing through the obstacles for international cooperation and financial support for research (Pillai & Jayasree, 2017). In order to overcome these problems, recently some initiatives and international collaboration protocols were created. This is the case of the international rare cancers initiative (IRCI), which functions as a platform to develop new international clinical trials in rare tumors (Pillai & Jayasree, 2017), thus getting more people involved and available to enter the trials. [108]

US NIH – National Cancer Research also has promoted the MyPART - My Pediatric and Adult Rare Tumor Network[109], a genomic and other molecular parameters database on rare tumors that include clinical data and patient-reported outcomes, and that is available to researchers as they are collected. In conclusion, research consortia integrated with international reference networks that gather multidisciplinary expert centers can encourage and offer some advantage to researchers, which may bring innovation to rare diseases investigation and drug discovery (Blay, Coindre, Ducimetiere, & Ray-Coquard, 2016; Boyd, Dancey, Gilks, & Huntsman, 2016; Komatsubara & Carvajal, 2016).

Private companies worldwide are having their take on research in orphan drugs. This is the case of the 'Labialfarma - Laboratório Produtos Farmacêuticos E Nutracêuticos, S.A' a Portuguese pharmaceutical company. Through funding from several European Union grants, they develop a drug based on cannabis to treat rare diseases symptoms ("Labialfarma compra antiga bafel e vai investir 20 milhões de euros," 2019). In similar contours, the drug tradename 'Sativex' (Nabiximols) by GW Pharmaceuticals to treat symptoms as spasms from multiple sclerosis was also developed from cannabis and is approved in several countries worldwide.[110] These drugs, however, do not treat or cure rare diseases; they help to control the symptoms.

In a recent turn, the US government made headlines in some Portuguese journals due to granting funds to Portuguese entities for research in a rare disease named Machado-Joseph Disease (MJD). This disease is also known as spinocerebellar ataxia type 3 (SCA3), the most common form of spinocerebellar ataxias in the world. This multisystem neurodegenerative disease affects 0.3 to 2.0 per 100,000 individuals in the world and it is more frequent in counties such as Brazil, Portugal (mostly occurs in Flores Island, in the Azores archipelago), Singapore, China, the Netherlands, Germany and Japan (Bettencourt & Lima, 2011). [111] A new drug designated by NLX-112 targets the serotonin release that is behind motor activity in the body. The drug will be tested in Portuguese laboratories and promises to delay the debilitating physical condition of this rare disease' patients (DN/Lusa, 2019; Redaçao, 2019). The project will also count with the contribution from Neurolix, a North American biotechnology company (Neurolixis, 2019). [112]

A newly develop molecular biology technique come to break many scientific barriers. The translational importance and clinical impact are yet to be shown. However, CRISPR gene editing has been shown to be promising in to understand and correct genetic abnormalities. Recently, researchers used CRISPR editing to correct a mutation in muscle stem cells in a model of Duchenne muscular dystrophy, a rare genetic disease characterized by muscle loss and physical impairment (Min et al., 2019; Nance et al., 2019). The long-term effects of using this technique are yet to be studied, however it may represent the start of groundbreaking treatments for muscular dystrophy. [113]

FUTURE RESEARCH DIRECTIONS

Most of the 400 million people affected by a rare disease across the world have no cure or treatment options. Many of these diseases are life-threating and very debilitating. Furthermore, many countries do not have policies to assist in the management of these conditions. Still, international policies and guidance have begun to emerge and to be updated. For instance, now many official entities include policies about including women and members of minority groups in research and in clinical trials. [114]

Further courses of action can, however, be undertaken. These include: implementation of strategies for recruiting underrepresented groups in research; education provided to patients, providers and researchers about the value and importance of participating in research, including by contributing with biological samples to biobanks (an example is how umbilical cord is typically medical waste that can have better use in research for, for example, stem cells isolation and propagation); genomic information on diverse patient populations accessible for researchers; databases with information on disease prevalence, disparities in disease morbidity and death and genetic factors involved, including ancestral information and ethnic or racial background (Mjoseth, 2018). Overcoming these barriers will allow precision medicine to quickly develop and to change the paradigm in clinical practice of rare diseases (Landry, Ali, Williams, Rehm, & Bonham, 2018). It is also important to empower patients and ensure that rare diseases become a health priority by assuring continued research and development, as well as equitable access to diagnosis, treatment and care. To answer this problematic, working groups have been created, most notably by the European Commission and by US National Institutes of Health (NIH). The progress in rare diseases research in the period from 2010 to 2016, including the contribute of international consortiums to rare diseases research advances has been reviewed elsewhere (Dawkins et al., 2018).

Concomitantly, there is a group of rare diseases often overlooked: parasitic and bacterial infections termed 'neglected tropical rare diseases". These infections affect millions of people, mostly in developing economies and with a particular toll in their children. Often, more than one parasite or contamination affect these people. Cost-effective strategies including medication accessible to people and non-medical staff could aid to control these infections and diseases.

Rare diseases have increasingly been discussed in the media over the past years, specially about new treatments and scientific findings. This can be easily identified by using search words on search engines as Google such as "rare disease patient hope" or "rare disease cure" and see the diversity of hits that are listed from official rare diseases institutions as NIH to online news pages and patient groups pages, and also videos on YouTube. Since the approval of the Orphan Drug Act in the US parliament, an initiative that was later followed by Japan and Europe, the number or approved new drugs for rare diseases has increased drastically. Just in 2017, the FDA approved 80 new orphan medications and, 57 in the first eight months of 2018. The FDA also granted orphan designations to over 429 unique drugs in 2017 (IQVIA, 2018). Therefore, the increased focus and interest from drug manufactures have resulted in the development of therapies for orphan indications and half of the new active substances found were not previously approved for any medicinal use or product. Clinical spending on drugs is shifting from traditional small molecules drugs towards specialty drugs or precise medicine. However, non-orphan drugs or medicine for non-rare diseases still represent much of the use and sales.

On the other hand, the gene therapy sector for rare diseases is fast growing. There is treatment for only a few hundred rare diseases amongst the several thousand registries. Gene therapy present a key tool as over 80% of rare diseases are caused by gene abnormalities (Development, 2010). Traditionally, small molecule medicines work to minimize symptoms rather than cure the diseases, which can mean frequent use of the drugs in order to manage the conditions. However, gene therapy has the potential to cure the abnormalities offering an actual cure to patients. Furthermore, this can be achieved in a single administration. The concept of gene therapy is simple: deliver nucleic acids / gene(s) to target cells to alter their function in a beneficial manner; usually a virus is used to the delivery. Patients life-quality would improve drastically as they would not require life-long treatments and therapies.

In 2018, a gene therapy product called Luxturna® (voretigene neparvovec-rzyl) got approved by FDA. It is used for the treatment of patients with inherited retinal disease due to mutations in both copies of the RPE65 gene. They must also have enough remaining cells in the retina (the thin layer of tissue in the back of your eyes). [115] Propelled by this, families of children with rare diseases decided to start crowdfunding to gather funds for research into diseases unknown for most people. Millions of dollars were raised in this way to fund basic research and clinical trials that can save children's lives. More about this phenomenon can be read at the online magazine 'The Scientist' under the title "Families of children with rare diseases fuel gene therapy research" (Yeager, 2018). Then, in 2019, Novartis got approval for Zolgensma®, a gene product administered by injection in patients' bloodstream to treat spinal muscular atrophy (SMA), a neurodegenerative rare disease that affects many newborns worldwide. This product got immense mediatic exposure and media attention due to its price tag. It was named the most expensive medicine in the world (Curran, 2019). [116]

Just recently, researchers also used gene therapy to alter patients' own blood stem cells. In this case, from children born with a rare genetic disorder called X-linked severe combined immunodeficiency. Early results resulted in the correction of these children abnormal immune cells (Mamcarz et al., 2019).

Gene therapies are promising and in fast evolution. Thus, to help accelerate the field of gene therapy, certain programs to incentivize multidisciplinary collaborations and pilot studies are in place. [117]

Concurrently, immunotherapy is also in a pivotal period in its evolution. Clinical immunology has been proven to be effective and safe in common immune-inflammatory diseases (e.g. rheumatoid arthritis and inflammatory bowel disease). But, newly developed antibodies and/or inhibitors can also result in clinical improvement for patients with rare immune-inflammatory diseases (Musters, Assaf, Gerlag, Tak, & Tas, 2015). Nonetheless, the side effects cannot be overlooked as they can be life-threating themselves. This unique spectrum of side effects is called immune-related adverse events or, adverse events of special interest and include dermatologic, gastrointestinal, hepatic, endocrine, and other inflammatory occurrences (Michael A. Postow, Callahan, & Wolchok, 2015; M. A. Postow, Sidlow, & Hellmann, 2018; Weber, Postow, Lao, & Schadendorf, 2016). Immunotherapy treatment in a cancer patient was also reported to have caused encephalitis (Johnson et al., 2019). This was reported in an online journal of research news (Center, 2019).

The number of outlets for health-related news has increased significantly. The lack of user friendliness of some internet sites and complicated language for the non-specialist creates some barriers between the public and information on rare diseases. These recent news outlets and social media facilitate public awareness as well as the retention and better adherence of people to funding campaigns and specific trials participation. Thus, health communication, particularly through online tools as with social media can improve both clinicians and public adherence to clinical trials facilitating pharma companies recruitment and, thus, interest into the pursuit of new marketable drugs for rare or orphan diseases. Overall, the potential of health e-tools and social media to change rare diseases lack of treatments is significant. Additionally, these tools can reach people unrestricted by geography. A considerable amount of work can still be done by stakeholders (from governmental institutions to research consortiums) in order to improve the promotion of their message.

CONCLUSION

Rare diseases are an extremely complex health challenge of our time. There are currently about 8,000 known rare diseases, half of which affect children. Most rare diseases are misdiagnosed and thus underrepresented in international databases. Rare diseases can virtually affect any component of a cell and tissue on the body. They can be categorized into autoimmune / autoinflammatory, hereditary, cancer, skin, vascular, amongst many others. A rare disease can belong to more than one category. And international conciliation of classification and clinical practice guidelines can improve equity in the access of patients to therapies and treatments.

The largest cause of rare diseases is genetic, directly caused by a change in a gene or chromosome. They can result from the combination of recessive genes thus appearing in children with parents asymptomatic. However, the understanding of these diseases is very limited due to the lack of research. There are diagnostic tests for a few rare diseases. But many can pass unknown until the symptoms start to appear and aggravate.

Diagnosis, screening, treatment or even prevention of rare diseases is completely put aside as the cost of research is considered a liability as the return may fall short. The lack of funds is, regardless, associated to a residing economic problem in health care systems worldwide. Institutional activities should create models of social support for patients and their families while also investing in gathering funds for public health and social initiatives. Public awareness is of the highest importance for progress in research in rare diseases. For example, rare cancers are common, yet they lack research funding. Several culprits have been found for this problem. One is the cost of research and development, and marketing for pharma investors. Thus, companies are now focusing in to develop drugs that target a mutation that may also appear in other three or four different cancers. Then, the impact of research in rare disorders (including cancer) must not be disregarded just because of the size of the population they affect.

Furthermore, researchers may want to find treatments and understand the mechanisms, but because of the condition 'rarity', samples to even constitute a cell line to use in *in vitro* studies do not come easily. For all these problems, awareness is important. So that clinicians, patients and other stakeholders can understand the importance of giving to research either in biological samples, funding, media and public awareness or just be open to participate in clinical trials.

Gene therapy and precision health or medicine are giving their first steps. But they seem promising. The development of comprehensive international databases as well as close collaborations among industry, academic, regulatory, clinical and patients' communities is essential for the success of precision medicine. Patients must also be able to access the best expertise and medicines available for their particular case. Collaborations are thus necessary to harness the maximum benefits from research in rare diseases and communication, namely through media and online forums, has been pivotal in this process.

ACKNOWLEDGMENT

This research received no specific grant from any funding agency in the public, commercial, or not-for-profit sectors.

REFERENCES

Al-Falki, Y. H., Alshehri, M. A., Joseph, M. R. P., & Hamid, M. E. (2018). Fungal keratitis caused by a rare ocular pathogen, Gjaerumia minor: A case report. *Saudi Journal of Ophthalmology*, *32*(2), 160–163. doi:10.1016/j.sjopt.2017.09.007 PMID:29942188

Albakri, A. (2018). Restrictive cardiomyopathy: A review of literature on clinical status and meta-analysis of diagnosis and clinical management. *Pediatric Dimensions*, *3*(2). doi:10.15761/pd.1000170

Ali, S. R., Bryce, J., Cools, M., Korbonits, M., Beun, J. G., Taruscio, D., ... Ahmed, S. F. (2019). The current landscape of European registries for rare endocrine conditions. *European Journal of Endocrinology*, *180*(1), 89–98. doi:10.1530/EJE-18-0861 PMID:30407922

Alves, C., & Oliveira, C. S. (2014). Hearing loss among patients with Turner's syndrome: Literature review1. *Revista Brasileira de Otorrinolaringologia (English Ed.)*, *80*(3), 257–263. doi:10.1016/j.bjorl.2013.08.002 PMID:25153112

Amano, M., & Shimizu, T. (2014). Emphysematous cystitis: A review of the literature. *Internal Medicine (Tokyo, Japan)*, *53*(2), 79–82. doi:10.2169/internalmedicine.53.1121 PMID:24429444

Assal, F. (2018). Diogenes Syndrome. *Frontiers of Neurology and Neuroscience*, *41*, 90–97. doi:10.1159/000475688 PMID:29145187

Au, P. Y. B., Innes, A. M., & Kline, A. D. (1993-2019). Au-Kline Syndrome. In M. P. Adam, H. H. Ardinger, R. A. Pagon, S. E. Wallace, L. J. H. Bean, K. Stephens, & A. Amemiya (Eds.), *GeneReviews((R))*. Seattle, WA: University of Washington, Seattle.

Baddini-Martinez, J., Baldi, B. G., Costa, C. H. d., Jezler, S., Lima, M. S., & Rufino, R. (2015). Update on diagnosis and treatment of idiopathic pulmonary fibrosis. Jornal brasileiro de pneumologia: publicacao oficial da Sociedade Brasileira de Pneumologia e Tisilogia, 41(5), 454-466. doi:10.1590/S1806-37132015000000152

Bamforth, I. (2010). Stendhal's Syndrome. *The British Journal of General Practice*, *60*(581), 945–946. doi:10.3399/bjgp10X544780

Bates, M. D., Bucuvalas, J. C., Alonso, M. H., & Ryckman, F. C. (1998). Biliary atresia: Pathogenesis and treatment. *Seminars in Liver Disease*, *18*(3), 281–293. doi:10.1055-2007-1007164 PMID:9773428

Bell, D. J., & Gaillard, F. (2019). Mondini malformation. Retrieved from https://radiopaedia.org/articles/mondini-malformation?lang=gb

Beltran-Quintero, M. L., Bascou, N. A., Poe, M. D., Wenger, D. A., Saavedra-Matiz, C. A., Nichols, M. J., & Escolar, M. L. (2019). Early progression of Krabbe disease in patients with symptom onset between 0 and 5 months. *Orphanet Journal of Rare Diseases*, *14*(1), 46. doi:10.118613023-019-1018-4 PMID:30777126

Berman, J. J. (2014). What are the Rare Diseases, and Why do we Care? In Rare Diseases and Orphan Drugs (pp. 3-8). doi:10.1016/B978-0-12-419988-0.00001-8

Biason-Lauber, A. (2003). Disorders of Steroid Synthesis and Metabolism. In Physician's Guide to the Laboratory Diagnosis of Metabolic Diseases. Berlin, Germany: Springer. doi:10.1007/978-3-642-55878-8_35

Biason-Lauber, A., Boscaro, M., Mantero, F., & Balercia, G. (2010). Defects of steroidogenesis. *Journal of Endocrinological Investigation, 33*(10), 756-766. doi:10.3275/6869 10.1007/bf03346683

Black, D. W. (2007). A review of compulsive buying disorder. *World Psychiatry; Official Journal of the World Psychiatric Association (WPA)*, *6*(1), 14–18. Retrieved from https://www.ncbi.nlm.nih.gov/pubmed/17342214 PMID:17342214

Blake, K. D., & Prasad, C. (2006). CHARGE syndrome. *Orphanet Journal of Rare Diseases*, *1*(1), 34. doi:10.1186/1750-1172-1-34 PMID:16959034

Blom, J. D. (2016). Alice in Wonderland syndrome: A systematic review. *Neurology. Clinical Practice*, *6*(3), 259–270. doi:10.1212/CPJ.0000000000000251 PMID:27347442

Blom, R. M., van Wingen, G. A., van der Wal, S. J., Luigjes, J., van Dijk, M. T., Scholte, H. S., & Denys, D. (2016). The Desire for Amputation or Paralyzation: Evidence for Structural Brain Anomalies in Body Integrity Identity Disorder (BIID). *PLoS One*, *11*(11). doi:10.1371/journal.pone.0165789 PMID:27832097

Boat, T. F., & Field, M. J. (Eds.). (2010). *Rare Diseases and Orphan Products: Accelerating Research and Development (Vol. 2)*. Washington, DC: National Academies Press.

Boermans, J., & Egger, J. (2010). Compulsive buying or oniomania: An overview. *Tijdschrift voor Psychiatrie*, *52*, 29–39. PMID:20054795

Borhani, A. A., Wiant, A., & Heller, M. T. (2014). Cystic Hepatic Lesions: A Review and an Algorithmic Approach. *AJR. American Journal of Roentgenology*, *203*(6), 1192–1204. doi:10.2214/AJR.13.12386 PMID:25415696

Bourget, D., & Whitehurst, L. (2004). Capgras syndrome: A review of the neurophysiological correlates and presenting clinical features in cases involving physical violence. *Canadian Journal of Psychiatry*, *49*(11), 719–725. doi:10.1177/070674370404901102 PMID:15633849

Brunelle, R., Baradaran, N., & Keeler, S. (2016). Iliac artery endofibrosis: Case study of an elite triathlete. *Canadian Family Physician Medecin de Famille Canadien*, *62*(4), 318–e184. Retrieved from https://www.ncbi.nlm.nih.gov/pubmed/27076542 PMID:27076542

Bull, L. N., Roche, E., Song, E. J., Pedersen, J., Knisely, A. S., van der Hagen, C. B., ... Freimer, N. B. (2000). Mapping of the Locus for Cholestasis-Lymphedema Syndrome (Aagenaes Syndrome) to a 6.6-cM Interval on Chromosome 15q. *American Journal of Human Genetics*, *67*(4), 994–999. doi:10.1086/303080 PMID:10968776

CDC. (2019). Hearing Loss in Children - Data & Statistics. Retrieved from https://www.cdc.gov/ncbddd/hearingloss/data.html

Chasset, F., Richez, C., Martin, T., Belot, A., Korganow, A.-S., & Arnaud, L. (2019). Rare diseases that mimic Systemic Lupus Erythematosus (Lupus mimickers). *Joint, Bone, Spine*, *86*(2), 165–171. doi:10.1016/j.jbspin.2018.10.007 PMID:30837156

Cipriani, G., Lucetti, C., Vedovello, M., & Nuti, A. (2012). Diogenes syndrome in patients suffering from dementia. *Dialogues in Clinical Neuroscience*, *14*(4), 455–460. PMID:23393422

Crum-Cianflone, N. F. (2008). Bacterial, fungal, parasitic, and viral myositis. *Clinical Microbiology Reviews*, *21*(3), 473–494. doi:10.1128/CMR.00001-08 PMID:18625683

Czaja, A. J. (2016). Diagnosis and Management of Autoimmune Hepatitis: Current Status and Future Directions. *Gut and Liver*, *10*(2), 177–203. doi:10.5009/gnl15352 PMID:26934884

Da Costa, L., O'Donohue, M.-F., van Dooijeweert, B., Albrecht, K., Unal, S., Ramenghi, U., ... MacInnes, A. W. (2018). Molecular approaches to diagnose Diamond-Blackfan anemia: The EuroDBA experience. *European Journal of Medical Genetics*, *61*(11), 664–673. doi:10.1016/j.ejmg.2017.10.017 PMID:29081386

Darwin, E., Hirt, P. A., Fertig, R., Doliner, B., Delcanto, G., & Jimenez, J. J. (2018). Alopecia Areata: Review of Epidemiology, Clinical Features, Pathogenesis, and New Treatment Options. *International Journal of Trichology*, *10*(2), 51–60. doi:10.4103/ijt.ijt_99_17 PMID:29769777

Dawkins, H. J. S., Draghia-Akli, R., Lasko, P., Lau, L. P. L., Jonker, A. H., Cutillo, C. M., ... Austin, C. P. (2018). Progress in Rare Diseases Research 2010-2016: An IRDiRC Perspective. *Clinical and Translational Science*, *11*(1), 11–20. doi:10.1111/cts.12501 PMID:28796411

DeLeve, L. D. (2003). Vascular liver diseases. *Current Gastroenterology Reports*, *5*(1), 63–70. doi:10.100711894-003-0011-0 PMID:12530950

DeLeve, L. D., Valla, D. C., & Garcia-Tsao, G. (2009). Vascular disorders of the liver. *Hepatology (Baltimore, Md.)*, *49*(5), 1729–1764. doi:10.1002/hep.22772 PMID:19399912

DeVrieze, B. W., & Hurley, J. A. (2019). Goodpasture Syndrome (Anti-glomerular Basement Membrane Antibody Disease). In *StatPearls*. Treasure Island, FL: StatPearls Publishing.

EASL Clinical Practice Guidelines. (2012). EASL Clinical Practice Guidelines: Wilson's disease. *Journal of Hepatology*, *56*(3), 671–685. doi:10.1016/j.jhep.2011.11.007 PMID:22340672

EASL Clinical Practice Guidelines. (2015). EASL Clinical Practice Guidelines: Autoimmune hepatitis. *Journal of Hepatology*, *63*(4), 971–1004. doi:10.1016/j.jhep.2015.06.030 PMID:26341719

EASL Clinical Practice Guidelines. (2016). Vascular diseases of the liver. *Journal of Hepatology*, *64*(1), 179–202. doi:10.1016/j.jhep.2015.07.040 PMID:26516032

Espinosa, P. S., Smith, C. D., & Berger, J. R. (2006). Alien hand syndrome. *Neurology*, *67*(12), E21. doi:10.1212/01.wnl.0000249303.88754.48 PMID:17190927

EURORDIS. (2005). Rare Diseases: Understanding this Public Health Priority.

EURORDIS. (2019). Rare Diseases Europe - The Voice of Rare Disease Patients in Europe. Retrieved from https://www.eurordis.org/about-rare-diseases

Fahy, T. A. (1989). Lycanthropy: A review. *Journal of the Royal Society of Medicine*, *82*(1), 37–39. doi:10.1177/014107688908200115 PMID:2647981

Fricker, Z. P., & Lichtenstein, D. R. (2019). Primary Sclerosing Cholangitis: A Concise Review of Diagnosis and Management. *Digestive Diseases and Sciences*, *64*(3), 632–642. doi:10.100710620-019-05484-y PMID:30725292

Fumeo, M., Manfredi, S., & Volta, A. (2019). Emphysematous cystitis: review of current literature, diagnosis and management challenges. Veterinary medicine (Auckland, NZ), 10, 77-83. doi:10.2147/VMRR.S210463

Gao, X., Li, B., Chu, W., Sun, X., & Sun, C. (2016). Alien hand syndrome following corpus callosum infarction: A case report and review of the literature. *Experimental and Therapeutic Medicine*, *12*(4), 2129–2135. doi:10.3892/etm.2016.3608 PMID:27698701

Gates, G. A. (2006). Ménière's Disease Review 2005. *Journal of the American Academy of Audiology*, *17*(1), 16–26. doi:10.3766/jaaa.17.1.3 PMID:16640057

Genetics Home Reference, N. (2019a). Alport syndrome. Retrieved from https://ghr.nlm.nih.gov/condition/alport-syndrome#sourcesforpage

Genetics Home Reference, N. (2019b). Donnai-Barrow syndrome. Retrieved from https://ghr.nlm.nih.gov/condition/donnai-barrow-syndrome

Genetics Home Reference, N. (2019c). Keratitis-ichthyosis-deafness syndrome. Retrieved from https://ghr.nlm.nih.gov/condition/keratitis-ichthyosis-deafness-syndrome

Germain, D. P. (2010). Fabry disease. *Orphanet Journal of Rare Diseases*, *5*(1), 30. doi:10.1186/1750-1172-5-30 PMID:21092187

Gravholt, C. H., Andersen, N. H., Conway, G. S., Dekkers, O. M., Geffner, M. E., Klein, K. O., ... International Turner Syndrome Consensus, G. (2007a). Clinical Practice Guidelines for the Care of Girls and Women with Turner Syndrome [TS]: Brief Synopsis for Turner Syndrome Girls and Women and for their Parents/Caregivers/Families. *European Journal of Endocrinology, 177,* G1-G70. Retrieved from http://www.eje-online.org/content/177/3/G1.full.pdf+html

Gravholt, C. H., Andersen, N. H., Conway, G. S., Dekkers, O. M., Geffner, M. E., Klein, K. O., ... International Turner Syndrome Consensus, G. (2007b). Clinical practice guidelines for the care of girls and women with Turner syndrome: Proceedings from the 2016 Cincinnati International Turner Syndrome Meeting. *European Journal of Endocrinology, 177*(3), G1-G70. doi:10.1530/EJE-17-0430

Hernandez, B. A. (2018). Neurophysiological and Images Studies in a Case of Foreign Accent Syndrome Secondary to Multiple Sclerosis. *Journal of Neurology and Neuroscience*, *09*(01). doi:10.21767/2171-6625.1000240

Hollenbach, J. A., & Oksenberg, J. R. (2015). The immunogenetics of multiple sclerosis: A comprehensive review. *Journal of Autoimmunity*, *64*, 13–25. doi:10.1016/j.jaut.2015.06.010 PMID:26142251

Huck, J. H. J., Verhoeven, N. M., Struys, E. A., Salomons, G. S., Jakobs, C., & van der Knaap, M. S. (2004). Ribose-5-Phosphate Isomerase Deficiency: New Inborn Error in the Pentose Phosphate Pathway Associated with a Slowly Progressive Leukoencephalopathy. *American Journal of Human Genetics*, *74*(4), 745–751. doi:10.1086/383204 PMID:14988808

Iulini, B., Costassa, E. V., Corona, C., Meloni, D., Favole, A., Mazza, M., . . . Casalone, C. (2017). Classical and Atypical Bovine Spongiform Encephalopathy: Epidemiology, Pathogenesis and Diagnosis. In Prion - An Overview. Edited by Yusuf Tutar. doi: . Retrieved from https://www.intechopen.com/books/prion-an-overview/classical-and-atypical-bovine-spongiform-encephalopathy-epidemiology-pathogenesis-and-diagnosis doi:10.5772/67332

Johnston, S. L., Lock, R. J., & Gompels, M. M. (2002). Takayasu arteritis: A review. *Journal of Clinical Pathology*, *55*(7), 481–486. doi:10.1136/jcp.55.7.481 PMID:12101189

Josephs, K. A. (2007). Capgras Syndrome and Its Relationship to Neurodegenerative Disease. *JAMA Neurology*, *64*(12), 1762–1766. doi:10.1001/archneur.64.12.1762 PMID:18071040

Karlsen, T. H., Folseraas, T., Thorburn, D., & Vesterhus, M. (2017). Primary sclerosing cholangitis - a comprehensive review. *Journal of Hepatology*, *67*(6), 1298–1323. doi:10.1016/j.jhep.2017.07.022 PMID:28802875

Knight, A. W., & Senior, T. P. (2006). The common problem of rare disease in general practice. *The Medical Journal of Australia*, *185*(2), 82–83. doi:10.5694/j.1326-5377.2006.tb00477.x PMID:16842062

Kothari, S. (2001). Takayasu's arteritis in children - a review. *Images in Paediatric Cardiology*, *3*(4), 4–23. Retrieved from https://www.ncbi.nlm.nih.gov/pubmed/22368604 PMID:22368604

Kruegel, J., Rubel, D., & Gross, O. (2013). Alport syndrome—insights from basic and clinical research. *Nature Reviews. Nephrology*, *9*(3), 170–178. doi:10.1038/nrneph.2012.259 PMID:23165304

Kruse-Jarres, R., Kempton, C. L., Baudo, F., Collins, P. W., Knoebl, P., Leissinger, C. A., ... Kessler, C. M. (2017). Acquired hemophilia A: Updated review of evidence and treatment guidance. *American Journal of Hematology*, *92*(7), 695–705. doi:10.1002/ajh.24777 PMID:28470674

Landry, L. G., Ali, N., Williams, D. R., Rehm, H. L., & Bonham, V. L. (2018). Lack Of Diversity In Genomic Databases Is A Barrier To Translating Precision Medicine Research Into Practice. *Health Affairs (Project Hope)*, *37*(5), 780–785. doi:10.1377/hlthaff.2017.1595 PMID:29733732

Laurindo, E. E., & Barros Filho, I. R. (2017). Encefalopatia espongiforme bovina atípica: Uma revisão. *Arquivos do Instituto Biológico*, *84*(0). doi:10.1590/1808-1657000392015

Lautenschlager, S., Kemp, M., Christensen, J. J., Mayans, M. V., & Moi, H. (2017). 2017 European guideline for the management of chancroid. *International Journal of STD & AIDS*, *28*(4), 324–329. doi:10.1177/0956462416687913 PMID:28081686

Lavigne, B., Hamdan, M., Faure, B., Merveille, H., Pareaud, M., Tallon, E., ... Calvet, B. (2016). Syndrome de Diogène et Hoarding disorder: Une même entité? *L'Encéphale*, *42*(5), 421–425. doi:10.1016/j.encep.2016.02.010 PMID:27017316

Lee, R. H. (2018). Acute fatty liver of pregnancy. Retrieved from https://www.uptodate.com/contents/acute-fatty-liver-of-pregnancy

Legroux, L., & Arbour, N. (2015). Multiple Sclerosis and T Lymphocytes: An Entangled Story. *Journal of Neuroimmune Pharmacology*, *10*(4), 528–546. doi:10.100711481-015-9614-0 PMID:25946987

Liberal, R., Vergani, D., & Mieli-Vergani, G. (2015). Update on Autoimmune Hepatitis. *Journal of Clinical and Translational Hepatology, 3*(1), 42-52. doi:10.14218/JCTH.2014.00032

Lin, S., Zhou, Y., Fang, Q., Wu, J., Zhang, Z., Ji, Y., & Luo, Y. (2016). Chromosome 10q26 deletion syndrome: Two new cases and a review of the literature. *Molecular Medicine Reports*, *14*(6), 5134–5140. doi:10.3892/mmr.2016.5864 PMID:27779662

Lindor, K. D., & Lee, R. H. (2019). Intrahepatic cholestasis of pregnancy. Retrieved from https://www.uptodate.com/contents/intrahepatic-cholestasis-of-pregnancy

Lippert-Gruener, M., Weinert, U., Greisbach, T., & Wedekind, C. (2005). Foreign accent syndrome following traumatic brain injury. *Brain Injury: [BI]*, *19*(11), 955–958. doi:10.1080/02699050500109506 PMID:16243750

Loddo, I., & Romano, C. (2015). Inflammatory Bowel Disease: Genetics, Epigenetics, and Pathogenesis. *Frontiers in Immunology*, *6*(551). doi:10.3389/fimmu.2015.00551 PMID:26579126

Mackenzie, G., & Will, R. (2017). Creutzfeldt-Jakob disease: Recent developments. *F1000 Research*, *6*, 2053–2053. doi:10.12688/f1000research.12681.1 PMID:29225787

Macri, A., Wilson, A. M., Shafaat, O., & Sharma, S. (2019). Osler-Weber-Rendu Disease (Hereditary Hemorrhagic Telangiectasia, HHT). In *StatPearls*. Treasure Island, FL: StatPearls Publishing.

Majumder, S., & Chari, S. T. (2016). Chronic pancreatitis. *Lancet*, *387*(10031), 1957–1966. doi:10.1016/S0140-6736(16)00097-0 PMID:26948434

Maloney, W. J. (2009). Hutchinson-Gilford Progeria syndrome: Its presentation in F. Scott Fitzgerald's short story 'The Curious Case of Benjamin Button' and its oral manifestations. *Journal of Dental Research*, *88*(10), 873–876. doi:10.1177/0022034509348765 PMID:19783794

Manix, M., Kalakoti, P., Henry, M., Thakur, J., Menger, R., Guthikonda, B., & Nanda, A. (2015). Creutzfeldt-Jakob disease: Updated diagnostic criteria, treatment algorithm, and the utility of brain biopsy. *Neurosurgical Focus*, *39*(5), E2. doi:10.3171/2015.8.FOCUS15328 PMID:26646926

Manohar, M., Verma, A. K., Venkateshaiah, S. U., Sanders, N. L., & Mishra, A. (2017). Pathogenic mechanisms of pancreatitis. *World Journal of Gastrointestinal Pharmacology and Therapeutics*, *8*(1), 10–25. doi:10.4292/wjgpt.v8.i1.10 PMID:28217371

Marcucci, G., Cianferotti, L., Beck-Peccoz, P., Capezzone, M., Cetani, F., Colao, A., ... Brandi, M. L. (2015). Rare diseases in clinical endocrinology: A taxonomic classification system. *Journal of Endocrinological Investigation*, *38*(2), 193–259. doi:10.100740618-014-0202-6 PMID:25376364

Mavilia, M. G., Pakala, T., Molina, M., & Wu, G. Y. (2018). Differentiating Cystic Liver Lesions: A Review of Imaging Modalities, Diagnosis and Management. *Journal of Clinical and Translational Hepatology*, *6*(2), 208–216. doi:10.14218/JCTH.2017.00069 PMID:29951366

McAdoo, S. P., & Pusey, C. D. (2017). Anti-Glomerular Basement Membrane Disease. *Clinical Journal of the American Society of Nephrology; CJASN*, *12*(7), 1162–1172. doi:10.2215/CJN.01380217 PMID:28515156

Mikolasevic, I., Filipec-Kanizaj, T., Jakopcic, I., Majurec, I., Brncic-Fischer, A., Sobocan, N., ... Milic, S. (2018). Liver Disease During Pregnancy: A Challenging Clinical Issue. *Medical Science Monitor*, *24*, 4080–4090. doi:10.12659/MSM.907723 PMID:29905165

Mjoseth, J. (2018). Genomic databases weakened by lack of non-European populations. Retrieved from https://www.genome.gov/news/news-release/Genomic-databases-weakened-by-lack-of-non-European-populations

Montastruc, F., Schwarz, N., Schmitt, L., & Bui, E. (2012). An Overview of the Symptoms and Typical Disorders Associated with Alice in Wonderland Syndrome. *Neuropsychiatry*, *2*(4), 281–289. doi:10.2217/npy.12.37

Morgan, T. (2007). Turner Syndrome. *Diagnosis and Management American Family Physician*, *76*(3), 405–410. PMID:17708142

Nasirian, M., Banazadeh, N., & Kheradmand, A. (2009). Rare variant of lycanthropy and ecstasy. *Addiction & Health*, *1*(1), 53–56. Retrieved from https://www.ncbi.nlm.nih.gov/pubmed/24494083 PMID:24494083

Network, H. H. (2019). Rare Endocrine Genetic Diseases | Hormone Health Network. Retrieved from https://www.hormone.org/your-health-and-hormones/rare-endocrine-genetic-diseases

Neumann, H. P. H., Young, W. F. Jr, & Eng, C. (2019). Pheochromocytoma and Paraganglioma. *The New England Journal of Medicine*, *381*(6), 552–565. doi:10.1056/NEJMra1806651 PMID:31390501

NHS. (2019). Idiopathic pulmonary fibrosis. Retrieved from https://www.nhs.uk/conditions/idiopathic-pulmonary-fibrosis/

NIH. (2016). Quick Statistics About Hearing. Retrieved from https://www.nidcd.nih.gov/health/statistics/quick-statistics-hearing

NIH. N. H., Lung, and Blood Institute. (2019). Idiopathic Pulmonary Fibrosis. Retrieved from https://www.nhlbi.nih.gov/health-topics/idiopathic-pulmonary-fibrosis

NIH, & GARD. (2019). Rare diseases: Endocrine diseases. Retrieved from https://rarediseases.info.nih.gov/diseases/diseases-by-category/8/endocrine-diseases

NINDS. (2018). Creutzfeldt-Jakob Disease Fact Sheet. Retrieved from https://www.ninds.nih.gov/Disorders/Patient-Caregiver-Education/Fact-Sheets/Creutzfeldt-Jakob-Disease-Fact-Sheet

Niraj, J., Färkkilä, A., & D'Andrea, A. D. (2019). The Fanconi Anemia Pathway in Cancer. *Annual Review of Cancer Biology*, *3*(1), 457–478. doi:10.1146/annurev-cancerbio-030617-050422 PMID:30882047

O'Farrell, N. (2002). Donovanosis. *Sexually Transmitted Infections*, *78*(6), 452–457. doi:10.1136ti.78.6.452 PMID:12473810

Oberman, B. S., Patel, V. A., Cureoglu, S., & Isildak, H. (2017). The aetiopathologies of Ménière's disease: a contemporary review. [L'eziopatogenesi della Sindrome di Ménière: stato dell'arte]. Acta otorhinolaryngologica Italica: organo ufficiale della Societa italiana di otorinolaringologia e chirurgia cervico-facciale, 37(4), 250-263. doi:10.14639/0392-100X-793

Ontaneda, D., & Fox, R. J. (2015). Progressive multiple sclerosis. *Current Opinion in Neurology*, *28*(3), 237–243. doi:10.1097/WCO.0000000000000195 PMID:25887766

Orsini, J. J., Escolar, M. L., Wasserstein, M. P., & Caggana, M. (1993). Krabbe Disease. In M. P. Adam, H. H. Ardinger, R. A. Pagon, S. E. Wallace, L. J. H. Bean, K. Stephens, & A. Amemiya (Eds.), *GeneReviews((R))*. Seattle, WA: University of Washington, Seattle.

Osio, A., Fraitag, S., Hadj-Rabia, S., Bodemer, C., de Prost, Y., & Hamel-Teillac, D. (2010). Clinical Spectrum of Tufted Angiomas in Childhood: A Report of 13 Cases and a Review of the Literature. *JAMA Dermatology*, *146*(7), 758–763. doi:10.1001/archdermatol.2010.135 PMID:20644037

Panageas, A. (2019). Disabled Characters in Movies: The Controversy and Science Behind the Screen. *D. U. Quark*, *3*(2). Retrieved from https://dsc.duq.edu/duquark/vol3/iss2/11

Pavan, S., Rommel, K., Mateo Marquina, M. E., Höhn, S., Lanneau, V., & Rath, A. (2017). Clinical Practice Guidelines for Rare Diseases: The Orphanet Database. *PLoS One*, *12*(1). doi:10.1371/journal.pone.0170365 PMID:28099516

Pillai, R. K., & Jayasree, K. (2017). Rare cancers: Challenges & issues. *The Indian Journal of Medical Research*, *145*(1), 17–27. doi:10.4103/ijmr.IJMR_915_14 PMID:28574010

Podolec, P. (2017). Rare cardiovascular diseases. *European Heart Journal*, *38*(43), 3190–3192. doi:10.1093/eurheartj/ehx611 PMID:29145662

Porciuncula, R., Spada, P., & Goulart, K. O. B. (2018). Leukoencephalopathy with Evanescent White Matter: A Case Report. *Revista Paulista de Pediatria: Orgao Oficial da Sociedade de Pediatria de Sao Paulo*, *36*(4), 515–518. doi:10.1590/1984-0462/;2018;36;4;00001 PMID:29995139

Rajabi, F., Drake, L. A., Senna, M. M., & Rezaei, N. (2018). Alopecia areata: A review of disease pathogenesis. *British Journal of Dermatology*, *179*(5), 1033–1048. doi:10.1111/bjd.16808 PMID:29791718

Rammos, A., Meladinis, V., Vovas, G., & Patsouras, D. (2017). Restrictive Cardiomyopathies: The Importance of Noninvasive Cardiac Imaging Modalities in Diagnosis and Treatment-A Systematic Review. *Radiology Research and Practice*, *2017*. doi:10.1155/2017/2874902 PMID:29270320

Rare chromosome disorder support group, R. C. (Producer). 10q25 and 10q26 deletions. Retrieved from https://www.rarechromo.org/media/information/Chromosome%2010/10q25%20and%2010q26%20deletions%20FTNP.pdf

Rawla, P., & Limaiem, F. (2019). Lymphogranuloma Venereum. In *StatPearls*. Treasure Island, FL: StatPearls Publishing.

Rihani, F. B. (2013). Cervico-oculo-acoustic (Wildervanck) syndrome: Clinicoradiological findings. *BMJ Case Reports*, *2013*(apr23 1). doi:10.1136/bcr-2013-009065 PMID:23616324

Ringrose, J. L. (2018). *Understanding and treating dissociative identity disorder (or multiple personality disorder)*. Routledge. doi:10.4324/9780429484483

Ritchie, H., & Roser, M. (2019). *Mental Health.* Retrieved from https://ourworldindata.org/mental-health

Sanchez, S., & Ewton, A. (2006). Essential Thrombocythemia: A Review of Diagnostic and Pathologic Features. *Archives of Pathology & Laboratory Medicine*, *130*(8), 1144–1150. doi:10.1043/1543-2165(2006)130[1144:Et]2.0.Co;2 PMID:16879015

SANE. (2019). Factsheet: Dissociative identity disorder. Retrieved from https://www.sane.org/information-stories/facts-and-guides/dissociative-identity-disorder

Sayar, G., Kagan, G., & Ozten, E. (2014). Man transforming into wolf: A rare case of clinical lycanthropy. *The Journal of Neurobehavioral Sciences*, *1*(2), 50. doi:10.5455/JNBS.1401371806

Scarpa, M.-G., Grazia, M. D., & Tornese, G. (2017). 46,XY ovotesticular disorders of sex development: A therapeutic challenge. *Pediatric Reports*, *9*(4), 7085–7085. doi:10.4081/pr.2017.7085 PMID:29285340

Sciascia, S., Radin, M., Roccatello, D., Sanna, G., & Bertolaccini, M. (2018). Recent advances in the management of systemic lupus erythematosus. *F1000 Research*, *7*(970). doi:10.12688/f1000research.13941.1 PMID:30026918

Shah, M. H., Goldner, W. S., Halfdanarson, T. R., Bergsland, E., Berlin, J. D., Halperin, D., ... Zuccarino-Catania, G. (2018). NCCN Guidelines Insights: Neuroendocrine and Adrenal Tumors, Version 2.2018. *Journal of the National Comprehensive Cancer Network*, *16*(6), 693–702. doi:10.6004/jnccn.2018.0056 PMID:29891520

Sitammagari, K. K., & Masood, W. (2019). Creutzfeldt Jakob Disease. In *StatPearls*. Treasure Island, FL: StatPearls Publishing.

Spinner, N. B., Leonard, L. D., & Krantz, I. D. (1993). Alagille Syndrome. In M. P. Adam, H. H. Ardinger, R. A. Pagon, S. E. Wallace, L. J. H. Bean, K. Stephens, & A. Amemiya (Eds.), *GeneReviews((R))*. Seattle, WA: University of Washington, Seattle.

Tabet, P., & Saliba, I. (2017). Meniere's Disease and Vestibular Migraine: Updates and Review of the Literature. *Journal of Clinical Medicine Research*, *9*(9), 733–744. doi:10.14740/jocmr3126w PMID:28811849

The Lancet Diabetes & Endocrinology. (2019). Spotlight on rare diseases. *The Lancet Diabetes & Endocrinology*, *7*(2), 75. doi:10.10162213-8587(19)30006-3

Tran, T. T., Ahn, J., & Reau, N. S. (2016). ACG Clinical Guideline: Liver Disease and Pregnancy. *The American Journal of Gastroenterology*, *111*(2), 176–194, quiz 196. doi:10.1038/ajg.2015.430 PMID:26832651

Trinidad, B., & Lala, V. (2019). Takayasu Arteritis. In *StatPearls*. Treasure Island, FL: StatPearls Publishing.

van Dijk, M. T., van Wingen, G. A., van Lammeren, A., Blom, R. M., de Kwaasteniet, B. P., Scholte, H. S., & Denys, D. (2013). Neural basis of limb ownership in individuals with body integrity identity disorder. *PLoS One*, *8*(8). doi:10.1371/journal.pone.0072212 PMID:23991064

Wamelink, M. M., Gruning, N. M., Jansen, E. E., Bluemlein, K., Lehrach, H., Jakobs, C., & Ralser, M. (2010). The difference between rare and exceptionally rare: Molecular characterization of ribose 5-phosphate isomerase deficiency. *Journal of Molecular Medicine (Berlin, Germany)*, *88*(9), 931–939. doi:10.100700109-010-0634-1 PMID:20499043

Wang, W., Wang, S. A., Medeiros, L. J., & Khoury, J. D. (2017). Pure erythroid leukemia. *American Journal of Hematology*, *92*(3), 292–296. doi:10.1002/ajh.24626 PMID:28006859

Watson, L., Richardson, A. R. W., Holt, R. C. L., Jones, C. A., & Beresford, M. W. (2012). Henoch Schonlein Purpura – A 5-Year Review and Proposed Pathway. *PLoS One*, *7*(1). doi:10.1371/journal.pone.0029512 PMID:22235302

White, J. J. (1990). An Overview of the Genitourinary System. In H. K. Walker, W. D. Hall, & J. W. Hurst (Eds.), *Clinical Methods: The History, Physical, and Laboratory Examinations*. Boston, MA: Butterworths, Butterworth Publishers.

Yılmaz, E., Afşarlar, Ç. E., Karaman, İ., Özgüner, İ. F., Karaman, A., & Hızlı, F. (2013). Congenital hemiscrotal agenesis: Report of a rare entity. *Journal of Pediatric Urology*, *9*(1), e76–e77. doi:10.1016/j.jpurol.2012.09.005 PMID:23044375

Yoon, P. W., Bresee, J. S., Olney, R. S., James, L. M., & Khoury, M. J. (1997). Epidemiology of biliary atresia: A population-based study. *Pediatrics*, *99*(3), 376–382. doi:10.1542/peds.99.3.376 PMID:9041292

Zamel, R., Khan, R., Pollex, R. L., & Hegele, R. A. (2008). Abetalipoproteinemia: Two case reports and literature review. *Orphanet Journal of Rare Diseases*, *3*(1), 19–19. doi:10.1186/1750-1172-3-19 PMID:18611256

Zuo, Z., Polski, J. M., Kasyan, A., & Medeiros, L. J. (2010). Acute erythroid leukemia. *Archives of Pathology & Laboratory Medicine, 134*(9), 1261–1270. doi:10.1043/2009-0350-ra.1 PMID:20807044

ADDITIONAL READING

An initiative of the Office of Rare Diseases Research (ORDR) and the National Center for Advancing Translational Sciences (NCATS) bridging The Gap Between Rare Diseases And Research: https://www.rarediseasesnetwork.org

Deticek, A., Locatelli, I., & Kos, M. (2018). Patient Access to Medicines for Rare Diseases in European Countries. *Value in Health, 21*(5), 553–560. doi:10.1016/j.jval.2018.01.007 PMID:29753352

EURORDIS-Rare Diseases Europe is a non-profit alliance of 869 rare disease patient organizations from 71 countries: https://www.eurordis.org

Evaluation Report on the European Joint Action Project RD-ACTION (Promoting Implementation of Recommendations on Policy, Information and Data for Rare Diseases). (2018). Retrieved from http://www.rd-action.eu/wp-content/uploads/2018/09/677024-Evaluation-report.pdf

National Organization for Rare Disorders. I. N. (2003). NORD Guide to Rare Disorders (3rd ed.). Philadelphia, PA: Lippincott Williams & Wilkins. ISBN-10: 0781730635

Orphanet Journal of Rare Diseases: https://ojrd.biomedcentral.com

Podolec, P. (2017, November 14). Rare cardiovascular diseases. *European Heart Journal, 38*(43), 3190–3192. doi:10.1093/eurheartj/ehx611 PMID:29145662

Rare Diseases Epidemiology. Update and Overview. (2017). (M. P. d. l. Paz, D. Taruscio, & S. C. Groft, Eds., Second ed.): Springer, Cham. doi:10.1007/978-3-319-67144-4

The portals for rare diseases and orphan drugs: www.orpha.net & https://rarediseases.org

ENDNOTES

1 Definitions at Orphanet go as follow: • A **rare disorder** is defined according to the European legislation defining a prevalence threshold of not more than

five affected persons per 10'000 (Regulation (EC) N°141/2000 of the European Parliament and of the Council of 16 December 1999 on orphan medicinal products) • **Disorders** – a set of entities including diseases, syndromes, anomalies and clinical situations. They are clinically homogeneous entities described in at least two independent individuals or patients, confirming that the symptoms or clinical signs are not random or associated by a fortuity. o **Disease:** Alteration of health resulting from a physio-pathological mechanism, with homogeneous clinical presentation and evolution and homogeneous therapeutic possibilities (i.e. presenting similar symptoms that can be treated identically); it excludes developmental anomalies. o **Malformation syndrome:** Set of morphological anomalies that result from errors or problems during development and involve more than one morphogenetic field, independently of what cause it; it excludes sequences and associations. o **Clinical syndrome:** Set of manifestations (symptoms) resulting from the change in the physiological state of a person and that can be present in various diseases. o **Morphological anomaly:** Set of anomalies that result from a developmental anomaly involving only one morphogenetic field; it includes isolated anomalies and variants. o **Biological anomaly:** Alteration of the normal biological values (e.g. congenital isolated thyroxine-binding globulin deficiency). o **(Particular) clinical situation:** Set of manifestations or symptoms presenting of a disease under certain circumstances (e.g. pneumonia caused by *Pseudomonas aeruginosa*) This applies to information via Orphadata (http://www.orphadata.org) and The Orphanet Rare Disease Ontology (ORDO).

2 Zolgensma, https://www.fda.gov/vaccines-blood-biologics/zolgensma (Access date: August 13, 2019)

3 Zolgensma Cost, https://www.medicaldevice-network.com/comment/zolgensma-cost-2019/ (Access date: August 13, 2019)

4 Occurrence and Transmission, https://www.cdc.gov/prions/cjd/occurrence-transmission.html (Access date: September 04, 2019)

5 Tay-Sachs Disease, https://ghr.nlm.nih.gov/condition/tay-sachs-disease (Access date: September 04, 2019)

6 Rare Neurological Disease Special Report 2019 published in Neurology Reviews and accessible at https://www.neurologyreviews-digital.com/neurologyreviews/nr_nord_march_2019/MobilePagedReplica.action?pm=1&folio=Cover (Access date: September 04, 2019)

7 Rare neurological diseases – A Pandora's box for neurology and neurosciences, https://www.ean.org/Rare-Diseases.2682.0.html (Access date: September 04, 2019)

8 Diagnostic and Statistical Manual of Mental Disorders (DSM), https://doi.org/10.1176/appi.books.9780890425596 (Access date: September 04, 2019)

9 International Classification of Diseases (ICD), https://www.who.int/classifications/icd/en/ (Access date: September 04, 2019)

10 National Alliance on Mental Illness, https://www.nami.org (Access date: September 04, 2019)

11 Behavioral and Mental Disorders, https://rarediseases.info.nih.gov/diseases/diseases-by-category/3/behavioral-and-mental-disorders (Access date: September 04, 2019)

12 Endocrine Web, https://www.endocrineweb.com (Access date: September 04, 2019)

13 Orphanet, https://www.orpha.net (Access date: September 04, 2019)

14 RD-Connect, https://rd-connect.eu (Access date: September 04, 2019)

15 Diseases by Category – Immune System Diseases, https://rarediseases.info.nih.gov/diseases/diseases-by-category/13/immune-system-diseases (Access date: September 04, 2019)

16 International Patient Organization for Primary Immunodeficiencies, https://ipopi.org (Access date: September 04, 2019)

17 Rare Diseases – Ashersons-Syndrome, https://rarediseases.org/rare-diseases/ashersons-syndrome/ (Access date: September 04, 2019)

18 Rare Cutaneous Lupus Erythematosus, https://www.orpha.net/consor/cgi-bin/OC_Exp.php?Lng=GB&Expert=535 (Access date: September 04, 2019)

19 Immune System Diseases, https://rarediseases.info.nih.gov/diseases/diseases-by-category/13/immune-system-diseases (Access date: September 04, 2019)

20 Syndromic Hearing Loss, www.babyhearing.org/syndromic-genetic (Access date: September 04, 2019)

21 American Thoracic Society, www.thoracic.org (Access date: September 04, 2019)

22 American lung association, www.lung.org (Access date: September 04, 2019)

23 Rare Lung Diseases Consortium, https://www.rarediseasesnetwork.org/cms/rld/Learn-More/Disorder-Definitions (Access date: September 04, 2019)

24 Rare Diseases Clinical Research Network (RDCRN), https://www.rarediseasesnetwork.org (Access date: September 04, 2019).

25 EU Clinical Trials Register, www.clinicaltrialsregister.eu/ctr-search/search (Access date: September 04, 2019).

26 US NIH, https://clinicaltrials.gov (Access date: September 04, 2019).

27 A list of rare heart diseases can be found at https://rarediseases.info.nih.gov/diseases/diseases-by-category/4/heart-diseases (Access date: September 04, 2019).

28 Brugada Syndrome, https://rarediseases.org/rare-diseases/brugada-syndrome/ (Access date: September 04, 2019).

29 Press Release – Researchers discover first treatment to improve survival in rare heart condition, https://www.escardio.org/The-ESC/Press-Office/Press-releases/Researchers-discover-first-treatment-to-improve-survival-in-rare-heart-condition (Access date: September 04, 2019).

30 More about the clinical trial for this orphan drug at https://clinicaltrials.gov/ct2/show/NCT01994889 (Access date: September 04, 2019)

31 Rare Diseases – Polyarteritis Nodosa, https://rarediseases.org/rare-diseases/polyarteritis-nodosa/ (Access date: September 04, 2019)

32 Rare Diseases – Lymphomatoid-Granulomatosis, https://rarediseases.org/rare-diseases/lymphomatoid-granulomatosis/ (Access date: September 04, 2019)

33 Rare Diseases – Hereditary Lymphemeda, https://rarediseases.org/RARE-DISEASES/HEREDITARY-LYMPHEDEMA/ (Access date: September 04, 2019)

34 VASCERN, a European Reference Network, https://vascern.eu (Access date: September 04, 2019)

35 Rare Liver, Clinical Perspective https://www.rare-liver.eu/index.php/clinical-perspective (Access date: September 04, 2019)

36 European Reference Network for Rare or Low Prevalence Complex Diseases > Hepatological Diseases Network, www.rare-liver.eu (Access date: September 04, 2019)

37 The European Association for the Study of the Liver, https://easl.eu accessed (Access date: September 04, 2019)

38 Rare Gastrointestinal Diseases, https://rarediseases.info.nih.gov/diseases/diseases-by-category/6/digestive-diseases (Access date: September 04, 2019)

39 Information about these diseases can be found at https://www.iffgd.org/other-disorders/rare-diseases.html by the International Foundation for Gastrointestinal disorders (Access date: September 04, 2019)

40 Kidney and urinary diseases, https://rarediseases.info.nih.gov/diseases/diseases-by-category/26/kidney-and-urinary-diseases (Access date: September 04, 2019)

41 Henoch Schonlein Purpura, https://rarediseases.info.nih.gov/diseases/8204/henoch-schonlein-purpura (Access date: September 04, 2019)

42 H Australia Henoch Schonlein Purpura, https://www.rch.org.au/clinicalguide/guideline_index/HenochSchonlein_Purpura/ (Access date: September 04, 2019)

43 Royal Berkshire NHS Foundation Trust, Henoch Schonlein Purpura Guideline – GL604, https://www.royalberkshire.nhs.uk/Downloads/GPs/GP%20protocols%20and%20guidelines/Paediatric%20handbook/Henoch%20Schonlein%20Purpura%20guideline.pdf (Access date: September 04, 2019)

44 NORD – National Organization of Rare Disorders, Arthirtis, Infectious, https://rarediseases.org/rare-diseases/arthritis-infectious/ (Access date: September 04, 2019)

45 Fungal Eye Infection, https://www.cdc.gov/fungal/diseases/fungal-eye-infections/index.html (Access date: September 04, 2019)

46 Bacterial Infections, https://rarediseases.info.nih.gov/diseases/diseases-by-category/2/bacterial-infections (Access date: September 04, 2019)

47 Viral Infections, https://rarediseases.info.nih.gov/diseases/diseases-by-category/25 (Access date: September 04, 2019)

48 Fungal Infections, https://rarediseases.info.nih.gov/diseases/diseases-by-category/11 (Access date: September 04, 2019)

49 Orphanet classification of rare infectious diseases, https://www.orpha.net/consor/www/cgi-bin/Disease_Classif.php?lng=EN&data_id=203&Disease_Disease_Classif_diseaseGroup=Rare-infectious-disease&PatId=10557&search=Disease_Classif_Simple&PatId_Search=17505&BranchId=10557_17505 (Access date: September 04, 2019)

50 Aquagenic Urticaria, https://rarediseases.info.nih.gov/diseases/10901/aquagenic-urticaria (Access date: September 04, 2019)

51 Exercise Induced Anaphylaxis, https://rarediseases.info.nih.gov/diseases/6392/exercise-induced-anaphylaxis (Access date: September 04, 2019)

52 Familial Dermographism, https://rarediseases.info.nih.gov/diseases/9480/familial-dermographism (Access date: September 04, 2019)

53 Elastoderma, https://rarediseases.info.nih.gov/diseases/12716/elastoderma (Access date: September 04, 2019)

54 A list of skin rare diseases as per NIH-GARD can be found at https://rarediseases.info.nih.gov/diseases/diseases-by-category/22 (Access date: September 04, 2019)

55 Musculoskeletal Diseases, https://rarediseases.info.nih.gov/diseases/diseases-by-category/15/musculoskeletal-diseases (Access date: September 04, 2019)

56 International Osteoporosis Foundation, https://www.iofbonehealth.org/skeletal-rare-diseases-working-group accessed (Access date: September 04, 2019)

57 Congenital and Genetic Disease, https://rarediseases.info.nih.gov/diseases/diseases-by-category/5/congenital-and-genetic-diseases (Access date: September 04, 2019)

58 Neurofibromatosis – Type 1 and 2, https://rarediseases.org/rare-diseases/neurofibromatosis-type-1-nf1/; https://rarediseases.org/rare-diseases/neurofibromatosis-2/ (Access date: September 04, 2019)

59 Schwannomatosis, https://ghr.nlm.nih.gov/condition/schwannomatosis#statistics (Access date: September 04, 2019)

60 For example, https://www.clinicaltrials.gov/ct2/results?cond=%22Neurofibromatosis%22 and https://clinicaltrials.gov/ct2/results?cond=%22schwannomatosis%2 (Access date: September 04, 2019)

61 SBSVICELAND, https://www.facebook.com/SBSVICELAND/videos/2719447908086781/ (Access date: September 04, 2019)

62 EU countries will cooperate in linking genomics databases across borders, https://ec.europa.eu/digital-single-market/en/news/eu-countries-will-cooperate-linking-genomic-databases-across-borders (Access date: September 04, 2019)

63 Newborn Screening, https://rarediseases.info.nih.gov/diseases/diseases-by-category/37/newborn-screening (Access date: September 04, 2019)

64 Genetic Disorders, https://www.genome.gov/For-Patients-and-Families/Genetic-Disorders (Access date: September 04, 2019)

65 See, for example, https://www.orphananesthesia.eu/en/rare-diseases/published-guidelines.html a project from the German society of Anesthesiology and Intensive care Medicine (Access date: September 04, 2019)

66 Blood Cancer Network Ireland (BCNI), https://www.cancer.ie/research/collaborative-research-centres/blood-cancer-network-ireland#sthash.aQdDRxsQ.dpbs (Access date: September 04, 2019)

67 EuroBloodNet - European Reference Network on Rare Hematological Diseases, http://www.eurobloodnet.eu/index/ (Access date: September 04, 2019)

68 Enerca - European Network for Rare and Congenital Anemias, https://www.enerca.org (Access date: September 04, 2019)

69 Primary Lymphedema, https://www.orpha.net/consor/cgi-bin/OC_Exp.php?lng=en&Expert=77240 (Access date: September 04, 2019)

70 Meige Disease, https://ghr.nlm.nih.gov/condition/meige-disease (Access date: September 04, 2019)

71 Castlemans Disease, https://rarediseases.org/rare-diseases/castlemans-disease/ (Access date: September 04, 2019)

72 Hodgkins Disease, https://rarediseases.org/rare-diseases/hodgkins-disease/ (Access date: September 04, 2019)

73 Nutritional Disease, https://rarediseases.info.nih.gov/diseases/diseases-by-category/18 (Access date: September 04, 2019)

74 See https://rarediseases.org/rare-diseases/rickets-vitamin-d-deficiency/; https://rarediseases.org/gard-rare-disease/8761/keshan-disease/ (Access date: September 04, 2019)

75 Tay-Sachs Disease, https://rarediseases.org/rare-diseases/tay-sachs-disease/ (Access date: September 04, 2019)

76 Tay-Sachs Disease – Causes, https://ghr.nlm.nih.gov/condition/tay-sachs-disease#genes (Access date: September 04, 2019)

77 Congenital Disorder of Glycosylation, https://www.orpha.net/consor/cgi-bin/OC_Exp.php?lng=EN&Expert=137 (Access date: September 04, 2019)

78 Portuguese news, https://www.eurordis.org/pt-pt/content/viver-com-cdg-duas-historias-uma-esperanca-partilhada (Access date: September 04, 2019)

79 For example, the Facebook page with the story of a little girl suffering from this disease, https://www.facebook.com/osorrisodamafalda/ (Access date: September 04, 2019)

80 Autosomal Systemic Lupus Erythematosus, https://www.orpha.net/consor/cgi-bin/OC_Exp.php?lng=EN&Expert=300345 (Access date: September 04, 2019)

81 HERNS Syndrome - Hereditary endotheliopathy with retinopathy, nephropathy, and stroke disease, https://www.orpha.net/consor/cgi-bin/OC_Exp.php?lng=EN&Expert=63261(Accessdate:September04,2019)

82 Retinal vasculopathy with cerebral leukoencephalopathy and systemic manifestations, https://www.orpha.net/consor/cgi-bin/OC_Exp.php?lng=EN&Expert=247691(Accessdate:September04,2019)

83 Female Reproductive Diseases, https://rarediseases.info.nih.gov/diseases/diseases-by-category/10 (Access date: September 04, 2019)

84 Rare Genetic Gynecological and Obstetrical Diseases, https://www.orpha.net/consor/cgi-bin/OC_Exp.php?lng=en&Expert=183731(Accessdate:September04,2019)

85 Cancer, https://www.who.int/news-room/fact-sheets/detail/cancer (Access date: September 04, 2019)

86 RARECARE Cancer List, http://www.rarecare.eu/rarecancers/rarecancers.asp (Access date: September 04, 2019)

87 "Families" and List of Rare Cancers, https://www.rarecancerseurope.org/About-Rare-Cancers/Families-and-List-of-Rare-Cancers (Access date: September 04, 2019)

88 The European Medical Society for Medical Oncology (ESMO) clinical practice guidelines for rare cancers, https://oncologypro.esmo.org/content/search?SearchText=*&dateFilter=&subtreeFilter=32370-32023-49570&sort=score&topic_filter%5B%5D=Rare%2520Cancers (Access date: September 04, 2019)

89 International Rare Cancer Initiative EORTC-UK-US ttps://www.eortc.org/blog/2011/11/23/international-rare-cancer-initiative-eortc-uk-us-global-collaboration-2/ (Access date: September 04, 2019)

90 Bosma Arhinia Microphthalmia Syndrome, https://rarediseases.org/rare-diseases/bosma-arhinia-microphthalmia-syndrome/ (Access date: September 04, 2019)

91 Breast implants scrutinized following cancer death, https://www.nhs.uk/news/cancer/breast-implants-scrutinised-following-cancer-death/ (Access date: September 04, 2019)

92 Silicone Gel Breast Implants, https://nwhn.org/silicone-gel-breast-implants/ (Access date: September 04, 2019)

93 Saline, Silicone Gel, and Alternative Gels, https://www.fda.gov/regulatory-information/search-fda-guidance-documents/saline-silicone-gel-and-alternative-breast-implants (Access date: September 04, 2019)

94 Risks and Complications of Breast Implants, https://www.fda.gov/medical-devices/breast-implants/risks-and-complications-breast-implants (Access date: September 04, 2019)

95 Heavy Metal Poisoning, https://rarediseases.org/rare-diseases/heavy-metal-poisoning/ (Access date: September 04, 2019)

96 Mercury Poisoning, https://www.orpha.net/consor/cgi-bin/OC_Exp.php?lng=en&Expert=330021 (Access date: September 04, 2019)

97 Asherson's Syndrome, https://rarediseases.org/rare-diseases/ashersons-syndrome/ (Access date: September 04, 2019)

98 Gerstmann Syndrome, https://rarediseases.org/rare-diseases/gerstmann-syndrome/ (Access date: September 04, 2019)

99 Central Pain Syndrome, https://rarediseases.info.nih.gov/diseases/5161/central-pain-syndrome (Access date: September 04, 2019)

100 Safe Sleeping, https://www.rch.org.au/rchcpg/hospital_clinical_guideline_index/Safe_sleeping/#Evidence%20Table (Access date: September 04, 2019)

101 Sudden infant death with dysgenesis of the testes syndrome, https://ghr.nlm.nih.gov/condition/sudden-infant-death-with-dysgenesis-of-the-testes-syndrome (Access date: September 04, 2019)

102 Congenital Zika Syndrome, https://rarediseases.info.nih.gov/diseases/13441/congenital-zika-syndrome (Access date: September 04, 2019)

103 Zika Virus Disease, https://www.orpha.net/consor/cgi-bin/OC_Exp.php?lng=en&Expert=448237 (Access date: September 04, 2019)

104 WHO ends Zika as a Public Health Emergency of International Concern, https://www.ecdc.europa.eu/en/news-events/who-ends-zika-public-health-emergency-international-concern (Access date: September 04, 2019)

105 AU-Kline Syndrome, https://ghr.nlm.nih.gov/condition/au-kline-syndrome#genes (Access date: September 04, 2019)

106 10q26 Deletion Syndrome, https://ghr.nlm.nih.gov/condition/10q26-deletion-syndrome (Access date: September 04, 2019)

107 Distal monosomy 10q, https://www.orpha.net/consor/cgi-bin/OC_Exp.php?lng=EN&Expert=96148 (Access date: September 04, 2019)

108 Research into rare cancers, https://www.cancerresearchuk.org/about-cancer/rare-cancers/research-clinical-trials/research-into-rare-cancers (Access date: October 26, 2019)

109 Challenges Rare Tumor Research, https://www.cancer.gov/pediatric-adult-rare-tumor/research/challenges-rare-tumor-research (Access date: October 26, 2019)

110 Sativex (Delta-9-tetrahidrocanabinol (THC PFV) + Canabidiol (CBD PFV), Prep de Fármacos Vegetais, ext Cannabis sativa) - Avaliação da comparticipação concluída https://www.infarmed.pt/web/infarmed/profissionais-de-saude/-/journal_content/56/15786/3210011 (Access date: October 26, 2019).

111 Further information in https://rarediseases.org/rare-diseases/machado-joseph-disease/; https://www.ninds.nih.gov/Disorders/Patient-Caregiver-Education/Fact-Sheets/Machado-Joseph-Disease-Fact-Sheet (Access date: October 26, 2019).

112 Neurolixis' Parkinson's Showcased by French Regional Business Accelerator, https://www.neurolixis.com/en/news.html (Access date: October 26, 2019).

113 The news about the application of this technique in a rare disease came in online outlets of science news as at https://www.sciencedaily.com/releases/2019/09/190917115430.htm and https://www.technologynetworks.com/genomics/news/researchers-use-crispr-to-correct-mutation-in-duschenne-muscular-dystrophy-model-324043 (Access date: October 26, 2019).

114 NIH Policy and Guidelines on The Inclusion of Women and Minorities as Subjects in Clinical Research, https://grants.nih.gov/grants/funding/women_min/guidelines.htm (Access date: October 26, 2019).

115 Could LUXTURNA be right for you?, https://luxturna.com/about-luxturna/ (Access date: October 26, 2019).

116 Zolgensma Approval History, https://www.drugs.com/history/zolgensma.html (Access date: October 26, 2019).

117 Gene Therapy Platform for Rare Diseases, https://ncats.nih.gov/trnd/projects/gene-therapy (Access date: October 26, 2019)

APPENDIX

Rare Neurological Disorders

Creutzfeldt-Jakob Disease (CJD): Fatal degenerative brain disorder caused by the buildup of a protein called prion. Only about 10% cases of CJD are hereditary and about 300 people are diagnosed with this disease each year (Mackenzie & Will, 2017; NINDS, 2018). It occurs in about 1 in every 1 million people worldwide. The disease can be caused by contact with infected brain or nervous system tissue or consuming infected beef and, has no cure. CJD is difficult to diagnose as its symptoms resemble those of dementia. The diagnose can only be confirmed through a brain biopsy or autopsy. Symptoms include failing memory, behavior changes, impaired coordination and vision problems, followed by the aggravation of mental deterioration, uncontrolled movements, blindness, weakness and sometime people go into a coma (Mackenzie & Will, 2017; Manix et al., 2015; NINDS, 2018).

Rare Behavioral and Mental Disorders

Alice in Wonderland Syndrome (AIWS): Also known as **Todd syndrome**, is a neurologic condition in which patients suffer from altered perception namely have hallucinations, sensory distortion and altered sense of velocity that makes them sense like their body image, space, and/or time is distorted. These symptoms often trigger panic and fear responses. AIWS is often associated with migraines, epilepsy, brain tumors or drug abuse (J. D. Blom, 2016; Montastruc, Schwarz, Schmitt, & Bui, 2012).

Alien Hand Syndrome: Patients with this mental disorder have normal sensation but feel their hand is autonomous or 'with a will of its own'. These patients may personify the hand or limb as a separate entity. This may arise from damage to the corpus callosum of the individuals, which connects the two cerebral hemispheres of the brain. Other possible causes include stroke and damage to the parietal lobe. The hands then act in opposition to one another, being in 'intermanual conflict' or 'ideomotor apraxia'(Espinosa, Smith, & Berger, 2006; Gao, Li, Chu, Sun, & Sun, 2016).

Apotemnophilia: Also known as the body integrity disorder and patients report an overwhelming desire to amputate health parts of their body. Some believe it to be neurological and patients have been reported to have attempt to amputate their own limbs or damage is so surgical amputation has to be performed. It has been associated with damage to the right parietal lobe in the brain (R. M. Blom et al., 2016; van Dijk et al., 2013).

Capgras Syndrome: This is one of the rarest mental disorders. Patients believe that people in their life, as a close friend, spouse or family member, have been replaced by an impostor. Patients with schizophrenia, dementia, epilepsy or traumatic brain injury can develop this disorder which, is often treated with antipsychotic medication. This delusion may come from the loss of emotional recognition of familiar faces which may be due to the disconnection of the visual recognition system and the affective memory (Bourget & Whitehurst, 2004; Josephs, 2007).

Diogenes Syndrome (DS): DS is a neurobehavioral syndrome characterized by the commonly known 'hoarding' behavior which includes lack of insight into the condition. It is often secondary in associating with psychosis, bipolar disorder or even early stages of dementia. Despite known by professionals ranging from medical, psychiatric, neurological, social, scientific and ethical, the mechanisms of the syndrome remain largely incompletely understood. There has been authors making some distinction between hoarding and the Diogenes syndrome associating it with dimensions of hoarding and squalor which may resume into a matter of a different expression of one central etiology (Assal, 2018; Cipriani, Lucetti, Vedovello, & Nuti, 2012; Lavigne et al., 2016).

Dissociative Identity Disorder (DID): previously called multiple personality disorder, this mental illness involves disruptions or breakdowns of memory, awareness, identity and/or perception is, thus part of a group of conditions called dissociative disorders. It can occur at any age, not gender exclusive and it is a very rare and complex psychological condition. An history of trauma (e.g. war) and/or severe physical, verbal, or sexual abuse during childhood is usually associated to this disorder (Panageas, 2019; Ringrose, 2018; SANE, 2019).

Foreign Accent Syndrome (FAS): This syndrome causes a change in language; as the name implies, patients start to speak their native language as if they are from another country. This disorder is very rare (affects about 80 people in the world at the present) and is caused by serious brain injury that led to the distortion of coordination and articulation planning processes (Hernandez, 2018; Lippert-Gruener, Weinert, Greisbach, & Wedekind, 2005).

Lycanthropy: This delusion is a psychiatric syndrome in which the individual believes that is a werewolf or, more rarely, that another person has been transformed into an animal. They grunt, claw and feel like their body is covered with hair and that their nails are elongated like they have been or are in the process of metamorphosis into a wolf (Fahy, 1989; Sayar, Kagan, & Ozten, 2014). This delusion was also identified to occur after ecstasy drug use, especially in patients susceptible to schizophrenia (Nasirian, Banazadeh, & Kheradmand, 2009).

Oniomania: Also known as compulsive buying (or shopping) disorder; this disorder is not officially described in the 'Diagnostic and Statistical Manual of Mental Disorders (DSM).' There is debate if it is an impulse control disorder, a behavioral addiction or possibly related to obsessive-compulsive disorder (OCD). There is no standard treatment and affects mainly women with a lifetime prevalence of about 6% in the USA population (Black, 2007; Boermans & Egger, 2010).

Stendhal Syndrome or Hypeculturemia: The patients experience panic attacks, anxiety, dissociative disorders, confusion and hallucinations when exposed to something as art that they perceive as particularly beautiful or if they are exposed to large quantities of art concentrated in a single place (Bamforth, 2010).

Immune System Disorders

Alopecia Areata: Complex inflammatory disease that causes non-scarring hair loss. There is still no cure and its cause may vary. For more see (Darwin et al., 2018; Rajabi, Drake, Senna, & Rezaei, 2018)

Lupus: Chronic autoimmune disease with heterogeneous clinical manifestations namely skin lesions that resemble other pathologies such as rosacea (Chasset et al., 2019). Age on set it not defined and affects mostly women. Symptoms include fever and malaise, but also dermatological, musculoskeletal, renal, respiratory, cardiovascular, hematological, and neurological manifestations. In the face of recent advances in research some new therapies are being developed but there is still no cure (Sciascia, Radin, Roccatello, Sanna, & Bertolaccini, 2018).

Multiple Sclerosis (MS): MS is another chronic immune mediated disease with neurodegenerative effects and common cause of non-traumatic neurological disability in young adults (Hollenbach & Oksenberg, 2015). It is defined as an inflammatory disease of the central nervous system characterized by multifocal areas of demyelination, axonal damage, activation of glial cells, and immune cell infiltration (Legroux & Arbour, 2015). The disease affects a significant number of people worldwide but incomplete understanding of the disease pathogenesis and lack of validated outcome measures as well as negative clinical trials results for new therapies (Ontaneda & Fox, 2015) keep patients hoping for no more than palliative care at the moment.

Mentioned in Rare Ear Diseases

Alport Syndrome: This syndrome affects about one in 50,000 babies and is a genetic condition that results in kidney malfunction, hearing loss and ocular abnormalities. Alport syndrome is caused by an inherited defect in type IV collagen, a structural protein that is found and needed for the normal function of different tissues, including ears, eyes and kidneys (Genetics Home Reference, 2019a; Kruegel, Rubel, & Gross, 2013).

Donnai-Barrow Syndrome: Hereditary genetic disorder that affect several tissues. Patients usually have prominent facial features, wide-set eyes with outer corners pointed downward, short bulbous nose and ears that rotate backward as well as severe hearing impairment due to abnormalities of the inner-ear, eyes problems with progressive vision loss, and intellectual disabilities and development delay. Patients often lack corpus collosum (tissue connecting the two halves of the brain) or it is underdeveloped; other structural brain abnormalities may occur (Genetics Home Reference, 2019b). Prevalence is unknown with less than 50 cases in 20 families reported (https://www.orpha.net/consor/cgi-bin/OC_Exp.php?lng=en&Expert=2143 accessed 08-10-2019; https://rarediseases.info.nih.gov/diseases/1899/donnai-barrow-syndrome accessed 08-10-2019).

KID Syndrome: Rare genetic multi-system disorder, **Keratitis-ichthyosis-deafness** (KID) syndrome is characterized by eye problems, skin abnormalities (include red, rough, thickened plaques that are sometimes scaling), and hearing impairment or loss. It is present at birth and less than 100 cases have been reported up to date; prevalence is unknown(Genetics Home Reference, 2019c), https://www.orpha.net/consor/cgi-bin/OC_Exp.php?Lng=GB&Expert=477 accessed 08-10-2019; https://rarediseases.org/rare-diseases/keratitis-ichthyosis-deafness-syndrome/ accessed 08-10-2019.

Krabbe Disease: Krabbe disease is a lysosomal disorder that affects the white matter of the central and peripheral nervous systems. It can range from Infantile-onset disease (i.e., onset of extreme irritability, spasticity, and developmental delay before age 12 months) to later-onset disease (i.e., onset of manifestations after age 12 months and as late as the seventh decade). Infantile-onset Krabbe disease is characterized by normal development in the first months followed by rapid severe neurologic deterioration; the average age of death is 24 months (range 8 months to 9 years) while, Later-onset Krabbe disease is variable in its symptoms and disease course (Orsini, Escolar, Wasserstein, & Caggana, 1993). Northern-European populations seem to be more affected with a prevalence of 1 in 100,000. Only mutation analysis can confirm the diagnosis. While fatal in infantile and juvenile forms of the disease, adult-onset patients often survive for many years after the symptoms start. Children with Krabbe disease lack an enzyme the body needs to make myelin which protects the nerves. This lead to muscle weakness or stiffness, trouble walking, hearing or vision loss, seizures, etc. (https://www.orpha.net/consor/cgi-bin/OC_Exp.php?Expert=487 accessed 08-10-2019, (Beltran-Quintero et al., 2019)).

Ménière's Disease: Multifactorial disease of the inner ear that causes episodic vertigo combined with fluctuating hearing loss. Its causes and pathophysiology are not consensual. In common with other rare diseases, the lack of a proper clinical trial, appropriate animal model and specific treatment, contribute for the controversy. Typically, the physicians treat patients with symptom-specific medication and therapies (Gates, 2006). Pathologies not specific to Meniere's disease may delay the proper diagnosis (for example, vestibular migraine) (Tabet & Saliba, 2017). Guidelines published by the Committee on Hearing and Equilibrium of the American Academy of Otolaryngology – Head and Neck Surgery (Oberman, Patel, Cureoglu, & Isildak, 2017) also require update and an united push for more research opportunities and funding.

Mondini Dysplasia: abnormality of the inner-ear due to cochlear malformation defining a specific type of cochlear hypoplasia. Patients have sensorineural hearing loss, which is usually bilateral. High-frequency hearing is generally preserved because the basal turn of the cochlea is intact. This malformation of the cochlea (has 1.5turns instead of 2.5) is thought to occur around the 7th week of the embryonic development ((Bell & Gaillard, 2019) https://rarediseases.info.nih.gov/diseases/8215/mondini-dysplasia accessed 08-10-2019).

Turner Syndrome (TS): Also known as Monosomy X, Bonnevie-Ullrich syndrome and Ullrich-Turner syndrome, is rare genetic condition that affects one out of every 2,000-4,000 female newborns (Gravholt et al., 2007a; Morgan, 2007). It results from the total or partial loss of an X chromosome, most likely soon after fertilization. This chromosomal disorder often prevents females from normal growth and maturity. Symptoms vary greatly and include down-turning eyelids, low set and prominent ears and a small jaw. Patients are more susceptible to chronic ear infections and that can lead to hearing loss (Alves & Oliveira, 2014). Despite efforts, international experts still are not able to improve recommendations for the care of patients as well-designed and large studies are scarce. As in almost all rare conditions, there is a lack of sufficient numbers of participants and not enough collaborative efforts amongst researchers to overcome the obstacles for the development of proper studies to better understand the disease and find therapeutic targets (Gravholt et al., 2007b).

Wildervanck Syndrome: Also known as cervico-oculo-acoustic syndrome, COA Syndrome or Cervico-oculo-acoustic dysplasia is a musculoskeletal, congenital genetic disease that affects the bones in the neck, the eyes, and the ears. It involves other diseases as the Klippel-Feil anomaly (in which the bones of the neck fuse together), the Duane syndrome (an eye movement disorder), and hearing loss, and affects mostly females. Its exact cause remains unknown but it is thought to be of epigenetic origin (https://rarediseases.info.nih.gov/diseases/5569/wildervanck-syndrome accessed 09-10-2019; https://www.orpha.net/consor/cgi-bin/Disease_Search.php?lng=PT&data_id=3038&Disease(s)/group%20of%20diseases=Wildervanck-syndrome&title=Wildervanck-syndrome&search=Disease_Search_Simple accessed 09-10-2019; (Rihani, 2013)).

Rare Pulmonary Diseases

Anti-basement Membrane Syndrome (anti-GBM): Autoimmune disorder also known as Goodpasture syndrome or disease. It involves both lungs and kidneys and often presents pulmonary hemorrhage (bleeding) and glomerulonephritis (kidney diseases in which the glomeruli are damaged and cannot remove waste and fluid like they should). It is characterized by the presence of circulating pathogenic autoantibodies directed against proteins in the glomerular (kidney) and alveolar (lung) basement membranes (DeVrieze & Hurley, 2019; McAdoo & Pusey, 2017).

Takayasu's Arteritis: Inflammatory condition also known as pulseless disease (because of being asymptomatic with impalpable pulses or bruits). It is characterized by damage of the medium and large arteries and their branches and is more prevalent in young Asian women. It involves blood vessels like the aorta and its major branches and the renal arteries, for example. Its etiology and prevalence remain incomplete. It seems to be originated from abnormalities in cell-mediated immunity and affects about 3 people *per* million *per* year in USA and about 1 person per million per year in Sweden (Kothari, 2001; Trinidad & Lala, 2019). It is also difficult to diagnose with non-specific features as fever, night sweats, mild anemia and weight loss and headaches. Complications vary and can result in neuronal impairment and vital organ failure. Nonetheless, women affected can still get pregnant and deliver (Johnston, Lock, & Gompels, 2002).

Rare Cardiac Diseases

Transthyretin Amyloid Cardiomyopathy (ATTR-CM): This heart disease is characterized by deposits of amyloid proteins in the walls of the left ventricle of the heart, the main pumping chamber. It can be an inherited disorder or not, and it is often underdiagnosed and potentially fatal. The deposition of the amyloid proteins causes the heart to become stiff, because of this the left ventricle cannot properly relax and fill with blood or squeeze pump the blood out of the heart (Dungu, Anderson, Whelan, & Hawkins, 2012; Ruberg, Grogan, Hanna, Kelly, & Maurer, 2019).

Heart Disease in Pregnancy: Some pregnancies are complicated by maternal disease. The data of prevalence and incidence in pregnancy-related heart disease is incomplete and/or unknown. But disorders as the sudden death syndrome, peripartum cardiomyopathy and myocardial infarction were registered to be common causes of maternal death. Thus, pregnancy and/or partum, may exacerbate malfunctions or disorders that were otherwise unknown. Heart disease patients also should know and be strictly followed by clinicians to better manage their health and that of the baby. The optimum treatment and care for both must be a concern. More data and registries are urgently needed to improve the current knowledge on the issue, either in epidemiology or in drug exposure during pregnancy. This group of diseases have specific guidelines from the European Society of Cardiology (ESC) for the management of cardiovascular diseases during pregnancy, where anything from epidemics, to differential diagnosis, different heart conditions and treatment recommendations are approached (www.escardio.org/guidelines, (Regitz-Zagrosek et al., 2018)). These guidelines help to standardize treatments to the different patients and improve quality criteria and clinical impact.

Rare Vascular Diseases

Wegener's Granulomatosis (WG): Now known as **Granulomatosis with polyangiitis (GPA)** is a rare multisystem autoimmune disease of unknown origin. It is characterized by necrotizing granulomatous inflammation (forming granulomas - collection of immune cells called macrophages) and inflammation of small and medium-size blood vessels thus, affecting organs as the lungs and kidneys. Often underdiagnosed, prevalence is unknown https://rarediseases.org/rare-diseases/granulomatosis-with-polyangiitis/ accessed 16-10-2019).

Kawasaki Syndrome: Multisystem children's disease also called mucocutaneous lymph node syndrome where the blood vessels throughout the body become inflamed causing rush, fever and swelling. Cause is uncertain and seems to be more prevalent in males but data on prevalence is rather incomplete (https://rarediseases.org/rare-diseases/kawasaki-disease/ accessed 16-10-2019).

Churg-Strauss Syndrome: Multiorgan disease marked by the inflammation of blood vessels and that affects mainly the lungs. Also known as Eosinophilic granulomatosis with polyangiitis (EGPA), asthma is the most common sign of the condition. Etiology is unknown, it has no cure and it has an estimated prevalence of 2-3 cases per million per year (https://rarediseases.org/rare-diseases/churg-strauss-syndrome/ accessed 16-10-2019).

Rare Hepatic Diseases

Alagille Syndrome: the main characteristic of this syndrome is liver damage caused by defects in the bile ducts. Due to defects as narrowing, malformation and reduced number, the bile (which helps to digest fats) carry by the bile ducts end up in the liver which causes its scarring and prevents the liver from properly eliminates 'wastes' from the bloodstream. This syndrome is also associated with heart problems, including impaired blood flow from the heart into the lungs (pulmonic stenosis). This syndrome affects about 1 in 70,000 newborns but data about a later diagnosis is missing. It is mostly of genetic origin and may have other names based on the prominent phenotype: Alagille-Watson Syndrome, Arteriohepatic Dysplasia

(AHD), Cardiovertebral Syndrome, Cholestasis with Peripheral Pulmonary Stenosis, Hepatic Ductular Hypoplasia, Hepatofacioneurocardiovertebral syndrome, Paucity of Interlobular Bile Ducts, Watson-Miller Syndrome (Spinner, Leonard, & Krantz, 1993), https://ghr.nlm.nih.gov/condition/alagille-syndrome, https://rarediseases.org/rare-diseases/alagille-syndrome/ accessed 10-10-2019)

Primary Sclerosing Cholangitis (PSC): This rare disorder is characterized by idiopathic (appears spontaneously or the cause is unknown) multi-focal bile duct strictures, typically leading to cirrhosis, end-stage liver disease, and colonic or hepatobiliary malignancy and often inter-related with inflammatory bowel disease and colorectal cancer. Etiology, therapeutic options and proper diagnosis and screening are lacking, and there is no cure to the moment (Fricker & Lichtenstein, 2019; Karlsen, Folseraas, Thorburn, & Vesterhus, 2017).

Autoimmune Hepatitis (AIH): Formerly known as lupoid hepatitis, this is a chronic autoimmune disease (the body's immune system attacks the liver) of unknown cause characterized by continuing liver bleeding and that cell death which, may lead to cirrhosis. Often, treatments fail, and various doses of different antibodies and drugs may attenuate treatment failure, incomplete response, drug intolerance or relapse. Autoimmune hepatitis was the first liver disease to have an effective therapeutic intervention, corticosteroid treatment. However, 50 years later AIH still remains a major diagnostic and therapeutic challenge. Further research into molecular, cellular and pharmacological therapies and interventions are promising but underexplored (Czaja, 2016; Liberal, Vergani, & Mieli-Vergani, 2015). Clinical practice guidelines have been provided for the improvement of autoimmune hepatitis diagnosis and quality treatment by the EASL (The European Association for the Study of the Liver - ("EASL Clinical Practice Guidelines: Autoimmune hepatitis," 2015)).

Biliary Atresia: Biliary atresia often manifests soon after birth and it is due (as the name suggests) to the absence or obstruction of the bile ducts. Many healthy infants have jaundice during the first postnatal weeks that resolves spontaneously (physiologic jaundice). However, when this is persistent after a couple of weeks and conjugated with high levels of bilirubin (compound that comes from the breakdown of red blood cells and is excreted by the liver) it should prompt further investigation. About 1 in 10,000 to 15,000 newborns are registered to suffer from biliary atresia. The diagnosis often includes blood tests, ultrasonography, liver biopsy, and hepatobiliary scan, and surgery is the only treatment. The cause of this inflammatory response is unknown, but several infectious microorganisms have been implicated and a genetic component may be involved (Bates, Bucuvalas, Alonso, & Ryckman, 1998; Yoon, Bresee, Olney, James, & Khoury, 1997).

Wilson Disease: Rare, genetic disorder in which copper builds up in the body, affecting mostly the brain and the liver. This disease is believed to affect one in 30,000 to 40,000 people worldwide. Wilson disease is progressive and often fatal if not recognized and treated when symptomatic. Treatment is life-long and aimed at reducing the amount of copper that has accumulated in the body and maintaining normal copper levels thereafter three types of medications. Treatment include three types of medications: to remove (chelate) copper from the body by urinary excretion, then zinc salts to prevent the gut from absorbing copper from the diet, and finally, tetrathiomolybdate which both prevents absorbing copper and binds up toxic copper in the blood making it nontoxic (https://rarediseases.org/rare-diseases/wilson-disease/ and https://ghr.nlm.nih.gov/condition/wilson-disease#genes accessed 10-10-2019). Clinical practice guidelines for Wilson Disease have also been released by the European Association for the Study of the Liver ("EASL Clinical Practice Guidelines: Wilson's disease," 2012).

Cystic Liver Disease: Cystic liver disease encompasses a heterogeneous group of fluid-filled lesions within the liver. Hepatic cysts are the most commonly encountered hepatic lesion. Cystic hepatic lesions can be of developmental, inflammatory, neoplastic or trauma-related causes. Although most cysts are benign, some are malignant. Ultrasounds can aid to diagnose simple hepatic cysts and polycystic liver disease, but other tests as CT scans or MRI are essential to establish differential diagnosis (Borhani, Wiant, & Heller, 2014; Mavilia, Pakala, Molina, & Wu, 2018).

Vascular Liver Disease: The liver has dual blood supply. The portal vein (rich in nutrients and relatively high in oxygen) provides two thirds of blood flow to the liver, and the hepatic artery (oxygen-rich) supplies the rest. When portal vein blood flow increases, hepatic artery flow decreases and vice versa (the hepatic arterial buffer response). This dual system provides some protection from hepatic ischemia (when tissues are not getting enough blood causing a shortage of oxygen that is needed to keep them alive) in healthy people. Finally, the hepatic veins drain the liver into the inferior vena cava. Hepatic vascular disorders occur when there is an obstruction in either veins or arteries. These include: *ischemia* (resulting from reduced blood flow, reduced oxygen delivery, increased metabolic activity, or all 3); insufficient venous drainage (as, for example, in *congestive hepatopathy*, or because of obstruction in the intrahepatic or extrahepatic veins (*Budd-Chiari syndrome*) or in the intrahepatic terminal hepatic venules and hepatic sinusoids (*veno-occlusive disease*)); and specific vascular lesions to the hepatic artery, hepatic vein, or portal vein. Vascular hepatic disorders affect less than 5 in 10,000 people, but altogether account for a significant number of rare diseases that represent an important health problem worldwide (DeLeve, 2003). Guidelines for Vascular Liver Disease have also been published by both the European Association for the Study of the Liver ("EASL Clinical Practice Guidelines: Vascular diseases of the liver," 2016), and the American Association for the Study Liver (DeLeve, Valla, Garcia-Tsao, & American Association for the Study Liver, 2009).

Liver Disease in Pregnancy: Liver diseases that occur during pregnancy have been considered in isolate. This is a common clinical scenario with an incidence of 3-5% of pregnant women being diagnosed with some form of liver disease (Tran, Ahn, & Reau, 2016). Certain diseases are associated with pregnancy, whereas others are unrelated. Management of this can be challenging because both mother and unborn fetus have to be considered in treatment decisions (Mikolasevic et al., 2018). Because of this, guidelines have been released and put in place. This is the case of the guidelines published by the American College of Gastroenterology (Tran et al., 2016). Liver disease such as acute viral hepatitis can occur in pregnancy, or a patient with underlying chronic liver disease (e.g. Cirrhosis - late stage of liver scarring) may get pregnant. Liver diseases unique to pregnancy include:

- *Hyperemesis gravidarum* (extreme form of morning sickness that causes severe nausea and vomiting).
- Acute fatty liver of pregnancy (potentially fatal complication that occurs in the third trimester or early postpartum period and is characterized by maternal liver dysfunction and/or failure that can lead to maternal and fetal complications, including death (more by: (Lee, 2018)).
- Intrahepatic cholestasis of pregnancy ('pruritus and an elevation in serum bile acid concentrations, typically developing in the late second and/or third trimester and rapidly resolving after delivery' (Lindor & Lee, 2019)) .
- HELLP syndrome (considered a variant of preeclampsia, it is a complication of pregnancy characterized by hemolysis - rupturing (lysis) of red blood cells and release of their contents -, elevated liver enzymes, and a low platelet count).

Rare Gastrointestinal (GI) Diseases

Inflammatory Bowel Disease: Group of inflammatory conditions of the colon and small intestine of unknown cause whose main conditions are Crohn's disease and ulcerative colitis. These are characterized by chronic inflammation of the gastrointestinal (GI) tract (Loddo & Romano, 2015). Crohn's disease is an autoimmune-related disorder that affect any segment of the gastrointestinal tract from the mouth to the anus. Symptoms include abdominal pain, diarrhea, fever, and weight loss. Ulcerative colitis is a long-term condition that results in inflammation and ulcers of the colon and rectum. The first symptoms are abdominal pain and diarrhea mixed with blood.

Pancreatitis: Inflammation of pancreas caused by the destruction of acinar cells (functional unit of the exocrine pancreas that synthesizes, stores, and secretes digestive enzymes) caused by a number of factors including pancreatic duct obstruction, alcoholism, and mutation in the cationic trypsinogen gene (Manohar, Verma, Venkateshaiah, Sanders, & Mishra, 2017). Epidemiology is poorly defined, but incidence worldwide seems to be on the rise (Majumder & Chari, 2016).

Celiac Sprue: Celiac disease is a long-term disorder of a gluten-sensitive digestive tract, where there is an immune reaction to eating gluten, a protein found in wheat, barley and rye.

Peutz-Jeghers Syndrome: Inherited disorder characterized the development of noncancerous growths called *hamartomatous* polyps in the gastrointestinal in association with a distinct pattern of skin and mucosal macular melanin deposition. Patients have a much higher risk of developing certain types of cancer. Because this growths can be confused with other non-cancerous tumors or masses, often patients face misdiagnosis and overtreatment increasing the death rates (https://ghr.nlm.nih.gov/condition/peutz-jeghers-syndrome#statistics accessed 13-10-2019).

Neuroendocrine Tumors: These tumors affect the release of hormones into the bloodstream (by targeting the neuroendocrine cells). Neuroendocrine tumors are rare and can develop in different parts of the body (e.g. lungs, pancreas, digestive tract, rectum). They can be cancerous (malignant) or non-cancerous (benign) and are usually of slow growth. Associations as the American Society of Clinical Oncology (ASCO), NIH and NHS maintain platforms online to inform the public and give information about the diseases (https://www.cancer.net/cancer-types/neuroendocrine-tumors/introduction; https://rarediseases.info.nih.gov/diseases/13445/neuroendocrine-tumor ; https://www.nhs.uk/conditions/neuroendocrine-tumours/ accessed 13-10-2019). Guidelines are also provided for example by the European Society For Medical Oncology (https://www.esmo.org/Guidelines/Endocrine-and-Neuroendocrine-Cancers) and the European Neuroendocrine Tumor Society (https://www.enets.org/current_guidelines.html) as well as the National Comprehensive Cancer Network (NCCN (Shah et al., 2018)).

Hereditary Hemorrhagic Telangiectasia (HTT): Also known as Osler–Weber–Rendu disease or Osler–Weber–Rendu syndrome. This inherited disorder is characterized by multiple abnormalities in the blood vessels that can result in bleeding. Lesions can affect the nasopharynx, central nervous system (CNS), lung, liver, and spleen, as well as the urinary tract, gastrointestinal (GI) tract, conjunctiva, trunk, arms, and fingers. HHT has been underdiagnosed, affecting more than a million people worldwide (https://rarediseases.org/rare-diseases/hereditary-hemorrhagic-telangiectasia/ accessed 13-10-2019; (Macri, Wilson, Shafaat, & Sharma, 2019)).

Menetrier's Disease (Hypertrophic Gastritis): rare disease in which the cells lining the stomach overgrow immensely. symptoms include pain, nausea/vomiting, weight loss, weakness, and diarrhea. the incidence, prevalence and cause remain unknown (https://www.orpha.net/consor/cgi-bin/oc_exp.php?lng=en&expert=2494

; https://rarediseases.info.nih.gov/diseases/2436/menetrier-disease accessed 13-10-2019).

Rare Genitourinary Diseases

Steroid Synthesis Disorder: All major classes of biologically active steroid hormones (progestins, mineralocorticoids, glucocorticoids, and sex steroids) are generally synthesized from cholesterol in the gonads and adrenal glands and changed into other steroids (steroidogenesis). Genetic mutations in the enzymes mediating these reactions result in abnormal effects. Both biochemical and genetic research have brought to light new disorders (Anna Biason-Lauber, 2003; A. Biason-Lauber, Boscaro, Mantero, & Balercia, 2010; White, 1990).

Androgen Insensitivity Syndrome (AIS) (complete (CAIS) and partial (PAIS)): Intersex condition that results in the partial or complete inability of the cells to respond to androgens. It affects sexual development before birth and during puberty. Formerly known as **testicular feminization**, it is usually found in males (genetically, with one X chromosome and one Y chromosome in each cell) that are unable to respond to some male sex hormones (androgens) thus they may exhibit many female external sex characteristics. This syndrome results from genetic defects in the X chromosome. In complete AIS (CAIS) external male gonads fail to develop (https://www.orpha.net/consor/cgi-bin/OC_Exp.php?Lng=EN&Expert=99429 accessed 14-10-2019). In Partial AIS (PAIS), males have different male traits and can include other disorders as hypospadias, a condition in which the opening of the urethra is on the underside of the penis, instead of at the tip (https://rarediseases.org/rare-diseases/androgen-insensitivity-syndrome-partial/ accessed 14-10-2019). CAIS affects 2 to 5 newborn males in 100,000. PAIS is thought to be at least as common while mild androgen insensitivity is much less common (https://ghr.nlm.nih.gov/condition/androgen-insensitivity-syndrome#statistics accessed 14-10-2019).

Ovotesticular Disorders of Sex Development: This is an extremely rare disorder characterized by ambiguous genitalia (both testis and ovaries in the same person). Gender assignment in newborns is a challenge thus recently it is recommended to postpone the surgery leaving a neutral gender until patients are able to participate to the decision (Scarpa, Grazia, & Tornese, 2017). The causes of this disorder are known in only a small portion of patients. Ovotesticular DSD is the rarest disorder of sex development in humans and less than 1 in 20,000 people are affected. At least 500 affected individuals have been reported (https://rarediseases.org/rare-diseases/ovotesticular-disorder-of-sex-development/ accessed 14-10-2019).

Turner Syndrome: Female-only genetic disorder in which a female is partly or completely missing an X chromosome. Affects about 1 in every 2,000 -2,500 baby girls. Medical and developmental problems include short height, underdeveloped ovaries and heart defects (https://www.nhs.uk/conditions/turner-syndrome/ ; https://ghr.nlm.nih.gov/condition/turner-syndrome accessed 14-10-2019).

CHARGE Syndrome: Rare genetic disorder characterized by a variable combination of multiple anomalies. Previously associated with newborn children with the congenital features of coloboma of the eye (hole in one of the structures of the eye such as the iris or the retina), heart defects, atresia of the nasal choanae, retardation of growth and/or development, genital and/or urinary abnormalities, and ear abnormalities and deafness. It is now recognized that not all individuals affected present these non-random association of anomalies. The reported incidence of CHARGE syndrome goes from 0.1–1.2 per 10,000 and depends on professional recognition. The syndrome has been thoroughly described in the Orphanet Journal of Rare diseases (Blake & Prasad, 2006) and by US NIH (https://ghr.nlm.nih.gov/condition/charge-syndrome and https://rarediseases.info.nih.gov/diseases/29/charge-syndrome accessed 14-10-2019).

Rare Bacterial, Viral and Fungal Infections

Lymphogranuloma Venereum (LGV): Uncommon sexually transmitted disease (STD) caused by *Chlamydia trachomatis*; An ulcerative disease of the genital area with three stages of infection. It is common in the tropical and subtropical regions but rare in countries like the United States of America (Rawla & Limaiem, 2019).

Chancroid: Extremely rare sexually transmitted infection caused by *Haemophilus ducreyi* and characterized by one or more soft and painful genital ulcers, and regional lymphadenitis (infection of lymph nodes), which may develop into buboes (symptom of an inflammatory swelling of a lymphatic gland, especially in the groin or armpit). Recommendations for the diagnosis and management of chancroid have been given by different institutions and guidelines have been published by different sources (e.g. (Lautenschlager, Kemp, Christensen, Mayans, & Moi, 2017)).

Donovanosis or Granuloma Inguinale: Chronic cause of genital ulceration; STD caused by *Klebsiella granulomatis* (previously named *Calymmatobacterium granulomatis*) bacteria and characterized by genital ulcers. There was some outbreaks namely in the Aboriginals of Australia but elimination programs appear to have been successful ((O'Farrell, 2002), https://www.health.nsw.gov.au/Infectious/factsheets/Pages/donovanosis.aspx accessed 15-10-2019).

Cytomegalovirus: Common herpes virus, usually harmless.

Bovine Spongiform Encephalopathy (BSE) or Mad Cow Disease: Group of diseases named Transmissible spongiform encephalopathies (now known as prion diseases) that affect humans and animals through spongy degeneration of the brain with severe and fatal symptoms. It has a long incubation period (of 4-5 years) and is caused by a transmissible agent called prion. For unknown reasons the protein known as prion change into a pathogenic (harmful) form that then damages the nervous system. With a major outbreak worldwide in the early 2000s, it is now thought that the infection was derived from feeding cattle with proteins derived from other ruminants, and people would get affected by eating infected meat (Iulini et al., 2017; Laurindo & Barros Filho, 2017).

Creutzfeldt-Jakob Disease (CJD): Rapidly progressive, rare, transmissible, fatal, neurodegenerative condition caused by prion proteins that have long incubation periods and progress inevitably once clinical symptoms appear. The infectious agent, prion (a protein) can be transmitted either by direct contact with contaminated tissue (iatrogenic) or via inheriting a mutation in the prion protein gene (familial). However, most cases of CJD are sporadic. Usually affects older people (60-75 years old) and affects about 1 person per million per year worldwide. About 350 cases are registered per year in the United States (Sitammagari & Masood, 2019).

Rare Musculoskeletal Diseases

Osteogenesis Imperfecta (OI): OI or **Brittle Bone Disease**, is a heterogeneous group of genetic disorders characterized by increased bone fragility, low bone mass, and susceptibility to bone fractures with variable severity (shorturl.at/nyi03, ORPHA:666, accessed 16-10-2019). It is estimated to affect 6 to 7 per 100,000 people worldwide, and age of diagnosis depends of when symptoms appear. There are five clinically distinct types of OI, and they range from lethal to mild severity of multiple spontaneous fractures. And most of them are caused by mutations in genes encoding collagen protein https://ghr.nlm.nih.gov/condition/osteogenesis-imperfecta#statistics; https://rarediseases.org/rare-diseases/osteogenesis-imperfecta/ accessed 16-10-2019).

Osteosarcoma: This is the most common type of bone cancer, with most being diagnosed in adolescence. The cause is unknown, although in some cases an hereditary link was found (https://rarediseases.info.nih.gov/diseases/7284/osteosarcoma accessed 16-10-2019). There are several variants of osteosarcoma, they are all however highly malignant tumors. The classic osteosarcoma is very rare (0.2% of all malignant tumors) with an estimated incidence of 3 cases per million per year worldwide (https://www.orpha.net/consor/cgi-bin/OC_Exp.php?Lng=GB&Expert=668, ORPHA:668, accessed 16-10-2019).

Progeria: also called **Hutchinson-Gilford Progeria Syndrome** (HGPS), is characterized by galloping aging starting in childhood. Babies born with this congenital e genetic condition start to show symptoms after the first year of life which include aged-looking skin, joint stiffness, hip dislocations and cardiovascular disease. The average lifespan is of about 13 years, with some patients reaching 20 years of age. It is, nonetheless, a fatal syndrome. It is reported in only 1 in 4-8 newborns worldwide (https://rarediseases.info.nih.gov/diseases/7467/progeria accessed 16-10-2019). Many people got familiar with this syndrome through F. Scott Fitzgerald's short story 'The Curious Case of Benjamin Button' (Maloney, 2009), and loosely based 2008 movie directed by David Fincher and with acting starts as Brad Pitt and Cate Blanchett.

Synovial Sarcoma: aggressive soft tissue malignant tumor that occurs more commonly in adolescents and young adults localized near the large joints of the extremities but also in the head and neck, mediastinum and viscera (lung, kidney, etc.). The name is misleading as the tumor origin is postulated to be multipotent mesenchymal cells and not in the synovium (soft tissue that lines a joint and mediates nutrient exchange between blood and joint fluid). Prevalence is unknown, and cause is also unclear although previously linked to genetic factors (shorturl.at/lwF56, ORPHA:3273; https://rarediseases.info.nih.gov/diseases/7721/synovial-sarcoma accessed 16-10-2019).

Rare Hematological Diseases

Aagenaes Syndrome: also called cholestasis lymphedema syndrome (CLS), it is a multi-system rare disease possibly caused by mutations in the LSC1 gene on chromosome 15q. It is a hereditary condition mainly found in Norwegian descent people (shorturl.at/htAX7 accessed 28-10-2019). And it is characterized by severe neonatal cholestasis (i.e. bile cannot flow from the liver to the duodenum) that usually lessens during early childhood and becomes intermittent with age, and chronic severe lymphedema (i.e. localized fluid retention and tissue swelling) that mainly affects the lower limbs (Bull et al., 2000)(shorturl.at/ejyU1 accessed 28-10-2019, ORPHA: 1414). It has a prevalence under one per 1,000,000 general population.

Abetalipoproteinemia: Hereditary rare disease also named **Bassen Kornzweig syndrome**. It is caused by a mutation in a transfer protein resulting in deficiencies in proteins used in the synthesis and exportation of chylomicrons (lipoprotein particles) and very-low-density lipoprotein (VLDL) thus, interferes with the normal absorption of fat and fat-soluble vitamins from food. Symptoms appear usually in the first months of life and include failure to thrive (to grow in infancy), diarrhea and fatty, pale stools of foul smell, protruding abdomen, but also impaired nervous system function with possible developmental delay or intellectual disability, eye disorders and muscle discoordination. More than a hundred cases have been reported but prevalence is unknown (https://ghr.nlm.nih.gov/condition/abetalipoproteinemia #inheritance accessed 28-10-2019)(Zamel, Khan, Pollex, & Hegele, 2008).

Acquired Hemophilia: Rare bleeding / autoimmune disorder that interferes with the clotting process. Affects mostly older people (between 60 and 67 years old), and symptoms include prolonged bleeding, frequent nosebleeds, easy bruising and hematomas, and gastrointestinal and urologic bleeding. In this condition, the body's immune system attacks and disables a protein involved in coagulation (coagulation factor VIII, associated to **F8 gene**). It is often associated with other conditions as pregnancy, cancer, skin diseases, allergic reactions to medications and autoimmune disease. It affects 1 to 2 people per 1,000,000 per year in the U.S.A. and U.K. (shorturl.at/qHTZ3; shorturl.at/DEJRZ accessed 28-10-2019). Experts have created clinical guidelines for the disease management (Kruse-Jarres et al., 2017).

Acute Erythroid Leukemia: Very rare acute myeloid leukemia (AML) type, representing less than 5% of all cases, and characterized by prevalent erythroid precursor cells (over 50% of bone marrow nucleated cells should be of erythroid origin) leading to a shortage of all types of blood cells and consequently symptoms as fatigue, infections, weight loss, fever, night sweats, mucocutaneous bleeding and anemia (Zuo, Polski, Kasyan, & Medeiros, 2010). Often very aggressive type of cancer / leukemia and with a median survival of 3 months after diagnosis (Wang, Wang, Medeiros, & Khoury, 2017).

Diamond-Blackfan Anemia (DBA): Congenital erythroid aplasia (decline of red blood cells (erythrocytes) produced by the bone marrow). This inherited blood disorder is caused by mutations in several genes and different subtypes exist but with similar features. These features include anemia (low red blood cells count), physical anomalies as small head size (microcephaly), specific facial features as cleft palate, cleft lip, short and webbed neck, small shoulder blades and defects of the hands as well as of the genitals, urinary tract, eyes and hear. However, 30% of the patients diagnosed with this disorder did not have genetic mutations (Da Costa et al., 2018). Diamond-Blackfan anemia affects about 5 to 7 per million newborn babies worldwide (shorturl.at/duwTZ; https://ghr.nlm.nih.gov/condition/diamond-blackfan-anemia#statistics accessed 29-10-2019).

Essential Thrombocythemia: rare bleeding disorder characterized by increased number of platelets or thrombocytes (thrombocythemia). It can be asymptomatic or lead to problems associated with the excess of platelets, as for example, abnormal blood clotting (thrombosis), and clots that form or go to the brain and block the blood flow causing strokes or temporary stroke-like episodes (transient ischemic attacks). It affects about 1 to 24 people per million worldwide (https://ghr.nlm.nih.gov/condition/essential-thrombocythemia#statistics accessed 28-10-2019; ORPHA:124)(Sanchez & Ewton, 2006).

Fabry Disease: inherited X-linked lysosomal rare disease that results from the accumulation of a certain type of fat (globotriaosylceramide) in the cells. With onset usually at childhood, it causes symptoms as pain particularly in the hands and feet, clusters of small, dark red spots on the skin (angiokeratomas), decreased ability to swear (hypohidrosis), corneal opacity, gastrointestinal problems, ringing in the ears and hearing loss. It can be life-threating with episodes of kidney damage, heart attack and stroke. It affects about 1 in 40,000 to 60,000 men; the prevalence in unknown in women (https://ghr.nlm.nih.gov/condition/fabry-disease#statistics accessed 28-10-2019)(Germain, 2010).

Familial Platelet Disorder with Associated Myeloid Malignancy (FPD/ AML): Dense granule disease characterized by moderate thrombocytopenia (abnormally low levels of thrombocytes or platelets in the blood), abnormal platelet function and propensity to develop myeloid malignancies (hematopoietic disorder characterized by excessive proliferation, abnormal self-renewal, and/or differentiation defects of hematopoietic stem cells (HSCs) and myeloid progenitor cells). The prevalence is unknown, and less than 20 cases have been reported. It is estimated that can affect less than one newborn per million worldwide. (shorturl.at/hpqJX accessed 28-10-2019; ORPHA:71290).

Fanconi Anemia: Genetic hereditary disorder characterized by genomic instability, bone marrow failure (BMF), congenital defects, inability to repair DNA inter-strand crosslinks (ICLs), and cancer predisposition namely to myeloid leukemia and epithelial malignancies (Niraj, Färkkilä, & D'Andrea, 2019). It affects about 1 in 160,000 individuals worldwide or have a prevalence of 1-9 per million individuals. It is more common among people of Ashkenazi Jewish descent, the Roma population of Spain, and black South Africans (https://ghr.nlm.nih.gov/condition/fanconi-anemia#statistics ; https://www.orpha.net/consor/cgi-bin/OC_Exp.php?Expert=84 accessed 28-10-2019; ORPHA:84).

(Primary) Myelofibrosis: Also known as chronic idiopathic myelofibrosis (cIMF), is a group of rare bone marrow/ blood cancer of unknown cause classified as myeloproliferative neoplasms. In this condition, the marrow is replaced by scar tissue and is not able to make healthy blood cells. The bone marrow produces either too many or too few of certain blood cells, most of which do not function properly (each disorder's name comes from the cells that are affected). It affects about 1 in 1 in 500,000 individuals worldwide (https://ghr.nlm.nih.gov/condition/primary-myelofibrosis accessed 28-10-2019; ORPHA: 824).

Paroxysmal Nocturnal Hemoglobinuria (PNH): Rare, acquired, chronic, and life-threating disorder that most frequently presents in early adulthood and is characterized by the destruction of red blood cells by the immune system. It results in the death of about half of the diagnosed patients due to thrombotic complication. The name of the disease comes from the breakdown of red blood cells with release of hemoglobin into the urine, which turns it dark-colored specially in the morning. This is caused by the absence of protective proteins in the red blood cells membrane. It is estimated to affect 1 to 5 individuals per million people (shorturl.at/emBR0 accessed 28-10-2019; ORPHA:447).

Polycythemia Vera: Genetic disease mostly non-hereditary characterized by an increased number of red blood cells in the bloodstream. Patients may also have excess white blood cells and platelets making them propense to blood clots. Prevalence varies worldwide and it affects about 44 to 57 individuals per 100,000 in the U.S. It is more common in males than in females (https://ghr.nlm.nih.gov/condition/polycythemia-vera#inheritance accessed 28-10-2019; ORPHA: 729).

Sickle cell (beta) Thalassemia: Inherited blood disorder disorders that results in the decreased synthesis or complete absence of the beta globin chains of hemoglobin. Low levels of hemoglobin lead to a lack of oxygen in many parts of the body. The clinical course is variable ranging from asymptomatic condition to a disorder identical with sickle-cell anemia. The condition is relatively common worldwide. thousands of babies with beta thalassemia are born each year. Beta thalassemia affects mostly people from Mediterranean countries, North Africa, the Middle East, India, Central Asia, and Southeast Asia (https://ghr.nlm.nih.gov/condition/beta-thalassemia#statistics accessed 28-10-2019; ORPHA: 251359).

Tufted Angioma: Previously known as "angioblastoma of Nakagawa", it is a benign tumor of the blood vessels that grows in and just below the skin. It affects mostly infants and young children. Tufted angioma gets its name from the characteristic "tufts" of capillaries seen when the tumor tissue is examined under a microscope (Osio et al., 2010).

Williams Syndrome: rare genetic multisystemic neurodevelopmental disorder characterized by mild to moderate intellectual disability or learning problems, unique personality characteristics, distinctive facial features, and heart and blood vessel (cardiovascular) problems. It is thought to affect about 1 in 10,000 individuals (https://ghr.nlm.nih.gov/condition/williams-syndrome#statistics accessed 28-10-2019; ORPHA:904).

Yellow Nail Syndrome: also known as "primary lymphedema associated with yellow nails and pleural effusion", is a very rare disease characterized by pleural effusions (excess of fluid in the pleural cavity, the fluid-filled space that surrounds the lungs), lymphedema (fluid retention and tissue swelling due to under development of the lymphatic vessels) and yellow dystrophic nails. The cause is unknown and it was reported in over a hundred individuals of middle-age but it can show in children too (https://rarediseases.org/rare-diseases/yellow-nail-syndrome/ accessed 28-10-2019; ORPHA:662)

Rare Metabolic Diseases

CDG Syndromes: Large group of congenital and inherited disorders of glycosylation or carbohydrate-deficient glycoprotein (CDG). Glycosylation is the process of adding sugar blocks, called glycans, to proteins. CDGs patients are unable to properly add glycans to proteins, and this is required by just about every tissue in the human body. Thus, patients display numerous health problems which, may include seizures, liver disease, ocular abnormalities, coagulation disorders, etc. Each CDG type is different and rare so clinical experience with CDG is very limited. Over 130 different genes have been identified to cause CDG. New types of CDG are discovered every year, through efforts from scientists, health professionals and parents. Prevalence and incidence is unknown (https://rarediseases.org/rare-diseases/congenital-disorders-of-glycosylation/ ; accessed 28-10-2019; ORPHA:137).

Rare Gynecological and Obstetrical Diseases

Gestational Trophoblastic Disease (GTD): Umbrella term for a complex family of disorders that includes any of the group of diagnoses that behave out of character from what is expected of gestational trophoblastic tissue. It can include benign or malign conditions. They all arise from trophoblasts, which are the group of cells responsible for the formation of the placenta, an essential organ for the delivery of nutrients and removal of waste from the growing fetus. There is a predisposition in groups of women with Asian, Hispanic and Native American ethnicity. Adolescents and women over forty years old also have higher risk (https://rarediseases.org/rare-diseases/gestational-trophoblastic-disease/ accessed 28-10-2019; ORPHA: 254685).

CHARGE Syndrome: multiple congenital anomaly. The name is an abbreviation for features common in the disorder: coloboma, heart defects, atresia choanae (also known as choanal atresia), growth retardation, genital abnormalities, and ear abnormalities. The pattern of malformations varies among patients with this syndrome, and they present several health problems that can be life-threatening in infancy. It affects about 1 to 9 newborns in 100,000 births (https://ghr.nlm.nih.gov/condition/charge-syndrome accessed 28-10-2019; ORPHA: 138).

HELLP Syndrome: rare liver and blood clotting disorder that can affect pregnant women. It usually occurs after labor, but it can appear any time after 20 weeks of gestation. The letters in the name refer to each conditions of the disease: hemolysis (red blood cells burst), elevated liver enzymes (in the blood stream they signal liver damage), and low platelet count (leading to abnormal clotting). And it can be life-threatening. This condition is probable multifactorial with some epigenetic predisposition but at the moment the exact cause and mechanisms remain unknown (https://rarediseases.info.nih.gov/diseases/8528/hellp-syndrome accessed 29-10-2019; ORPHA: 244242).

BRCA Hereditary Breast and Ovarian Cancer Syndrome: inherited cancer-predisposition syndrome mostly, in the breast (in both men and women) and in the ovaries (in women). Mutations in the genes BRCA1 and BRCA2 are associated with increased risk to develop these cancers. But, some people with mutations in these genes may never be affected by any cancer. Thus, the syndrome represents a predisposition or tendency. The risk for ovarian cancer in the general population is approximately 1-2%, but 39-63% with BRCA1 gene variations and 16.5-27% with BRCA2 variations. The prevalence this syndrome is about 1 to 5 per 10,000 people in the general population, but it can affect certain populations more than others. It is estimated to occur in about 1 in 200 to 1in 800 people in the general population (https://rarediseases.org/rare-diseases/hereditary-breast-ovarian-cancer-syndrome/ accessed 30-10-2019; ORPHA: 145).

Chapter 2
Health-Related Communication and Rare Diseases:
A Passport for the Patient Journey

Michaela Liuccio
https://orcid.org/0000-0002-6091-2285
Sapienza University Rome, Italy

ABSTRACT

Rare diseases are often characterized as diseases with low prevalence in population that stem from genetic disorders or environment conditions. As a result of its low prevalence and lack of knowledge of its causes, symptoms, and/or treatment, patients' access to healthcare, and their quality of life may be affected. A key challenge is also the physician-patient interaction that differs from traditional medical care settings by demanding physicians' experience in dealing, for example, with psychological problems associated with the diagnosis process. Information and Communication Technologies can facilitate the interaction between the sources of information and patients, overcoming geographical distances. This chapter discusses the role of Information and Communication to extract health data in rare diseases and reinforce physician-patient interactions. It argues that Information and Communication are crucial to meet patients' needs, drivers, and decision-making that tend to occur during the patient's journey (pre-diagnosis, diagnosis, and post-diagnosis).

DOI: 10.4018/978-1-7998-2088-8.ch002

INTRODUCTION

Rare diseases impact negatively upon on patients' access to high-quality healthcare and both patients and care-givers' quality of life (Hesselgrave, 2003; Huyard, 2009; Pasculli, Resta, Guastamacchia, Suppressa, Sabbà, 2004; Schieppati, Henter, Daina, & Aperia, 2008). Part of this impact may be owing to the uncertainty often associated to this kind of diseases and, subsequently, have an impact on trust in physicians and healthcare systems.

Lack of certainty is, indeed, one of the greatest challenges that is likely to predominate in disease diagnosis and treatment. Babrow, Kasch and Ford (1998) point out that uncertainty can result from complex situations (e.g. multicausal or contingent pathways to outcomes), properties of information (e.g. clarity, completeness, volume, or consistency), probabilistic thinking (e.g. belief in a single probability or a range of probabilities), the structure of information (e.g. how or whether information is integrated with other information), and lay epistemology (e.g. individual beliefs about the nature of knowledge).

In health-related communication, investigating the way uncertainty is managed by patients (Brashers, Goldsmith, & Hsieh, 2002; Martin, Stone, Scott, & Brashers, 2010) and their social network members (Donovan-Kicken & Bute, 2008) has been a continuing concern within socio-medical context. Patients and caregivers usually rely on community social support to help with information seeking (Brashers, Neidig, & Goldsmith, 2004; Cline & Haynes, 2001), coping skills and disease management (Patsos, 2001), reinforcing perceived relational stability and changes in the patient's perspective on the disease impact (Doyle, 2015).

Provider-patient relationships can be also fundamental to aid in uncertainty management; however, they can also exacerbate certain moments of uncertainty when dealing with the dualism of a "credible authority" and information scarcity. In fact, Mishel (1988) draws our attention to the fact that a "credible authority" (i.e, trust and confidence in health care providers) are important predictors of uncertainty. If, on the one hand, they can be a valuable source of information or advice and facilitate decision-making, on the other hand, they may express uncertainty towards incidence (i.e. number of newly diagnosed cases) of rare diseases (Brashers, Hsieh, Neidig, & Reynolds, 2006; Gordon, Joos, & Byrne, 2000).

In health provider-patient interactions, mirroring uncertainty (Clayton, Dudley, & Musters, 2008) can also occur, having an impact on patient's satisfaction and anxiety (Blanch, Hall, Roter, & Frankel, 2009). It can be manifested through the following ways: (a) Question asking (Eggly et al., 2006); and (b) Information sharing (Nakash, Dargouth, Oddo, Gao, & Alegría, 2009). Given that this process may be amplified with the use of Information and Communication Technologies (Lewis, Gray, Freres, & Hornik, 2009) and affect patients' attitudes (Parrott, 2009) and health (Pecchioni,

Thompson, & Anderson, 2006), understanding the role of communication among different stakeholders (i.e. patients, caregivers, physicians, policy-makers) in rare diseases is of utmost importance.

The aim of this chapter is to discuss the role of information and communication to extract health data in rare diseases, and the implications in the patient's journey (pre-diagnosis, diagnosis and post-diagnosis).

HEALTH-RELATED COMMUNICATION AND RARE DISEASES IN THE DIGITAL AGE

Although a precise definition of health-related communication is lacking, it is undeniable the importance of the transdisciplinary involving both health and social sciences (Lambert, & McKevitt, 2002; Schiavo, 2007). The Centers for Disease Control and Prevention (2019) defines it as:

The study and use of Communication strategies to inform and influence individual decisions that enhance health.

The interpersonal and intrapersonal interactions (Ruesch, 1951) may involve different channels (e.g. letters, newspapers, mass media, mobile media, VR, games) and health stakeholders (e.g. physician, patient, caregivers). Alongside the advances in health with the emergence of ehealth (Eysenbach, 2001), digital and smart health (Kostkova, 2015; Solanas, et al., 2014), mhealth (Fiordelli, Diviani, & Schulz, 2013), VR or Gamified Health (Johnson, et al., 2016; Riva, 2002) and communication have also evolved from the linear source-message-receiver process (Lasswell, Lerner & Pool, 1952; Shannon & Weaver, 1949) to an increasingly multimodal, interactive (Robinson, & Stivers, 2001), peer-to-peer and complex one.

Patient empowerment (Aujoulat, d'Hoore, & Deccache, 2007; Holmström & Röing, 2010; Rifkin, 2006) involves a demand for information and both participation in active (and interactive) health management and shared responsibilities with health stakeholders. In fact, such empowerment is considered very important to those cases in which not only compliance with pharmacological treatment is required, but also a radical change in lifestyle (Rifkin, 2006). As a result, it can impact on advocacy for health, through the combination of individual and social actions aimed to support policies for a particular health goal or program (Maibach, & Holtgrave, 1995). In addition, in the health context, the role of communication is closely connected to trust (Hou, & Shim, 2010), i.e. trust is an important component of the relationship between people and health information, and between people and healthcare professionals; it may vary because the same health information/communication would be perceived differently; and this variance may affect health communication outcomes.

Media advocacy has been of particularly value to divulgate the patients' needs and unite different health stakeholders (e.g. patients, politicians, public opinion, those who organize and provide health services- physicians, nurses, caregivers, professional associations, pharmaceutical industry) (Walker, 2013; Wallack, Dorfman, Jenigan, & Themba-Nixon, 1993).

In the individual-health-society relationships, it is worth noting that the cultural "building" power of the media can be centered on the following levels (Liuccio, & Giorgino, 2019):

- **Media-action:** Production of cultural products, often stereotyped that may have an impact on social effects;
- **Mediation:** Bridge the gap between expert knowledge, medical-scientific, and undifferentiated audiences;
- **Disintermediation process:** Diminish the power of media culture, thanks to the spread of new media.

In a digital age, patient-citizen-consumers have access to many sources of information (Adams, 2011; Biehl, 2016) and tend to be less faithful to the uniqueness of medical assistance and adherence to paternalism in physician-patient relationships (McKinstry, 1992). Through the use of digital platforms, they can (Lupton, & Jutel, 2015; Swan, 2009):

a. Plan, decide, interact and monitor their health;
b. Search and choose their own physician;
c. Choose freely between public and private services; and
d. Demonstrate advocacy skills and strategically affect health policies, especially through patient's associations.

In all, patients are the decision-makers and the co-producers of their own health (Bopp, 2000; Fotaki, 2011). Amongst the possible actions that patients can perform with the use of digital media, information search is the most influential on patients' decision-making and reliability of the source, being trust a constant concern (Impicciatore, Pandolfini, Casella, & Bonati, 1997). In addition, mobile technologies have been used over the years to get georeferenced information on patients' health, diagnosis and self-care; surveil and self-monitor diseases, and send short messages towards health (Kahn, Yang, & Khan, 2010). Mobile media is recognized as an important source of health information, but it is unclear whether people from different social groups use mobile media to seek health information.

Some studies have shown that used sources of health information may vary by ethnicity (O'Malley, Kerner, & Johnson, 1999), race (Nicholson, Grason, & Powe, 2003) and socioeconomic status (Hesse et al., 2005).

Relatively few studies (e.g. Budych, Helms, & Schultz, 2012; Coulson, Buchanan, & Aubeeluck, 2007; Glenn, 2015; Lasker, Sogolow, & Sharim, 2005; Patsos, 2011) have deeply considered the role-set of communication in rare diseases (Liuccio, Belotti, Comune, Zambito, & Schulz, 2015). Most of the studies are focused on the interpersonal communication between patient and care givers (e.g. Budych, Helms, & Schultz, 2012; Bensing, 1991), and on psycho-social support (e.g. Coulson, Buchanan, & Aubeeluck, 2007; Kaplan, Cassel, & Gore, 1977).

Furthermore, there are studies on the information patients extract from the media (new and mass media) (Rekatsinas, et al., 2015), but no adequate attention has been paid to patients' health information seeking behaviors. The term HISB (Health Information Seeking Behaviors) (Lambert, & Loiselle, 2007) is used to refer to the type and amount of information sources consulted and, subsequently, one's decision-making and actions performed. When applied to rare diseases, HISB are likely to be of interest to health professionals in that informational interventions are tailored to individuals' needs and preferences (Liuccio, et al., 2015).It would be, therefore, important to promote studies on patients' health information seeking behaviors, information reliability and divulgation channels, and non-alarmist data that are easy to decode regarding rare diseases.

Relative to the source of medication information and other disease information (Web-based information, pharmacists, physicians), patients diagnosed with rare diseases often perceive physicians and Web-based information as credible sources and information mediators concerning such topics as side effects and drug effectiveness (Liuccio et al., 2015).

Web-based information can be beneficial for patients with rare diseases by:

- **Connecting with other patients diagnosed with the same/similar diseases:** This connection can help patients to cope with their disease, obtaining knowledge and support from who share the same symptoms and are challenged with similar obstacles/difficulties on a daily basis (Doyle, 2015);
- **Helping with screening prevention, diagnosis and treatment of the disease:** Web-based information enables early identification, personalized treatment, and health management (Dwyer, Quinton, Morin, & Pitteloud, 2014; Kowalski, Kahana, Kuhr, Ansmann, & Pfaff, 2014; Schumacher, et al., 2014);
- **Overpassing the limitations of the patient-physician communication:** Patients may be more open to express their concerns in web communities rather than with their physician (Hilton-Kamm, Sklansky, Chang, 2014);

- **Searching information and reaching online communities:** Web-based interventions and online communities may be helpful to decode clinical information, explore new therapeutic modalities and provide new insights about certain disease relevant for health providers-patients interactions. These are relevant to ensure patients' empowerment (Aymé, Kole & Groff, 2008);
- **Ensuring the effectiveness of patient advocacy groups for rare diseases and raise public awareness** in general (Morgan et al. 2014). When individuals access accurate and reliable information, they can make informed decisions (Liuccio et al. 2015).

Regarding patients' illnesses and health needs, three elements play a determinant role: (a) the individual's illness; (b) medical entities (e.g. physicians, nurses, health professionals…); and (c) society as a whole (with collective symbolic representations, strategies or political visions, economic maneuvers). A disease pathology is dependent on the individual, cultural and subjective perspective or experience of a physical and mental discomfort. A disease also refers to how the social system represents and interprets a disease, an experience of illness and, therefore, rights, duties and insured practices associated to it (disease) (Giarelli, & Venneri, 2009). In the specific case of rare diseases, the patients' perception of illness severity also varies with their attitude towards the disease and others' recognition (socio-cultural aspects) (Augè, & Herzlich, 1986; Liuccio, 2018), and the media plays in that way an essential role.

PATIENT-PHYSICIAN INTERACTIONS

In Patient-Physician Interactions, communication is mainly affected by the role of behavior of both the patient and health care providers. Previous studies on patients with rare diseases (Aymé, Kole, & Groff, 2008; Bronstein, & Kakki, 2016; Mavris & Cam, 2012) have shown that patients often become experts in their own diseases and health providers have to recognize the active role of the patient as an informed, engaged and interactive partner in the therapeutic process. This is a change in mind-set of the traditional healthcare systems.

Physicians do not have always enough knowledge and experience in all rare diseases and, therefore, patients are faced with deep uncertainty. In particular, most of the treatments are considered experimental, hence the concern about their safety and effectiveness (Aartsma-Rus et al., 2011; Abrahamyan, et al., 2016). Thus, the information passed on by different health professionals may be inconsistent or controversial, and the patient is confronted with conflicting opinions and different treatment options from the top experts involved. Ambiguity, variety and unpredictability of the symptoms are then major problems. Nevertheless, patients' experience would, probably, get better if health professionals were capable of meeting their moral expectations more often, especially in terms of diagnosis disclosure and information (Liuccio et al. 2015).

Patient-Physician interactions encompass two dimensions of communication: content (sometimes referred to as task/instrumental) and affective/relational. Beach, Keruly and Moore (2006) advocate that patients want to be regarded as individuals by health stakeholders and not merely as patients. For that, positive affect from care providers and encouragement of question-asking are also crucial (Ong, Visser, Lammes, & De Haes, 2000; Pieterse, Van Dulmen, Beemer, Bensing, & Ausems, 2007).

For many years, physician-patient relationships were hierarchical, in which physicians were the entities who had all the knowledge and transmitted it to a 'passive' patient. These interactions have been changed within a socio-cultural setting and living condition and the patient role has also involved in a much more sympathetic and emphatic approach (Greenfield, Kaplan, & Ware, 1985; Warne, & McAndrew, 2007).

The current advancements on the digital age tend to lead to a dematerialization of the physical contact between physician and patients and representation of these interactions through images, videos and simulacra. The Parsonian's role of a passive agent relative to health and self-care is likely to have evolved to an active agent responsible for their health (Armstrong, 2014), who understand his/her own pathology and is able to exchange information with the physician and negotiate treatments and drug intake.

In the view of the interrelationship between illness and social life, Parsons (1996) highlights that the sickness condition and its severity is more than a subjective dimension, but a socio-cultural one. The role of the patient is described as temporary and closely related to the condition of the disease, as an alternative to the normality of the roles played in life based on cultural and social variables.

Living and coping with a disease is also part of one's identity and culture context. Indeed, individuals live the condition of illness as a modification of physical, social and moral harmony. In many cases, they come to think that the change in their body, due to the pathology, has irremediably changed their identity, and it has developed a post-diagnosis identity.

In this regard, Frank (1998) has identified three different types of disease "storytelling": the restitution story, the chaos story and the quest story. These are characterized as follows:

- **Restitution story:** The restitution story is the popular disease storytelling in Western cultures, especially in North America, Australia and Great Britain. It is characterized by its optimistic approach that emphasizes the individual's ability to control the disease. The pathology is an enemy to be fought and the biomedicine is the weapon of defense against the enemy.
- **Chaos story:** The Chaos story represents a completely opposite storytelling that emphasizes the physical individual decline, the lack of effectiveness of the treatments and all the consequent economic and social problems that involve patients and their family.
- **Quest story:** The quest story refers to illness as a condition of 'research', a state in which something could be learned. This is a more optimistic view focused on how the disease and the changes that it necessarily entails in individuals' lives. There is an opportunity to reflect on one's own existence and also make choices that go in different directions, perhaps thanks to the rediscovery of neglected values.

In recent years, medical testing has been regarded as a providential solution to assist the birth and the evolution of a pathology. However, medical testing may increase individuals' waiting state for a test result, marked by anxiety and fear (Uhlenbusch et al., 2019). In addition, individual health living has been defined as a condition of potential ill (Lupton, 2012), leading to certain obligation to screening and testing in the medical activities. Medicalization gave rise to "patients-in-waiting" (Annandale, 2014; Timmermans, & Buschbinder, 2010) for a test result or a piece of information relative to a certain pathology that can affect their life. Alongside medicalization, current advances in biotechnology paved the way to a "techno-scientific" patients' identity and risk management based on technological screening (Sulik, 2009; Waring, 2009). As a result, some individuals may discover their pre-pathological identity even in the complete absence of symptoms (Sulik, 2009).

When coping with disease and its impact on daily basis, three groups of social actors are often involved: people affected by the disease; the doctors with whom patients interact with; and the patients' family members or caregivers (Liuccio et al., 2015). In the light of the progressive increase in chronic and chronic-degenerative diseases, the "normalization" of a pathology must be added to the cultural construction of the contemporary illness. The term "normalization" is used to refer to the patients and caregivers' attitudes and actions in daily life, regardless of the disease and inherent changes in identity and social relationships. Compliance becomes, therefore, indispensable – i.e. the patients' adherence of such behaviors as taking drugs, self-care and change lifestyles, following the physicians' orders. In case of non-compliance, patients and caregivers' attitudes are regarded as a sign of uncooperative personality trait from the medical community, being more difficult to accept it when dealing with chronic diseases (Giarelli, & Venneri, 2009). Bury (1982) identifies the following features that are associated to these diseases:

- **Indeterminacy:** Difficulty in identifying the beginning of the pathology and diagnosis, in comparison with an acute pathology;
- **Unpredictability:** The chronic disease has often a fluctuating and unpredictable trend;
- **Uncertainty:** Individuals are faced with the prospect of a cohabitation with the pathology. Whereas acute pathology is focused on survival, the focus of chronic diseases lies in living with the pathology and rethinking its own existence.

In the same vein, the changes of the "physician-patient relationship", the types of "disease storytelling", the "medicalization" and the "normalization" affect intensely in rare diseases (Liuccio, 2018).

In terms of the psycho-social support in rare diseases, patients and caregivers tend to be negatively affected by the scarcity of information and lack of access to a social and psychological support (Anderson, Elliot, & Zurynski, 2013; Pati, 2010; Pelentsov, Laws, & Esterman, 2015). Access to medical services is frequently described as a tedious and a tangled process, and for the family, the behavioral symptoms are the most difficult to manage because of their high impact on daily life (Anderson, Elliott, & Zurynski 2013; Griffith et al. 2011). Nowadays, self-care extends the traditional health systems, aided by family and other caregivers and patient associations. These latter may offer an important contribution, providing their members the most accurate and reliable information on the disease and possible treatments while providing relevant social, legal and financial services.

In view of all that has been mentioned relative to patient-physician interactions in rare diseases, one may suppose that a set of networks configure the context in which patients weave social relationships and have an effect on individual's health and access to healthcare resources. These networks can be of three types (Giarelli, & Venneri, 2009):

- **Primary/Informal networks:** These networks comprise face-to-face relationships, mainly referring to natural ties (family or friends) that also constitute health protectives systems;
- **Secondary/informal networks:** These networks rely on self-mutual-aid groups, such as voluntary or patient associations.
- **Secondary/formal networks:** These networks are represented by the institutions responsible for care and by the professionals involved in the provision of services (hospitals, health companies, doctors, nurses etc.).

Having discussed the role of communication to extract health data in rare disease and in patient-physician interactions, the next section addresses the implications of communication in the patient's journey divided into pre-diagnosis and post diagnosis.

IMPLICATIONS OF COMMUNICATION IN THE PATIENT'S JOURNEY

The patient's journey encompasses a certain level of complexity in which the patient responds to a disease over time (Nanton, Docherty, Meystre, & Dale, 2009; Trebble, et al., 2010), being influenced by the availability of information. These responses to the disease can be not only physical, but also cognitive, emotional and social. Two major steps can be found in a patient journey. These are: a) the pre-diagnosis stage; and b) the post-diagnosis stage. It is, therefore, necessary to know in depth the experience of the patients before and during the illness: the life before the illness, the onset of symptoms, the progression of the disease, the repercussions on the family and on the job. Each stage is accompanied by specific health, pharmacological and psychological services.

From the author's perspective (Liuccio, 2018), patients with rare diseases have a two-step journey: 1. A journey before diagnosis; and 2. Post-diagnosis journey.

1. **A journey before diagnosis:** In the first journey, the family has the main role. Patients, once labeled as "rare patients", they may be ready to leave the family nest and move around in search of relationships that can help to take on and solve their health problems. The family plays a fundamental role because it is the communicative mediator with the outside world, and is the only source, emotional and cognitive, to face the physical and psychological difficulties.
2. **Post-diagnosis journey:** In the second journey, or post-diagnosis, the physician, social networks, and reference communities become the protagonists. It is known that family members of patients play a significant role in patients' socialization and practical and emotional support. They are often mediators between the patient and physicians and health professionals, transmitting and validating information and sources. The focus on patients with rare diseases confirms this aspect, especially for the complex supporting role that the family must have in the long and difficult phase of identification of a diagnosis.

As shown in these journeys, the communicative actors involved are family-doctors-network (off-line and online) and they have different roles in the two steps.

Family is at the center of the informal health care ecosystem that includes self-care and family care (Giarelli & Venneri, 2009). Indeed, domestic care management (home care) is basically entrusted to the family that provides care work through three components (Bulmer, 1987): 1. Materially caring, or helping the patient in their daily activities; 2. Psychological and emotional support through advice and comfort; and 3. Financial support, aimed at the patients' physical and mental well-being. Family care is often based on the work of a caregiver who, in most cases, is played by a woman. This is obviously an unpaid informal work, which is, precisely for these reasons, often called "work of love" (Graham, 1991).

To support the family, there is a community of care that consists in informal and formal secondary networks. The informal ones are made up of services, organizations, associations and groups of the third sector, based on a non-profit logic; those of a formal nature refer to public sector or private sector services, based, however, on the logic of profit.

The activation of formal networks is usually mediated by a health professional (the family doctor, a nurse, etc.), who acts as a gatekeeper for access to the system of available care and services (Kilbride & Joffe, 2018).

The informal secondary networks mainly include three types: service volunteering; advocacy organizations; and self-help groups. When compared to formal networks, informal networks can intervene in three different ways: substitute because their action is a substitute for the inaction of formal networks; complementarity because they support additional services compared to those of the formal network services; and competition because they provide alternative services in competition with the formal sector.

When facing with long-term care needs, most appropriate responses necessarily lie in primary care in collaboration with family care and the informal sector of community care. Family also plays a fundamental role in helping to deal with the pathology and mediate the relationship in the patient-physician- care structure.

The doctor-patient relationship still is, with reference to rare diseases, critical for several reasons: (a) the physician often knows little about the rare pathology; (b) the physician underestimates the patient's symptoms; and (c) the physician hardly takes care of the patient continuously over time. All of this obviously affects the trust agreement and creates communication difficulties and a low compliance. Physicians do not always have enough specific knowledge and experience, and therefore patients are faced with deep uncertainties. Besides that, most treatments are considered experimental, so they often generate concern for their safety and effectiveness. In general, information transmitted by different health professionals can be inconsistent or controversial and the patient is confronted with conflicting opinions and conflicting treatment options.

This picture is even more critical if we consider that, in a modern society, part of the intimacy of the personal relationship between doctor and patient had been lost, which was instead constant and customary in pre-modern societies. In the Information and Communication society, the physician-patient relationship has evolved from the consensual model to the evolutionary model, passing through the conflict model. In the evolutionary model, mediation has become relational (Liuccio et al., 2015), since the analysis of the body as an object text left the place to the study of the cognitive, affective and value framework of the person.

Such elements as empathy (Ardigò, 1997), attention to the "determinants" of health and the "interpersonal care" have become more important, although these aspects do not always find concrete and adequate value. In specific, patients often find it difficult to communicate their daily disease-difficulties to social relations, internal and external to the family or labor context. From the physicians' perspective, these elements enable to understand the impact of the patient's disease syndrome and facilitate their rehabilitation.

On the contemporary physician-patient relationship impacts also the medical dominance crisis. The medical dominance crisis, more generally, must also be read through the "de-professionalization", i.e. the decline of the monopoly of medical knowledge due above all to the entry of the media, new media and of the technology applied to diagnostics. In particular, it should be emphasized that the patient is not only a potential good patient, who is "passive" and welcoming with respect to the recognition of the physician's domain (i.e. experience, knowledge), but he/she is also a consumerist patient, that uses the material and immaterial health products on the market according to its economic-social and cultural capital.

The "control" exercised by the patient-consumer necessarily forces physicians to be more cautious in making decisions, undermining the authority. The democratization enabled by the Internet made it possible for patients and caregivers to have access to the disease information that was once exclusive of the health professionals. In some cases, physicians are regarded as mere executors of prescriptions that the patient has already decided, and this position of resistance, non-cooperation and lack of trust is also a result of the absence of attention to interpersonal communication in medical class training.

The idea that there is a diagnosis for each pathological condition and that for each diagnosis there is a set of specific treatment strategies continues to prevail in medical teaching. An example of this view is in the student's assessments, in which they are assessed on the basis of the speed with which they are able to process the diagnosis and follow a therapeutic protocol. The problem lies in the universalistic relationships (based on general norms, which do not recognize the specificities of the individual interlocutors) that are favored, in which performance, specificity (i.e. being specialist in a field) and affective neutrality (i.e. no emotional involvement with the patient and his condition). Although the condition of objective physical, psychological and relational weakness, in which the patient finds himself/herself, the patient affective journey from emotional shock to anxiety for his/her own future has been overlooked within the medical community. A condition that inevitably makes it difficult to act with rationality and rely on certain beliefs and practices, trough fake news or what Freidson (1960) called "profane reference system" (the known person who suffered the same symptoms, the trusted pharmacist, an acquaintance who was once a nurse, etc.).

In the patient's journey, even in that of rare disease patient, four main elements can profoundly affect the relationship between the physician and patient (Rubinelli, Camerini, Schulz, 2010): the "anonymous" process, the "new diagnostics" and the "juridical and economization" process. Each element is detailed below:

- **"Anonymous" process:** A Physician who is a mere specialist in the area and its interaction with the patient and caregivers are from solely a technical intervention, with no social contact;
- **The "new diagnostics":** Changes in the "diagnostic procedures" applied by the doctor also affected the doctor-patient relationship. They interact on the basis of different perspectives: the doctor tries to analyze the condition of the patient in order to follow a "standardized" diagnostic process and the patient wishes to receive information as much "personalized" as possible. This distance increases the difficulty of communication and understanding between the two agents in the communication process.
- **The "juridical and economization" process:** On the legal level, the "informed consent", which is a mandatory, provides for the patient's written acceptance of any examination, test or intervention. The physicians and other health professionals must now compulsorily sign an insurance to cover the costs of any legal action. It is evident that this juridical process can affect the choices of the physicians, who can opt for a type of treatment that exposes them less to the risk of legal actions even knowing that it may not be the most adequate and effective, and undermine the fiduciary agreement between the physician and the patient, making communication between the two less spontaneous.

Different forms of relationship between physicians and patients can also affect the patient's journey before and after disease diagnosis, mainly with rare disease diagnosis. These are (Matteucci, 2015; Roter & Hall, 2006; Rubinelli, Camerini, Schulz, 2010):

- **Paternalism:** The "paternalistic" form provides an asymmetrical structure of the relationship based on a relationship of trust and on the responsibility that the healthcare professional assumes towards the patient. The mediation put in place by the doctor provides an authoritarian modality, with little involvement of the patient. The risk in this case is that the professional is not able to give the right weight to the information that the patient tells him/her about the disorder and, therefore, misunderstands the patient's health conditions, in some cases even make a wrong diagnosis. This type of authoritarian mediation can compromise adherence and compliance by the patient, when he/she does not recognize the expert sufficient authority to support validity of some choices (Taylor, 2009).
- **Consumerism:** Mediation based on consumerism starts from the assumption of the patient's reached autonomy and responsibility, relative to that stage which is most commonly entitled the "patient empowerment." In this case, the relationship between patient and healthcare professional is transformed into the relationship between consumer and seller. This model of mediation usually attracts patients of medium-high culture, who have an active role in determining health costs, who seek information also by consulting technical texts and developing independent thoughts about their health conditions and their pathology.
- **Reciprocity:** The third form of relationship, that based on reciprocity, relationship-centered care, can be defined as an ideal relationship. Both the patient and the professional are oriented towards a critical discussion of the problems and neither plays an absolute role. To encourage this type of relationship, the professional should implement some forms of mediation (Brody, 1995): 1) create an atmosphere of openness, in which the patient perceives that the professional is willing to listen to him/her; 2) tune in to the patient's expectations; 3) educate the patient on the nature of his/her problem, explaining the "expert" point of view in detail; and 4) understand the patient's preferences and look for ways to negotiate.
- **Carelessness:** The model of "carelessness" refers to an interaction in which roles and goals are not clear. There is no will to reconcile dialogue between the two actors involved, doctors and patients, (Rubinelli, Camerini, Schulz, 2010).

In a nutshell, these different elements and interactions that occur among the different health stakeholders are essential to close or enlarge the gap established between "to cure" and "to care". Whereas "to cure" means that the healthcare professional assumes the commitment and responsibility only for the patient's physical health, "to care" embodies the patient's psycho-social well-being. In fact, the expression "to care" expresses the commitment and the personal involvement of the health worker with the person suffering. An involvement that is also expressed through compassion, care, encouragement and emotional support. At the base of this difference, there is certainly an evolution of the relational, informational and managerial aspect of the professional towards the patient.

CONCLUSION

This chapter discussed the role of information and communication to extract health data in rare diseases and reinforce physician-patient interactions. It argued that information and communication are crucial to meet patients' needs, drivers and decision-making that tend to occur during the patient's journey. In the author's perspective, patients with rare diseases have a two-step journey: 1. A journey before diagnosis; and 2. Post-diagnosis journey. Whereas in the first journey, the family has the main role being a communicative mediator with the outside world, in post-diagnosis, the physician, social networks, and reference communities become the protagonists.

In addition, patient-physician interactions in rare diseases were addressed and its implications in the patient's journey. Indeed, a relationship between health professionals, patients and family members are likely to be key to overcome the lack of access to health services, the discontinuity of care, or the "empty" care, sometimes perceived as abandonment, which is likely to occur especially when more interlocutors or more assistance modalities are necessary for the treatment.

Taken together, communication in rare disease emerges as a passport for the patient journey. Communication imposes itself transversally through the patient journey, in the phases of pre-diagnosis and post-diagnosis. Moreover, it has become a concrete lever for intervention in various areas such as the provision and management of correct information through new and old means; "empathic" intermediation in the doctor-patient relationship, and, finally, as participation and support in the networks.

Continued efforts are still needed to make health-related communication more accessible to patients with rare diseases.

REFERENCES

Aartsma-Rus, A., Furlong, P., Vroom, E., van Ommen, G. J., Niks, E., Straathof, C., ... Karcagi, V. (2011). The risks of therapeutic misconception and individual patient (n= 1)“trials” in rare diseases such as Duchenne dystrophy. *Neuromuscular Disorders*, *21*(1), 13–15. doi:10.1016/j.nmd.2010.09.012 PMID:21051233

Abrahamyan, L., Feldman, B. M., Tomlinson, G., Faughnan, M. E., Johnson, S. R., Diamond, I. R., & Gupta, S. (2016, December). Alternative designs for clinical trials in rare diseases. In American Journal of Medical Genetics Part C: Seminars in Medical Genetics, 172(4), pp. 313-331. Doi:10.1002/ajmg.c.31533

Anderson, M., Elliott, E. J., & Zurynski, Y. A. (2013). Australian families living with rare disease: Experiences of diagnosis, health services use and needs for psychosocial support. *Orphanet Journal of Rare Diseases*, *8*(1), 22. doi:10.1186/1750-1172-8-22 PMID:23398775

Annandale, E. C. (2014). *The Sociology of Health and Medicine: A Critical Introduction*. Cambridge, UK: Polity Press.

Ardigò, A. (1997). *Società e salute*. Milano, Italy: Franco Angeli.

Armstrong, D. (2014). Actors, patients and agency: A recent history. *Sociology of Health & Illness*, *36*(2), 163–174. doi:10.1111/1467-9566.12100 PMID:24372176

Augè, M., & Herzlich, C. (a cura di). (1986). Il senso del male. Antropologia, storia e sociologia della malattia, Milano, Italy: Il Saggiatore.

Aujoulat, I., d’Hoore, W., & Deccache, A. (2007). Patient empowerment in theory and practice: Polysemy or cacophony? *Patient Education and Counseling*, *66*(1), 13–20. doi:10.1016/j.pec.2006.09.008 PMID:17084059

Aymé, S., Kole, A., & Groft, S. (2008). Empowerment of patients: Lessons from the rare diseases community. *Lancet*, *371*(9629), 2048–2051. doi:10.1016/S0140-6736(08)60875-2 PMID:18555918

Babrow, A. S., Kasch, C. R., & Ford, L. A. (1998). The many meanings of uncertainty in illness: Toward a systematic accounting. *Health Communication*, *10*(1), 1–23. doi:10.120715327027hc1001_1 PMID:16370987

Beach, M. C., Keruly, J., & Moore, R. D. (2006). Is the quality of the patient-provider relationship associated with better adherence and health outcomes for patients with HIV? *Journal of General Internal Medicine*, *21*(6), 661. doi:10.1111/j.1525-1497.2006.00399.x PMID:16808754

Bensing, J. (1991). Doctor-patient communication and the quality of care. *Social Science & Medicine, 32*(11), 1301–1310. doi:10.1016/0277-9536(91)90047-G PMID:2068614

Biehl, J. (2016). Patient-Citizen-Consumers: Judicialization of health and metamorphosis of biopolitics. *Lua Nova: Revista de Cultura e Política*, (98), 77-105. Doi:10.1590/0102-6445077-105/98

Blanch, D. C., Hall, J. A., Roter, D. L., & Frankel, R. M. (2009). Is it good to express uncertainty to a patient? Correlates and consequences for medical students in a standardized patient visit. *Patient Education and Counseling*, *76*(3), 300–306. doi:10.1016/j.pec.2009.06.002 PMID:19604663

Bopp, K. D. (2000). Information services that make patients co-producers of quality health care. In *Studies in health technology and informatics* (Vol. 76, pp. 93–106). Information Technology Strategies from the United States and the European Union; doi:10.3233/978-1-60750-920-2-93

Brashers, D. E., Goldsmith, D. J., & Hsieh, E. (2002). Information seeking and avoiding in health contexts. *Human Communication Research*, *28*(2), 258–271. doi:10.1111/j.1468-2958.2002.tb00807.x

Brashers, D. E., Hsieh, E., Neidig, J. L., & Reynolds, N. R. (2006). Managing uncertainty about illness: Health care providers as credible authorities. In R. M. Dailey, & B. A. Le Poire (Eds.), *Applied interpersonal communication matters: Family, health, and community relations* (pp. 219–240). New York: Peter Lang.

Brashers, D. E., Neidig, J. L., & Goldsmith, D. J. (2004). Social support and the management of uncertainty for people living with HIV or AIDS. *Health Communication*, *16*(3), 305–331. doi:10.1207/S15327027HC1603_3 PMID:15265753

Brody, H. (1995). Relationship-centered care: Beyond the finishing school. *The Journal of the American Board of Family Practice*, *8*, 416–418. doi:10.3122/jabfm.8.5.416 PMID:7484233

Bronstein, M. G., & Kakkis, E. D. (2016). Patients as key partners in rare disease drug development. *Nature Reviews. Drug Discovery*, *15*(11), 731. doi:10.1038/nrd.2016.133 PMID:27444223

Budych, K., Helms, T. M., & Schultz, C. (2012). How do patients with rare diseases experience the medical encounter? Exploring role behavior and its impact on patient–physician interaction. *Health Policy (Amsterdam)*, *105*(2-3), 154–164. doi:10.1016/j.healthpol.2012.02.018 PMID:22464590

Bulmer, M. (1987). *The Social Basis of Community Care*. London, UK: Routledge.

Bury, M. (1982). Chronic illness as biographical disruption. *Sociology of Health & Illness*, *4*(2), 167–182. doi:10.1111/1467-9566.ep11339939 PMID:10260456

Centers for Disease Control and Prevention. (2019). *Health Communication. Gateway to Health Communication & Social Marketing Practice*, Centers for Disease Control and Prevention; 2019. Available at http://www.cdc.gov/healthcommunication/healthbasics/whatishc.html (Accessed August 7th 2019).

Clayton, M. F., Dudley, W. N., & Musters, A. (2008). Communication with breast cancer survivors. *Health Communication*, *23*(3), 207–221. doi:10.1080/10410230701808376 PMID:18569050

Cline, R. J., & Haynes, K. M. (2001). Consumer health information seeking on the Internet: The state of the art. *Health Education Research*, *16*(6), 671–692. doi:10.1093/her/16.6.671 PMID:11780707

Coulson, N. S., Buchanan, H., & Aubeeluck, A. (2007). Social support in cyberspace: A content analysis of communication within a Huntington's disease online support group. *Patient Education and Counseling*, *68*(2), 173–178. doi:10.1016/j.pec.2007.06.002 PMID:17629440

Donovan-Kicken, E., & Bute, J. J. (2008). Uncertainty of social network members in the case of communication-debilitating illness or injury. *Qualitative Health Research*, *18*(1), 5–18. doi:10.1177/1049732307309005 PMID:18174531

Doyle, M. (2015). Peer support and mentorship in a US rare disease community: Findings from the cystinosis in emerging adulthood study. *The Patient-Patient-Centered Outcomes Research*, *8*(1), 65–73. doi:10.100740271-014-0085-9 PMID:25231828

Dwyer, A. A., Quinton, R., Morin, D., & Pitteloud, N. (2014). Identifying the unmet health needs of patients with congenital hypogonadotropic hypogonadism using a web-based needs assessment: Implications for online interventions and peer-to-peer support. *Orphanet Journal of Rare Diseases*, *9*(1), 83. doi:10.1186/1750-1172-9-83 PMID:24915927

Eggly, S., Penner, L. A., Greene, M., Harper, F. W. K., Ruckdeschel, J. C., & Albrecht, T. L. (2006). Information seeking during "bad news" oncology interactions: Question asking by patients and their companions. *Social Science & Medicine*, *63*(11), 2974–2985. doi:10.1016/j.socscimed.2006.07.012 PMID:16962218

Eysenbach, G. (2001). What is e-health? *Journal of Medical Internet Research, 3*(2), e20. doi:10.2196/jmir.3.2.e20 PMID:11720962

Fiordelli, M., Diviani, N., & Schulz, P. J. (2013). Mapping mHealth research: A decade of evolution. *Journal of Medical Internet Research, 15*(5), e95. doi:10.2196/jmir.2430 PMID:23697600

Fotaki, M. (2011). Towards developing new partnerships in public services: Users as consumers, citizens and/or co-producers in health and social care in England and Sweden. *Public Administration, 89*(3), 933–955. doi:10.1111/j.1467-9299.2010.01879.x PMID:22165151

Frank, A. (1998). *The Wounded Storyteller: Body, Illness, and Ethics*. Chicago, IL: University of Chicago Press.

Freidson, E. (1960). Client Control and Medical Practice. *American Journal of Sociology, 65*, 374–382. doi:10.1086/222726

Giarelli, G., & Venneri, E. (2009). *Sociologia della salute e della medicina*. Milano, Italy: Franco Angeli.

Glenn, A. D. (2015). Using online health communication to manage chronic sorrow: Mothers of children with rare diseases speak. *Journal of Pediatric Nursing, 30*(1), 17–24. doi:10.1016/j.pedn.2014.09.013 PMID:25316198

Gordon, G. H., Joos, S. K., & Byrne, J. (2000). Physician expressions of uncertainty during patient encounters. *Patient Education and Counseling, 40*(1), 59–65. doi:10.1016/S0738-3991(99)00069-5 PMID:10705065

Graham, H. (1991). The concept of caring in feminist research: The case of domestic service. *Sociology, 25*(1), 61–78. doi:10.1177/0038038591025001004

Greenfield, S., Kaplan, S., & Ware, J. E. (1985). Expanding patient involvement in care. Effects on patient outcomes. *Annals of Internal Medicine, 102*(4), 520–528. doi:10.7326/0003-4819-102-4-520 PMID:3977198

Griffith, G. M., Hastings, R. P., Nash, S., Petalas, M., Oliver, C., Howlin, P., ... Tunnicliffe, P. (2011). "You have to sit and explain it all, and explain yourself." Mothers' experiences of support services for their offspring with a rare genetic intellectual disability syndrome. *Journal of Genetic Counseling, 20*(2), 165–177. doi:10.100710897-010-9339-4 PMID:21203808

Hesse, B. W., Nelson, D. E., Kreps, G. L., Croyle, R. T., Arora, N. K., Rimer, B. K., & Viswanath, K. (2005). Trust and Sources of Health Information: The Impact of the Internet and Its Implications for Health Care Providers – Findings from the First Health Information National Trends Survey. *JAMA Internal Medicine*, *165*(22), 2618–2624. doi:10.1001/archinte.165.22.2618 PMID:16344419

Hesselgrave, B. L. (2003). Helping to manage the high cost of rare diseases. *Managed Care Quarterly*, *11*(1), 1–6. PMID:12790059

Hilton-Kamm, D., Sklansky, M., & Chang, R. K. (2014). How not to tell parents about their child's new diagnosis of congenital heart disease: An internet survey of 841 parents. *Pediatric Cardiology*, *35*(2), 239–252. doi:10.100700246-013-0765-6 PMID:23925415

Holmström, I., & Röing, M. (2010). The relation between patient-centeredness and patient empowerment: A discussion on concepts. *Patient Education and Counseling*, *79*(2), 167–172. doi:10.1016/j.pec.2009.08.008 PMID:19748203

Hou, J., & Shim, M. (2010). The role of provider–patient communication and trust in online sources in Internet use for health-related activities. *Journal of Health Communication, 15*(sup3), 186-199. Doi:10.1080/10810730.2010.522691

Huyard, C. (2009). What, if anything, is specific about having a rare disorder? Patients' judgements on being ill and being rare. *Health Expectations*, *12*(4), 361–370. doi:10.1111/j.1369-7625.2009.00552.x PMID:19840131

Impicciatore, P., Pandolfini, C., Casella, N., & Bonati, M. (1997). Reliability of health information for the public on the World Wide Web: Systematic survey of advice on managing fever in children at home. *BMJ (Clinical Research Ed.)*, *314*(7098), 1875. doi:10.1136/bmj.314.7098.1875 PMID:9224132

Johnson, D., Deterding, S., Kuhn, K. A., Staneva, A., Stoyanov, S., & Hides, L. (2016). Gamification for health and wellbeing: A systematic review of the literature. *Internet interventions, 6,* 89-106. Doi:10.1016/j.invent.2016.10.002

Kahn, J. G., Yang, J. S., & Kahn, J. S. (2010). 'Mobile' health needs and opportunities in developing countries. *Health Affairs*, *29*(2), 252–258. doi:10.1377/hlthaff.2009.0965 PMID:20348069

Kaplan, B. H., Cassel, J. C., & Gore, S. (1977). Social support and health. *Medical Care*, *15*(5), 47–58. PMID:853781

Kilbride, M. K., & Joffe, S. (2018). The new age of patient autonomy: Implications for the patient-physician relationship. *Journal of the American Medical Association*, *320*(19), 1973–1974. doi:10.1001/jama.2018.14382 PMID:30326026

Kostkova, P. (2015). Grand challenges in digital health. *Frontiers in Public Health*, *3*, 134. doi:10.3389/fpubh.2015.00134 PMID:26000272

Kowalski, C., Kahana, E., Kuhr, K., Ansmann, L., & Pfaff, H. (2014). Changes over time in the utilization of disease-related Internet information in newly diagnosed breast cancer patients 2007 to 2013. *Journal of Medical Internet Research*, *16*(8), e195. doi:10.2196/jmir.3289 PMID:25158744

Lambert, H., & McKevitt, C. (2002). Anthropology in health research: From qualitative methods to multidisciplinarity. *BMJ (Clinical Research Ed.)*, *325*(7357), 210–213. doi:10.1136/bmj.325.7357.210 PMID:12142313

Lambert, S. D., & Loiselle, C. G. (2007). Health information—seeking behavior. *Qualitative Health Research*, *17*(8), 1006–1019. doi:10.1177/1049732307305199 PMID:17928475

Lasker, J. N., Sogolow, E. D., & Sharim, R. R. (2005). The role of an online community for people with a rare disease: Content analysis of messages posted on a primary biliary cirrhosis mailing list. *Journal of Medical Internet Research*, *7*(1), e10. doi:10.2196/jmir.7.1.e10 PMID:15829472

Lasswell, H. D., Lerner, D., & Pool, I. D. S. (1952). *Comparative study of symbols: An introduction*. Palo Alto, CA: Stanford University Press.

Lewis, N., Gray, S. W., Freres, D. R., & Hornik, R. C. (2009). Examining Cross-Source Engagement With Cancer-Related Information and Its Impact on Doctor–Patient Relations. *Health Communication*, *24*(8), 723–734. doi:10.1080/10410230903264030 PMID:20183381

Liuccio, M. (2018). Le malattie rare: informazione e comunicazione nel patient journey, *Sociologia della comunicazione*, 58, 30-47. Doi:10.3280/SC2018-055003

Liuccio, M., Belotti, R., Comune, A., Zambito, V., & Schulz, J. (2015). Communication in Rare Diseases: A Literature Review. *Journal of Communications Research*, *7*(3), 1–9.

Liuccio, M., & Giorgino, F. (2019). *La sanità medi@ta, Salute, società e comunicazione nell'era delle fake news*. Milan, Italy: Mondadori Università.

Lupton, D. (2012). *Medicine as Culture: Illness, Disease and the Body*. London, UK: Sage.

Lupton, D., & Jutel, A. (2015). 'It's like having a physician in your pocket!' A critical analysis of self-diagnosis smartphone apps. *Social Science & Medicine*, *133*, 128–135. doi:10.1016/j.socscimed.2015.04.004 PMID:25864149

Maibach, E., & Holtgrave, D. R. (1995). Advances in public health communication. *Annual Review of Public Health*, *16*(1), 219–238. doi:10.1146/annurev.pu.16.050195.001251 PMID:7639871

Martin, S. C., Stone, A. M., Scott, A. M., & Brashers, D. E. (2010). Medical, personal, and social forms of uncertainty across the transplantation trajectory. *Qualitative Health Research*, *20*(2), 182–196. doi:10.1177/1049732309356284 PMID:19955227

Matteucci, I. (2015). Social determinants of health inequalities: Moving toward a socio-constructivist model supported by information and communication technologies. *Global Bioethics*, *26*(3-4), 206–217. doi:10.1080/11287462.2015.1101213

Mavris, M., & Le Cam, Y. (2012). Involvement of patient organisations in research and development of orphan drugs for rare diseases in Europe. *Molecular Syndromology*, *3*(5), 237–243. doi:10.1159/000342758 PMID:23293582

McKinstry, B. (1992). Paternalism and the doctor-patient relationship in general practice. *The British Journal of General Practice*, *42*(361), 340–342. PMID:1457157

Mishel, M. H. (1988). Uncertainty in illness. *Image--the Journal of Nursing Scholarship*, *20*(4), 225–232. doi:10.1188/17.ONF.645-649 PMID:3203947

Morgan, T., Schmidt, J., Haakonsen, C., Lewis, J., Della Rocca, M., Morrison, S., ... Kaphingst, K. A. (2014). Using the internet to seek information about genetic and rare diseases: A case study comparing data from 2006 and 2011. *JMIR Research Protocols*, *3*(1), e10. doi:10.2196/resprot.2916 PMID:24565858

Nakash, O., Dargouth, S., Oddo, V., Gao, S., & Alegría, M. (2009). Patient initiation of information: Exploring its role during the mental health intake visit. *Patient Education and Counseling*, *75*(2), 220–226. doi:10.1016/j.pec.2008.10.010 PMID:19062233

Nanton, V., Docherty, A., Meystre, C., & Dale, J. (2009). Finding a pathway: Information and uncertainty along the prostate cancer patient journey. *British Journal of Health Psychology*, *14*(3), 437–458. doi:10.1348/135910708X342890 PMID:18718111

Nicholson, W. K., Grason, H. A., & Powe, N. R. (2003). The relationship of race to women's use of health information resources. *American Journal of Obstetrics and Gynecology*, *188*(2), 580–585. doi:10.1067/mob.2003.15 PMID:12592275

O'Malley, A. S., Kerner, J. F., & Johnson, L. (1999). Are we getting the message out to all?: Health information sources and ethnicity. *American Journal of Preventive Medicine, 17*(3), 198–202. doi:10.1016/S0749-3797(99)00067-7 PMID:10987635

Ong, L. M., Visser, M. R., Lammes, F. B., & De Haes, J. C. (2000). Doctor–patient communication and cancer patients' quality of life and satisfaction. *Patient Education and Counseling, 41*(2), 145–156. doi:10.1016/S0738-3991(99)00108-1 PMID:12024540

Parrott, R. (2009). *Talking about health. Why communication matters*. Chichester, UK: Wiley-Blackwell.

Parsons, T. (1996). *Sistema sociale*. Ed. Comunitá.

Pasculli, G., Resta, F., Guastamacchia, E., Suppressa, P., & Sabbà, C. (2004). Health-related quality of life in a rare disease: Hereditary hemorrhagic telangiectasia (HHT) or Rendu–Osler–Weber Disease. *Quality of Life Research: An International Journal of Quality of Life Aspects of Treatment, Care, and Rehabilitation, 13*(10), 1715–1723. doi:10.100711136-004-7865-y PMID:15651542

Pati, A. (2010). *Scarce support changes lives*. Nursing Standard (through 2013), 24(48), 18.

Patsos, M. (2001). The Internet and medicine: Building a community for patients with rare diseases. *Journal of the American Medical Association, 285*(6), 805–805. doi:10.1001/jama.285.6.805-JMS0214-2-1 PMID:11176922

Pecchioni, L. L., Thompson, T. L., & Anderson, D. J. (2006). Interrelations between family and health communication. In L. H. Turner, & R. West (Eds.), *The family communication sourcebook* (pp. 447–468). Thousand Oaks, CA: Sage.

Pelentsov, L. J., Laws, T. A., & Esterman, A. J. (2015). The supportive care needs of parents caring for a child with a rare disease: A scoping review. *Disability and Health Journal, 8*(4), 475–491. doi:10.1016/j.dhjo.2015.03.009 PMID:25959710

Pieterse, A. H., Van Dulmen, A. M., Beemer, F. A., Bensing, J. M., & Ausems, M. G. (2007). Cancer genetic counseling: Communication and counselees' post-visit satisfaction, cognitions, anxiety, and needs fulfillment. *Journal of Genetic Counseling, 16*(1), 85–96. doi:10.100710897-006-9048-1 PMID:17295054

Rekatsinas, T., Ghosh, S., Mekaru, S. R., Nsoesie, E. O., Brownstein, J. S., Getoor, L., & Ramakrishnan, N. (2015, June). SourceSeer: Forecasting rare disease outbreaks using multiple data sources. In *Proceedings of the 2015 SIAM International Conference on Data Mining* (pp. 379-387). Society for Industrial and Applied Mathematics. DOI:10.1137/1.9781611974010.43

Rifkin, S. B. (2006). Patient Empowerment: Increased Compliance or Total Transformation? In F. Porzsolt, & R. M. Kaplan (Eds.), *Optimizing health: Improving the value of healthcare delivery* (pp. 66–73). Boston, MA: Springer.

Riva, G. (2002). Virtual reality for health care: The status of research. *Cyberpsychology & Behavior*, *5*(3), 219–225. doi:10.1089/109493102760147213 PMID:12123244

Robinson, J. D., & Stivers, T. (2001). Achieving activity transitions in primary-care consultations: From history taking to physical examination. *Human Communication Research*, *27*, 253–298. doi:10.1111/j.1468-2958.2001.tb00782.x

Roter, D. L., & Hall, J. A. (2006). *Doctor talking with patients/Patients talking with doctors*, Praeger Publishers, Westport.

Rubinelli, S., Camerini, L., & Schulz, P. (2010). *Comunicazione e salute*. Milano, Italy: Apogeo.

Ruesch, J. (2006). Values, Communication, and Culture: An Introduction. In J. Ruesch, & G. Bateson (Eds.), *Communication – The Social Matrix of Psychiatry* (pp. 3–20). New York, NY: W. W. Worton & Company.

Schiavo, R. (2007). *Health communication: From theory to practice* (2nd ed.). San Francisco, CA: John Wiley & Sons.

Schieppati, A., Henter, J. I., Daina, E., & Aperia, A. (2008). Why rare diseases are an important medical and social issue. *Lancet*, *371*(9629), 2039–2041. doi:10.1016/S0140-6736(08)60872-7 PMID:18555915

Schumacher, K. R., Stringer, K. A., Donohue, J. E., Yu, S., Shaver, A., Caruthers, R. L., ... Russell, M. W. (2014). Social media methods for studying rare diseases. *Pediatrics*, *133*(5), e1345–e1353. doi:10.1542/peds.2013-2966 PMID:24733869

Shannon, C. E., & Weaver, W. (1998). *The mathematical theory of communication*. Urbana, IL: University of Illinois Press.

Solanas, A., Patsakis, C., Conti, M., Vlachos, I. S., Ramos, V., Falcone, F., ... Martinez-Balleste, A. (2014). Smart health: A context-aware health paradigm within smart cities. *IEEE Communications Magazine*, *52*(8), 74–81. doi:10.1109/MCOM.2014.6871673

Sulik, G. A. (2009). Managing biomedical uncertainty: The technoscientific illness identity. *Sociology of Health & Illness*, *31*(7), 1059–1076. doi:10.1111/j.1467-9566.2009.01183.x PMID:19619153

Swan, M. (2009). Emerging patient-driven health care models: An examination of health social networks, consumer personalized medicine and quantified self-tracking. *International Journal of Environmental Research and Public Health*, *6*(2), 492–525. doi:10.3390/ijerph6020492 PMID:19440396

Taylor, K. (2009). Paternalism, participations and partnership-the evolution of patient centeredness in the consultation. In V. Kalitzkus, & P. L. Twohig (Eds.), *Bordering biomedicine*. Amsterdam, The Netherlands: Rodopi; doi:10.1016/j.pec.2008.08.017

Timmermans, S., & Buchbinder, M. (2010). Patients-in-waiting: Living between sickness and health in the genomics era. *Journal of Health and Social Behavior*, *51*(4), 408–423. doi:10.1177/0022146510386794 PMID:21131618

Trebble, T. M., Hansi, N., Hydes, T., Smith, M. A., & Baker, M. (2010). Process mapping the patient journey: An introduction. *BMJ (Clinical Research Ed.)*, *341*. doi:10.1136/bmj.c4078 PMID:20709715

Uhlenbusch, N., Löwe, B., Härter, M., Schramm, C., Weiler-Normann, C., & Depping, M. K. (2019). Depression and anxiety in patients with different rare chronic diseases: A cross-sectional study. *PLoS One*, *14*(2). doi:10.1371/journal.pone.0211343 PMID:30785907

Walker, K. K. (2013). Rare disease-specific social media sites: An opportunity for collaboration. *Journal of Communication in Healthcare*, *6*(1), 71–76. doi:10.1179/1753807612Y.0000000026

Wallack, L., Dorfman, L., Jernigan, D., & Themba-Nixon, M. (1993). *Media advocacy and public health: Power for prevention*. Newbury Park, CA: Sage.

Waring, J. J. (2009). Constructing and re-constructing narratives of patient safety. *Social Science & Medicine*, *69*(12), 1722–1731. doi:10.1016/j.socscimed.2009.09.052 PMID:19883965

Warne, T., & McAndrew, S. (2007). Passive patient or engaged expert? Using a Ptolemaic approach to enhance mental health nurse education and practice. *International Journal of Mental Health Nursing*, *16*(4), 224–229. doi:10.1111/j.1447-0349.2007.00471.x PMID:17635621

KEY TERMS AND DEFINITIONS

HISB (Health Information Seeking Behaviors): The type and amount of information sources consulted and one's decision-making and actions performed.

Normalization: The patients and caregivers' attitudes and actions in daily life, regardless of the disease and inherent changes in identity and social relationships.

Paternalism (Physician-Patient Relationships): An asymmetrical structure of the relationship based on a relationship of trust and on the responsibility that the healthcare professional assumes towards the patient.

Patient Empowerment: The patient demand for information and both participation in active (and interactive) health management and shared responsibilities with health stakeholders.

Patient Journey: The patient responds to a disease over time, being influenced by the availability of information. These responses are physical, cognitive, emotional and social.

Reciprocity (Physician-Patient Relationships): A form of relationship based on reciprocity and relationship-centered care, which can be defined as an ideal relationship.

Chapter 3
Designing Sustainable Social Media Health Communication Campaigns for Promoting Rare Diseases

Isabell Koinig
University of Klagenfurt, Austria

Sandra Diehl
University of Klagenfurt, Austria

ABSTRACT

The third goal of the United Nations Sustainable Development Agenda aims to ensure individual's wellbeing and a long and healthy life. As such, health is perceived as an essential part of sustainable development. While progress has been made over the past decades, far too little attention has been paid to misdiagnosed and rare diseases. In the context of promoting "health for all", communication is of uttermost importance. By means of a content analysis for selected rare disease campaigns, the present contribution seeks to highlight the way the UN's health goal is communicated as part of health campaigns for rare diseases. Amongst others, this chapter sets out to understand how the goal is communicated, which aspects are stressed, and whether there are differences in message strategies across different platforms relative to rare diseases. Ultimately, the potential of social media for communicating rare diseases is carved out. Research limitations and directions for future research are also addressed.

DOI: 10.4018/978-1-7998-2088-8.ch003

INTRODUCTION

In the light of the third objective of the United Nations Sustainable Development Goals (SDGs), individual's life-long health, well-being and quality of life has been regarded as one of the most relevant indicators of the sustainable development of society (UN, 2019). In detail, Goal 3 sets out to end the epidemic of infectious and noncommunicable diseases as well as reduce malnutrition rates amongst others by 2030 (UN, 2019). While improvements have been made over the past decades in the health sector, especially in the area of infant and maternal mortality, HIV/AIDS and malaria, other diseases – amongst them "rare" or "orphan" diseases – continue to be life-threatening (Denis, Margaret, Fostier, Cleemput, & Simoens, 2010). Rare diseases are defined as diseases that only affect a small number of the total population (Orpha.net, 2012; WHO, 2018, World Economic Forum, 2017). Due to the fact that they do not affect a large number of people, they often remain under the public's awareness threshold and are not part of people's agenda, as they are mainly unknown to the large public.

Achieving the goal of "health for all" in a mediatized world poses new challenges and opportunities for all stakeholders involved, including governments, communities and patients (Schiavo, 2007). Indeed, communication plays an important and sometimes decisive role in raising awareness, promoting individual acceptance and creating legitimization to achieve "health for all." In this context, health communication campaigns are of uttermost importance, because they are concerned with "influencing, engaging and supporting individuals, communities, health professionals [...] to champion, introduce, adopt, or sustain a behavior, practice or policy that will ultimately improve health outcomes" (Schiavo, 2007, p.xxi). Moreover, health campaigns are concerned with providing guidance as to how to address and improve social problems (Rossmann & Ziegler, 2013).

By means of a content analysis of selected campaigns addressing selected rare diseases (exemplified through Ataxia, and Epidermolysis Bullosa EB) as well as campaigns for Rare Disease Day, this chapter aims to understand how the UN's Sustainable Development Goal 3 is communicated in a "sustainable" way, as part of national and international health campaigns. For the purpose of this paper, we define sustainable health campaigns as promotional material that provides individuals with the right information, at the right time, in a comprehensible, appealing, and engaging manner, in order to bring about lasting (behavioral) change.

Sustainable health campaigns are concerned with educating the public about and creating permanent awareness for diseases, further calling upon individuals to become involved in their health or assist others in seeking help. At the same time, stigmatization of diseases and/or people affected should be reduced (Schiavo, 2007).

This chapter addresses the following research questions:

- **RQ1:** Which channels are used to promote rare diseases?
- **RQ2:** Which message appeals or design elements are used to attract attention? Is the reasoning rather rational or emotional?
- **RQ3:** To which extent are elements of selected health theories integrated into these messages and inasmuch are they used to achieve audience engagement?
- **RQ4:** Do messages differ across platforms, as well as across rare diseases?
- **RQ5:** Inasmuch are the criteria of a "sustainable" health campaign fulfilled?

This chapter is structured as follows: The next section introduces the concept of rare diseases and the importance of health campaigns to create awareness for rare diseases. Then, ad appeals in health communication, cross-media (health) campaigns and the use of social media in health communication are discussed. Finally, different campaigns used to create awareness for rare diseases are analyzed (i.e. Rare Disease Day, Ataxia and Epidermolysis Bullosa). In conclusion, the previously proposed questions are answered for all three campaigns. Afterwards, results are compared and both limitations and directions for future research are addressed.

DEFINITION OF RARE DISEASES

Despite the importance of "health for all" as presented in the SDGs (UN, 2019), not all diseases were given equal importance. The third goal is predominantly concerned with tackling the "big players" in the health field, including epidemic diseases and child or maternal deaths (UN, 2019). Nonetheless, this does not mean that rare diseases are any less important or do have less fatal consequences – they are simply smaller in scope (Rare Disease Day, 2019a; Eurodis, 2017).

"Rare diseases" or "orphan diseases" are defined as diseases that only affect a small number of the total population – they do have low prevalence. In Europe, for instance, a rare disease only affects 1 out of 2,000 people (Orpha.net, 2012), while in the U.S. the ratio is 1:200,000. The most affected age group tends to be the children (World Economic Forum, 2017). In most instances, rare diseases are brought forth through either genetic defects, environmental influences or bacterial infections (Rare Disease Day, 2019a). Furthermore, they are not only degenerating and progressive, but can also result in death (Eurordis, 2017). To date, more than 6,000 forms of rare diseases have been identified, with each and every one of them posing a significant threat not only to individuals and communities, but also the economic and the healthcare system (World Economic Forum, 2017).

The World Health Organization (2018) advocates the importance of rare diseases, as illustrated in the statement for the Rare Disease Day: *Rare diseases present fundamentally different challenges from those of more common diseases, especially for diagnosis. The small number of patients, the logistics involved in reaching widely dispersed patients, the lack of validated biomarkers and surrogate end-points, and the lack of clinical expertise and expert centers all present significant barriers (WHO, 2018).*

While developing cures for other diseases might require one single form of treatment, each rare disease case is unique in itself; likewise, rare diseases are often accompanied by rather general symptoms, which might keep the rare disease in disguise (Eurordis, 2017). In brief, rare diseases represent an increasing threat as they are still under-researched, when compared to diseases that affect larger sections of the population and for which major breakthroughs were possible in the last years due to intensive research and funding (e.g., as demonstrated by the ALS Ice Bucket Challenge; ALS, 2019).

CREATING AWARENESS FOR RARE DISEASES

One common problem that is claimed to result in a delayed diagnosis of rare diseases is the "lack of scientific knowledge and quality information" (Rare Disease Day, 2019a). Given this problem, health communication campaigns are essential in creating awareness for (rare) diseases.

HEALTH COMMUNICATION CAMPAIGNS

Communication is a viable asset to the health domain and also encompasses communication encounters in the health-care setting (i.e. patient-provider interactions) (Dutta, 2008; Thompson, 2000). From a rather practical perspective, health communication is conceptualized as "the study and use of communication strategies to inform and influence individual and community decisions that enhance health" (Center for Disease Control and Prevention - CDC, 2001; U.S. Department of Health and Human Services, 2005). While health messages can take multiple forms (e.g. public or commercial health campaigns, health education materials) (Schiavo, 2007), these materials are concerned with "informing, influencing, and motivating individual, institutional, and public audiences about important health issues" (U.S. Department of Health and Human Services, 2000). Health communication is also used to achieve "disease prevention through behavior modification" (Freimuth et al., 2000, p.337).

Health campaigns are "an essential part of health promotion, [and] can be defined as a systematic effort to change health behaviors [...] within a target population of people who are at risk for a health problem" (Bennett & Murphy, 1997; Salmon & Atkin, 2003; Wright et al., 2008, p. 233). As such, health campaigns are goal-oriented, directed at a relatively large, well-defined audience (Rogers & Storey, 1988; Snyder, 2001) and consist of a series of coordinated activities over a given period of time, and across a variety of media channels (Wakefield et al., 2010).

Up until now, campaign research has predominantly focused on major social issues, such as HIV (Niebel & Davidson, 2012), smoking or drug abuse or cancer screening (Jones & Owen, 2006) and has also investigated campaigns success, e.g., by increasing immunization rates (Paunio et al., 1991; Porter et al., 2000), elevating knowledge on vaccines (McDivitt et al., 1997), motivating individuals to do cancer screenings (Ramirez et al., 1999), and enhancing people's disease coping abilities respectively their adherence with either nutrition or fitness regimes (PEW Internet and American Life Project, 2007). Two meta-analyses on health campaigns also support this assumption (Derzon & Lipsey, 2002; Snyder & Hamilton, 2002).

In general, health campaigns "utilize three basic communication processes to move the target audience toward the desired response: awareness, instruction, and persuasion" (Salmon & Atkin, 2003, p. 455). Awareness messages educate people about what to do and identify who should adopt a defined behavior, offering recipients cues on the time and place of engagement. Instruction messages afford recipients with instructional "how-to-do-it" information (Salmon & Atkin, 2003), while persuasion messages offer reasons as to why message recipients should take up an advocated action (Salmon & Atkin, 2003). This path is eased once useful information is provided, since "an important objective of health campaigns is getting audiences to seek information, for this indicates that they found campaign content personally relevant enough to take active steps to obtain additional information" (Parrott, 2003, p. 446). Different ad appeals can be utilized in the process and have been applied in the area of health communication.

Ad Appeals in Health Communication

Ad appeals describe the way in which advertisers or other commercial parties want to trigger attention in recipients, influencing and shaping their interests and behaviors towards a message in a favorable manner (Belch and Belch, 1993). Two main forms can be distinguished: informative appeals that are explicit and based on hard facts, and emotional appeals that rely on visual stimuli to tell appealing stories and create favorable images in consumers' minds (Okazaki et al., 2010). Especially when convincing individuals to change their behaviors, **emotional appeals** are likely to be the most effective (Andsager et al., 2006), Thereby, positive emotional appeals and negative emotional appeals need to be distinguished. Via joy, happiness, humor and entertainment amongst others (Nabi, 2002), *positive emotional appeals* try to draw in recipients and provoke behavioral change. For instance, humor has been excessively used in health campaigns, as humorous appeals are more frequently recalled than other appeals given their arousing nature (Lang, 1995). In combination with attractive models or stimulating music, these appeals have even proven to be more successful than conventional (informative) ad appeals (Batra & Ray, 1986).

Negative emotional appeals, on the other hand, include disgust, shame as well as fear (Dobrenova et al., 2019; Nabi, 2002). One common form used in health communication is fear appeals, defined as "persuasive messages designed to scare people by describing the terrible things that will happen to them if they do not do what the message recommends" (Witte, 1992, p.329). Thereby, consequences can be both physically (*e.g.,* degrading health) or socially harmful (e.g., stigmatization) (Hale and Dillard, 1995). These appeals are prominently employed as research has found them to lead consumers to change their attitudes – and ultimately behaviors (Eagly and Chaiken, 1993).

Emotional appeals are renowned to also use **metaphors** (Lazard et al., 2016; Weiss, 1997). Metaphors describe one concept through another, slightly dissimilar concept (Palmer-Wackerly & Krieger, 2015), informing schemas and mental models for how individuals perceive and deal with often complex health issues (Palmer Wackerly & Krieger, 2015). They are commonly used in patient-provider communication, but also for promotional purposes (Weiss, 1997), such as in HIV/AIDS or anti-drug campaigns (Reinarman & Levine, 1995). When paired with visuals, metaphors take the form of **visual metaphors** (Lazard et al., 2016), conceptualized as "rhetorical figures that creatively merge two visuals and can be instrumental for messages that must be appealing and efficiently convey complex information" (Messaris, 1997; cf. Lazard et al., 2016, p.1260). Respondents are asked to match up those two concepts to derive the intended meaning (Scott, 1994). Visuals are not only more appealing, but also encourage recipients to engage in more elaborate thought processes (Gkiouzepas & Hogg, 2011). Additionally, both evaluations of and attitudes towards the message are claimed to be more favorable for pleasant images (Delbaere et al., 2011). In combination with textual elements, these rhetoric figures have been found to improve attitudes towards the message as well as message comprehension (Phillips, 2000). As part of health education messages, metaphors can thus aid in grabbing consumers' attention, making promotions stick out of the crowd due to the "novel" appeal they deploy (Smith et al., 2007).

In the health context, advertising executives have been advised to only use fear-evoking devices selectively (Piller, 2001), keep their ads' textual components rather short by focusing on the most relevant information, and stress how this information can benefit recipients (Piller, 2001). Textual and visual elements should be geared to each other (Batra & Ray., 1986), while textual elements alone have to build upon and complement each other (Piller, 2001).

Since research on the use of fear appeals is contradictory, as suggested by a 2015 meta-analysis (Tannenbaum et al., 2015), advertisers have started to look for alternatives, choosing positive over negative emotions (Dobrenova et al., 2019). Inasmuch this trend has been taken up when promoting awareness for rare diseases (both textually and visually) will be illustrated later on.

Integrating Health Theory and Audience Segmentation

In order to achieve lasting and positive effects, health communication messages need to be carefully crafted. According to Yzer (2012), successful messages can either be based on established health communication theories (following a theory-based message design) or take audience specifics into account instead (in line with an audience-based message design; Cho, 2012). We would like to argue that both strategies can be utilized at once. In terms of theory-based message design, the most commonly consulted theories concern the Health Belief Model (Rosenstock, 1974), Protection Motivation Theory (Rogers, 1975, 1983), the Theory of Planned Behavior (Ajzen, 1991), the Theory of Reasoned Action (Fishbein & Ajzen, 1975), as well as the Extended Parallel Process Model (Witte, 1998). In the present paper, the focus will, however, only be put on core variables as derived from the Health Belief Model (HBM; Rosenstock, 1974). Integrating selected health-theory elements into messages is highly recommended since studies have determined that health messages that are based on theory can actually influence recipients to change their behaviors (Yzer, 2012). Researchers (e.g. Becker, 1974; Becker, 1978; Glanz et al., 2002; Rogers, 1975; Rosenstock, 1974) have come to suggest that only a small number of variables needs to be considered when predicting, changing or reinforcing a particular behavior in the target audience. Amongst them, the most prominent ones in the message design context for rare diseases are: perceived severity, self-efficacy and cues to action (Rogers, 1975; Becker, 1978; Glanz et al., 2002).

- **Perceived severity** describes an individuals' estimation of both the condition's seriousness and its consequences (Rogers, 1975; Rosenstock, 1974) and can be enhanced through the provision of detailed information on both the risks and potential side effects.
- **Self-efficacy,** the most relevant element of the HBM, highlights the necessity to appeal to individuals' abilities and skills, as this confidence can encourage individuals to undertake a recommended behavior (Becker, 1978; Rogers, 1983). Only if individuals feel that they are in the position to bring about

change, they will form intentions to adopt a specific behavior. Thus, training and guiding messages are most effective in this context (Glanz et al., 2002).

- **Cues to action** can take multiple forms, all of which are intended to engage individuals (Becker, 1974). Ideally, through providing information or continuous reminders, individuals feel inclined to take up a specific behavior.

Another important theoretical construct is **social support**. In the context of social media, the scope of social support has been broadened (Kim et al., 2015). While Barnes (1954) discovered that social relationships also take up aspects outside of an individual's immediate family and work environment – a concept he referred to as social support – it was not until Cassel (1976) that the concept was also utilized in the health realm, where social networks offered support in terms of easing individuals' vulnerability to health-related stress respectively distress, positively affecting people's well-being. According to House (1981), four forms of support can be differentiated:

- **Emotional support** is concerned with showing empathy and concern for peoples' experiences, providing them with guidance and reassurance in times of need. This form of support can involve assistance from people in one's immediate environment, but also stretches to the online world, e.g., receiving support from individuals on social media (House, 1981).
- **Instrumental support** refers to actively providing support to the people dealing with a specific health condition. For instance, people on a person's immediate (physical) environment might help out with daily routines, relieving the burden on the individual person (House, 1981).
- **Informational support** entails providing individuals with concrete ways of becoming active by filling an informational need, e.g., giving out instructions, offering advice or suggesting alternatives. While doctors might pass on relevant information on medications and treatment options, family members might provide guidance on alternative treatments (House, 1981). Moreover, informational support might be offered by the online-community, including individuals on social media who provide access to additional resources or share their personal health stories (Glanz et al., 2002).
- **Appraisal support** centers on the provision of information that serves self-evaluation purposes, including constructive feedback and affirmative messages (House, 1981). For instance, information might assist people in building up their self-esteem and skills to cope with a difficult health situation. This appraisal support can be provided either by a close friend who has had a similar experience, or a cancer survivor on social media, who wants to

encourage others to keep fighting by sharing their personal stories (Glanz et al., 2002).

In the case of audience-based message design, which aims at reducing health disparities and improve health outcomes amongst a defined target audience by gaining a deep level of understanding and developing the intention to act upon the suggestions provided in the message (Davis & Resnicow, 2012), two concepts are commonly discussed: message targeting and message tailoring. While both are based on audience segmentation (Hawkins et al., 2008), **message targeting** is defined as the use of group-level data to customize health messages for a specific audience (target) group or segment that is relatively homogenous with regard to determinants affecting a specific health outcome (Davis & Resnicow, 2012). **Message tailoring**, on the other hand, follows the same rationale as targeting but consists of a higher degree of customization, whereby each audience member (or group) receives a unique combination of health messages based on individual- or group-level data (Davis & Resnicow, 2012). Research suggests that tailoring is more effective than targeting (Noar et al., 2007), as individuals are presumed to behave in certain ways to remain consistent with both their in-group norms and social roles (Harwood & Giles, 2005). Generally, targeting's effectiveness is subject to each audience members' attentiveness to health messages, their cognitive and emotional processing of these messages and self-referential thinking (Hawkins et al., 2008).

CROSS-MEDIA (HEALTH) CAMPAIGNS

The term cross-media refers to the distribution of content via different media channels (Sjurts, 2011). With consumer preferences gradually shifting and especially moving towards the Internet, consistent customer communication utilizing different distribution channels can be effective; at the same time, content can not only be used efficiently across a variety of platforms, but also references to other media channels and formats are enabled as part of an "active-user guidance" (Schweiger, 2002). This caters to users' varying interests, allowing them to make selections that are reflective of their individual media consumption patterns. By utilizing messages via multiple-channels, new target audiences can be reached; at the same time, new content can be continuously added in innovative ways or deepened through offerings on different platforms (e.g., cross-media storytelling). As such, communication efficacy can be increased (due to synergy effects) (Hass, 2006).

In the health context, individuals have also been renowned to use a variety of sources to gather health-related information (O'Keefe et al., 1998). With the rise of Health Information Technology (HIT) (Buntin et al., 2010), health information is available in abundance, both in digital (online) and traditional (offline) form. As a consequence, the manner of how health information is consumed has changed drastically over the past years (Smith, 2013; Simou, 2015). These alterations also have to be taken into account when designing health communication campaigns for an offline and online environment.

SOCIAL MEDIA IN HEALTH COMMUNICATION

Previous research found that patients have come to rely not only on the Internet but also on Social Networking Sites (SNS) respectively Social Media Sites when it comes to researching health information (Sarasohn-Kahn, 2008; Vance et al., 2009). By 2015, almost half of all people used social media for health education purposes, following a 2015 iTriage survey. Amongst respondents, 73% reported to consult social media in search of relevant health articles, while 16% requested medical advice. An additional 12% sought social support from their peers (Aetna, 2015). This is indicative of the fact that almost half of all respondents believe that social media and digital health information sources enable them to achieve a better health outcome (Aetna, 2015).

Calls to integrate social media into health-care respectively health communication have increased over time, with Dr. Parkins announcing: "The infrastructure of health care needs a total repair from the ground up. It needs to be Facebook-ed [and] wiki-ed" (Hawn, 2009, p. 362). Amongst the plethora of social networking sites available, the present outlets have already received academic attention in the context of health communication (Hawn, 2009):

- **Facebook**: To date, this social networking site has been found to assist users in gathering information on numerous health topics, the site thus fulfilling a "counseling" function (Kofinas et al., 2014; Morris et al., 2011). Moreover, Facebook's informative page character has been investigated in the context of diabetes (Greene et al., 2011) or concussions (Ahmed et al., 2010), allowing users to share, discuss as well as reflect on their very personal health experiences (Gajaria et al., 2011). At times, even calls to fund specific health projects are spread via Facebook (De La Torre Diaz et al., 2012; Farmer et al., 2009).
- **Twitter:** While messages are limited in space, this social media platform holds the potential to rapidly provoke responses from users (Vance et al., 2019). As such, Twitter can be used as a form of social support forum (e.g., for diabetes patients) (Pagoto et al., 2014; Winston et al., 2012) as well as to rapidly spread news (Hawn, 2009). For instance, during the H1N1 health

Figure 1. Conceptual framework (own illustration)

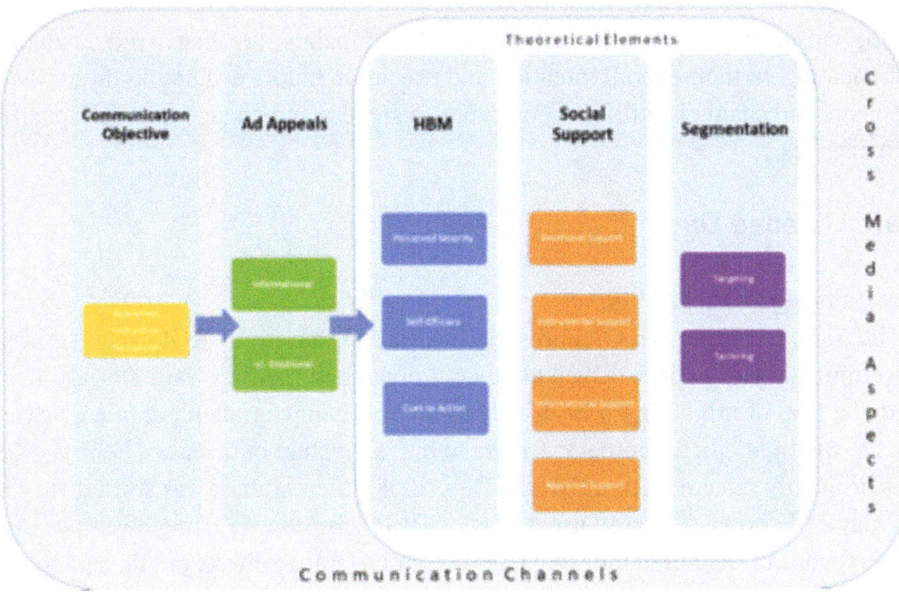

epidemic, the government relied on twitter to provide the public with relevant information (e.g., wait times for flu vaccinations) (CDC, 2009). As McNab (2009, p. 566) postulates: "After all, one fact sheet or an emergency message about an outbreak can be spread through Twitter faster than any influenza virus". This holds especially true for interesting and useful information (Zhao & Rosson, 2009). At the same time, funding campaigns using this social network have proven to be successful as in the case of the earthquake in Haiti (Sample Ward, 2011).

- **YouTube:** This video-hosting platform has mostly been used for health education purposes (Stellefson et al., 2014) as well as to spread smoking cessation or pro-vaccination messages (Ache & Wallace, 2008; Keelan et al., 2007; Freeman & Chapman, 2007). At the same time, this platform allows users to share their personal experiences with a broad crowd (Vance et al., 2009).

Figure 1 depicts the study's conceptual framework. Based on the current use of social media to divulgate health messages, this study aims to investigate which channels are utilized in raising awareness and engagement for rare diseases, as well as work out the potentials of social media for this particular group of diseases.

COMUNICATING RARE DISEASES

In the subsections that follow, three health campaigns are discussed in detail, commenting on their overall intention and execution before evaluating the stylistic elements and channels utilized to promote awareness and engagement for specific rare diseases.

Rare Disease Day

The Campaign

In 2008, the European Organization for Rare Diseases (EURORDIS) – a non-governmental and patient-driven alliance – organized the first Rare Disease Day, with the goal of initiating a world-wide awareness campaign that put rare diseases "in the spotlight". In order to pay tribute to the rare nature of diseases, February 29 was originally selected (Rare Disease Day, 2008); thereafter, it was shifted "to the last day of February" (Rare Disease Day, 2019b). Besides creating awareness for the existence of the number of rare diseases amongst the general public and policy makers, the impact of rare diseases on individual lives was highlighted to encourage donations to advance research on rare diseases (Rare Disease Day, 2019b, 2019c).

Campaign Theme and Execution

While the campaigns for Rare Disease Day have slightly changed their focus over the years (see Rare Disease Day, 2019d), engagement and participation have increased each time. Whereas in 2008 and 2009 rare diseases were meant to be pushed on the public agenda, 2010 emphasized the need to conduct more research in the field of rare diseases. After 2011 and a call to end health inequalities, solidarity was chosen as an overarching theme for both 2012 and 2013, before the need to increase health care for people living with rare medical conditions was emphasized in 2014. The living conditions of patients with rare disease were put at the center of the 2015 campaign, before directing attention towards their individual (patient) voices in 2016. In 2017 and 2018, the necessity to conduct research and potentials of research were put centerstage. A collection of themes, slogans for and participation in each Rare Disease Day can be found in Table 1.

Reviving the 2018 slogan "Show your rare. Show you care" (Rare Disease Day, 2019c; 2019e) but combining it with the theme of "Bridging health and social care", the 2019 initiative thematized the hardships individuals living with rare diseases have to take on besides their daily activities. Their daily care routine does not only involve their immediate family, but also extends to their community; for this reason, it is of uttermost importance to improve the communication and efficiency of the

Table 1. Overview of the Rare Disease Day themes and slogan

Year	Theme	Slogan	Participating Countries
2008	Rare Diseases as a Public Health Priority	A rare day for very special people.	18
2009	Rare Diseases as a Public Health Priority	Patient Care: A Public Affair!	30
2010	Bridging patients and Researchers	Patients and Researchers: Partners for Life!	45
2011	Rare Diseases and Health Inequalities.	Rare but Equal	55
2012	Solidarity	Rare but Stronger Together!	63
2013	Solidarity	Rare Disorders without Borders	72
2014	Care	Join Together for Better Care!	84
2015	Living with a rare disease	Day-by-day, hand-in-hand	85
2016	Patient voice	Join us in making the voice of rare diseases heard	85
2017	Research	With research, possibilities are limitless	94
2018	Research	Show your rare. Show you care.	90
2019	Bridging health and social care	Show your rare. Show you care.	90+

services involved in treating and caring for people living with rare diseases (Rare Disease Day, 2019c). In 2019, more than 90 nations worldwide participated in Rare Disease Day, including first-time participants Lesotho, Montenegro, Namibia, Qatar, Sri Lanka, and the Dominican Republic (Rare Disease Day, 2019e).

It was due to the use of Social Media that the number of participants continued to grow every year. Already before the actual event, the website served as an anchor site. The motto "Show your rare. Show you care" – reflected through a variety of colors and individual hand prints – guided the website design. Besides the extensive campaign material that was available for download – including web and print material such as logos, flyers, and banners – the website also directed users to the individual social media platforms. Figure 2 shows a number of posters used to promote Rare Disease Day.

Rare Disease Day is represented through two hashtags throughout the world (#ShowYourRare and #RareDiseaseDay); in the United States, a third hashtag (#ShowYourStripes) – in tribute to the zebra, the U.S. symbol of rare diseases – is used this year for the very first time (Gaucher Disease News, 2019). In terms of platforms, Facebook[1], Twitter[2] as well as YouTube[3] are employed. Rare Disease Day 2019 also comprises of a number of events that are scheduled to take place

Figure 2. Posters promoting Rare Disease Day (Rare Disease Day, 2019d)
Source: https://www.rarediseaseday.org/article/overview-of-past-rare-disease-days

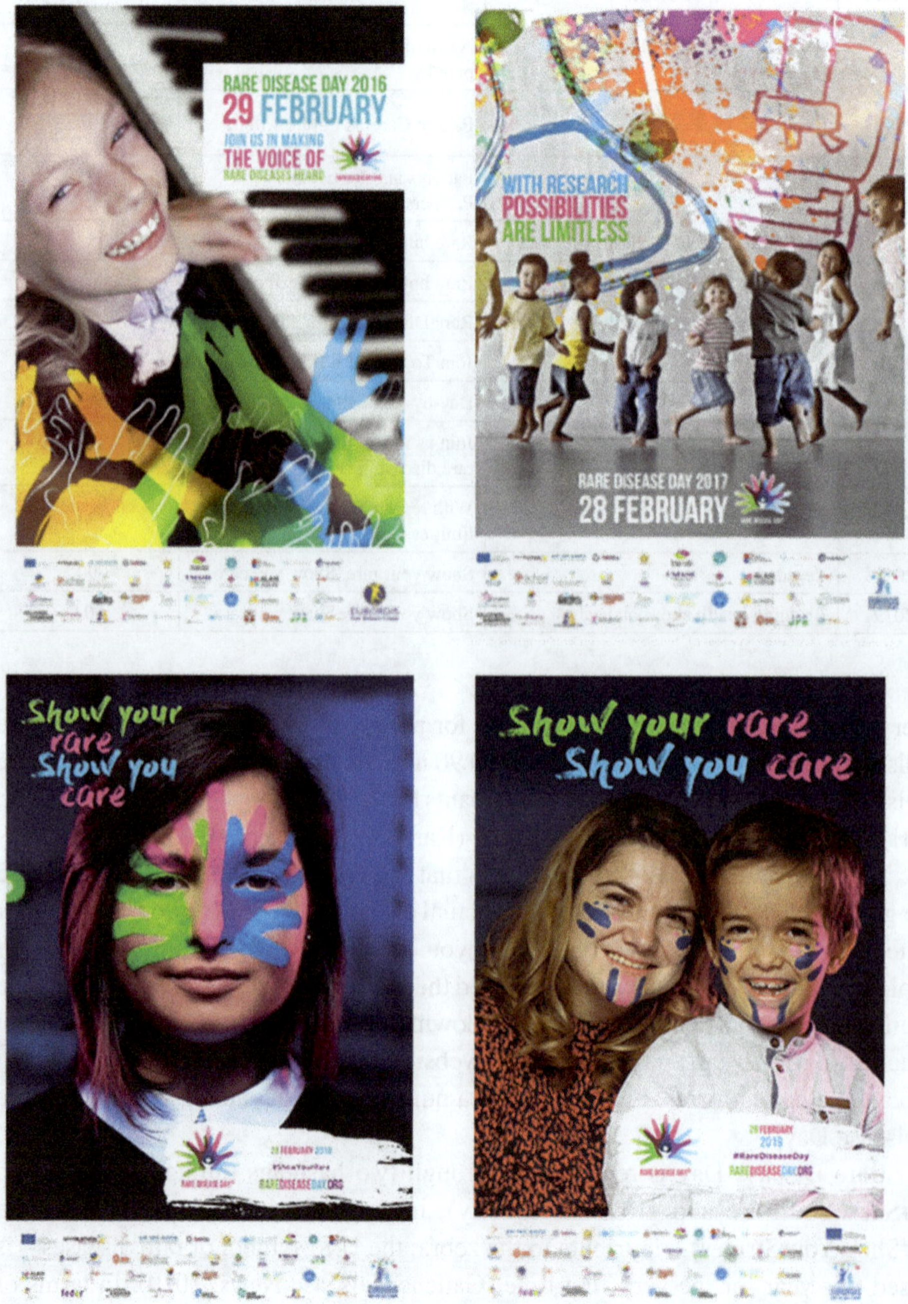

worldwide (Gaucher Disease News, 2019), where the general public as well as policy makers will unite with faces painted in bright colors to host community discussions or fundraisers (Rare Disease Day, 2019c).

In line with the campaign posters of previous years, the 2019 event used a personalized approach to rare diseases. The poster featured a young mother with her son, who is suffering from a rare disease; their faces are painted in an individual way, reflective of the fact that rare diseases present individual(ized) experiences and require individual(ized) treatments. The use of colors – as indicated in the poster of 2018 – is also reflective of the disease's uniqueness. Painting one's face in support of rare disease is also put centerstage on the campaign website, where message recipients are called upon to take an individual picture or group photo with painted faces and share it on social media throughout February together with the two campaign hashtags. Moreover, profile picture frames to be used on Facebook and Twitter are provided as well (Rare Disease Day, 2019e).

In total, four patient testimonial videos were produced as part of the 2019 campaign. The highlighted patient testimonial video on YouTube features Karlo, a young man living with neurofibromatosis type 1, and was filmed in Zagreb, Croatia, his home town. While the video shows Karlo to engage in a number of ordinary activities (e.g., like running), it also takes up the hardships of living with a rare disease (e.g the impact on his immediate environment or the surgeries he had to undergo). His family members comment on their efforts to support Karlo but stress the difficulty of living with a disease that cannot be cured. The video stresses Karlo's will to not let the disease defeat him. Overall, the relevance of social support (through family, friends and health organizations) is regarded as a valuable resource. As of 5 March 2019, the video (originally in Croatian with English subtitles) was viewed more than 2,000 times. In total, more than 30 versions of the video exist.

Campaign Evaluation

The overall purpose, as highlighted on the campaign website as well as across different media channels, is to create *awareness* for the existence of rare diseases as well as their impact on people living with rare diseases. In order to spread awareness amongst both policy makers and the general public, a variety of material is available for download. The campaign slogan itself "Show your rare. Show you care." includes a clear and *persuasive* call, inviting message recipients to not only donate but also to show their support by painting their faces in bright colors and tagging it with two pre-defined hashtags. As such, involvement and engagement are created across different social media outlets.

In terms of message appeal, a very *positive emotional image* is created. Even though the people affected have to suffer some tremendous pain, they are hopeful and manage to master the challenges associated with their daily lives, with the help of both their families and their immediate environments. Also, the campaign posters highlight the life-affirming message Rare Disease Day is meant to send. Instead of giving in to the pressures and struggles associated with living with a rare condition, a positive picture is painted, showing that in spite of being incurably ill, life is still worth living.

As it is concerned with raising awareness, the campaign itself addresses the *general public*. A moderate form of *targeting* can be observed, as the website, as well as campaign materials – including posters and campaign videos – are available in multiple languages in order to appeal to a world-wide audience. Content is also tailored to the requirements of the different platforms, which makes for an easy spreading of the overall message across a variety of media outlets.

With regard to health-message elements, the *perceived severity* of rare diseases is especially highlighted in the four campaign videos, in which people living with rare diseases provide insights into their daily routines. Throughout the campaign, however, *cues to action* dominate, inviting individuals to not only support research in the area of rare diseases by inviting to share images and tag these on social media. These calls also extend to offline activities, further pleading recipients to support research on rare diseases financially through donations.

The campaign does not only have a complex and elaborate website, it also utilizes a variety of social media platforms: Twitter (30,200 followers), Facebook (105,800 group members), and YouTube (4,000 subscribers). The inclusion of these platforms enables different forms of social support. *Emotional support* is provided through people indicating empathy for individuals living with rare conditions. Videos and images depicting people with painted faces can be seen as one form of emotional support, as can – for instance – the Empire State Building, whose rocket was illuminated in bright colors to pay tribute to rare disease day (ESB, 2019). The individual campaign videos highlight the relevance of *instrumental support*, suggesting that while the largest burden lies with the patient and their families, communities can help the individual respectively their loved ones by stepping in and fulfilling selected chores. *Informational support* is met through filling people's information needs, which might concern information on events that are hosted as part of Rare Disease Day as well as general information on their health condition. Hence, social media benefits these people in collecting and sharing information that might be useful in managing rare illnesses and symptoms. Increasingly, this informational support is also met by the various organizations intending to advance research on rare diseases, such as EURODIS, who shared a live broadcast of the Rare Disease Day Policy Event at the United Nations (NGO CRD, 2019). *Appraisal support* is best described through the "tell your story" feature, which invites people to discuss their or a relative's story with a broader audience, enabling like-minded people to connect. Moreover, the #RareBarometer survey, which is available in 23 languages, asks the people affected to share their personal experiences, especially if treatment options are available for their condition. This exchange is also useful in creating hope amongst affected peer group members, highlighting that with the correct treatment, life can be manageable.

Overall, it is worth noting that the interactive potential of web applications, as implemented on both the website and across the different social media channels, is exploited, enabling engagement on various levels and with differing purposes.

Ataxia

The Campaign

Friedreich's Ataxia – short Ataxia – is a progressive, genetic and neurodegenerative disorder that literally throws people "off balance". Initial signs of the disease may include unsteady posture, frequent falling, and progressive difficulty in walking due to an impaired ability to coordinate movements. As the degenerative state continues, further symptoms might include slurred speech, foot deformities and irregularly curved spines. Throughout the world, approximately 1 in 40,000 people are affected by Ataxia (Rare Disease Day, 2019a).

Campaign Theme and Execution

In an attempt to draw public attention towards this rare disease, Ataxia UK joined forces with star photographer Rankin for the charity's very first campaign in 2014 (Mortimer, 2014). This visually-oriented campaign set out to increase the public's knowledge for Ataxia, "one of the UK's least recognized neurological illnesses" (Mortimer, 2014). Instead of creating hopeful images, the campaign takes a "slice of life" approach by featuring "real people" and providing insights into the minds of people living with Ataxia (Figure 3), their suffering and their problems, including a loss of balance or co-ordination, slurred speech, or blurred vision (Smith, 2014).

The pictures capture people's struggles visually, while the accompanying text blocks indicate peoples' frustration and hopelessness of dealing with this rare condition (Little Black Book Online, 2014). The campaign's purposely black-and-white images are distorted to make people's message more powerful (Mortimer, 2014), while the textual elements are full of anger and despair: "Ataxia. It's like Multiple Sclerosis ganged up with Parkinson's and played a dirty trick on Cerebral Palsy." Or: "We're not one of the big names in diseases. But trust us, we can ruin

Figure 3. Rankin's blurred photos show what it is like to suffer from Ataxia (Eleftheriou-Smith, 2014)
Source: https://www.campaignlive.co.uk/article/rankins-blurred-photos-show-its-suffer-ataxia/1289566

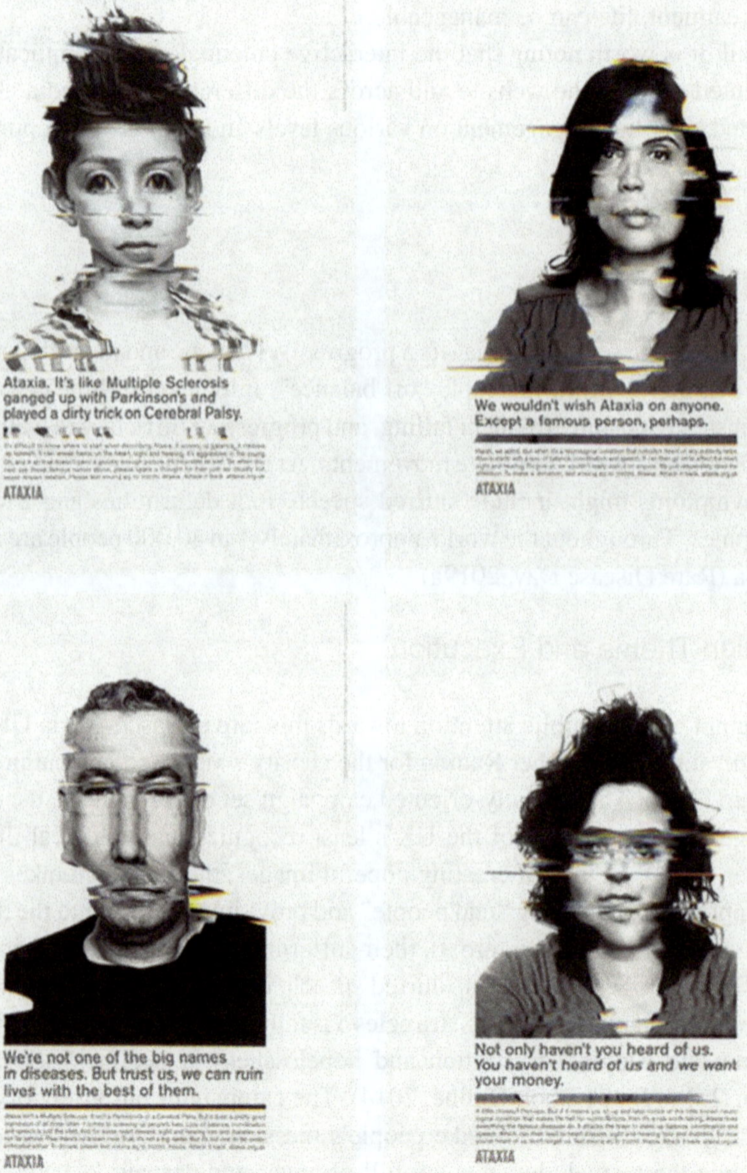

lives with the best of them." Through these powerful messages, not only awareness is meant to be raised but financial support is encouraged to advance research for people living with Ataxia (Little Black Book Online, 2014).

Campaign Evaluation

Rankin's slightly disturbing black-and-white campaign primarily intends to create *awareness* for Ataxia as well as the disease's symptoms. By use of a visual metaphor – blurring and distorted images – the photographer highlights how Ataxia can literally throw the people affected "off balance". Coupled with powerful headlines and text blocks that highlight people's frustration with this rare condition, *persuasion* is meant to be achieved by paying attention to people's real-life struggles with this rare condition. Consequently, a *negative emotional, fear-evoking appeal* serves as the campaign's theme. Powerful images express the disease's "disturbing character", which are backed up by strong (negative) emotional statements of people affected (e.g., "playing a dirty trick", "ruining lives", or "We wouldn't wish Ataxia on anyone"). These statements are *instructional*, trying to convince individuals of the need to financially support research on this disease. With regard to target audience, the message is directed at the general public and does not contain elements addressing a particular target segment. The campaign also incorporates health-theory elements, yet only selectively: on the one hand, individuals are called upon to donate and support research on Ataxia (*cues to action*), while, on the other hand, the *perceived severity* as indicated through both the visual illustrations and the verbal statements by people affected is stressed. No reference to *social support* is included.

Since the analysis of the campaign was conducted in retrospect, no indication of social media use could be detected. Nonetheless, there is a clear potential to also take this offline campaign online, where personalized stories could be used to draw in message recipients.

Epidermolysis Bullosa (EB)

The Campaign

With about 1 infection in every 50,000 people, epidermolysis bullosa (EB) qualifies as a rare disease that affects both men and women from all ethnicities; though, it predominantly is found in children. EB is a painful genetic skin disorder, whereby blisters are caused as a result of friction (Rare Disease Day, 2019b). In consequence, children living with this disease are commonly referred to as "butterfly children" on grounds of their skin being as fragile as butterfly wings (Isles, 2005).

Campaign Theme and Execution

While DEBRA, an international organization standing up for people living with a genetic skin condition, is highly active throughout the world, even utilizing the same campaign content in most countries, the following discussion will focus on campaign content from the German-speaking area, where the "Butterfly children" campaign has been implemented far longer than in other parts of the world. The organization itself wants to enable medical care for children living with EB (Debra Austria, 2013), and by raising funds to guarantee for high quality research, DEBRA's priority is to promote the development of effective treatments and cures for EB (Debra International, 2013). Internationally (2005-2015), and specifically in Austria (2005-present), a cross-media campaign has been employed, which consisted of a number of images featuring objects that pose a threat to butterfly children. Part of an award-winning campaign (Debra International, 2016), the threat potential of each object is visually emphasized, by equipping it with "teeth" that could hurt the fragile skin of children living with EB. A car seat can become a bear trap, walking in shoes feels like walking on nails. Everyday objects that children usually entertain themselves with or that are meant to protect them do the opposite: they pose harm. The visual's message is supported by an accompanying slogan: "This is what life feels like to butterfly children." A short body copy explains the disease and familiarizes people with the condition, for which most people lack awareness. The message then ends with a call to action – asking people to donate money to advance research that can safe a precious child's life. Similar content is also available in video-form on YouTube.[4] Figure 4 and 5 show selected posters of the global EB campaign.

Campaign Evaluation

This long-running cross-media campaign with varying yet mostly identical visual appeals, first and foremost, is concerned with raising *awareness* for the suffering and the specific accompanying symptoms that affect butterfly children. The visuals are expressive of the fact that these children's daily routines are strained by the threat basic objects pose to their health. Since the campaign has been consistent in terms of message presentation for more than a decade, it wants to achieve *persuasion* regarding the severity of Epidermolysis Bullosa.

In terms of message appeal, powerful visuals are metaphorically used, while text elements are reduced to a minimum. The visuals depict the harmful character of everyday– i.e. combing one's hair with a normal hairbrush feels like running through it with nails, as the disease comes with immense, piercing pain. The images might be appealing and colorful as such, but upon taking a closer look, the individual

Figure 4. Fear-evoking posters that create awareness to EB (Debra Institutional, 2016)
Source: http://www.debra-international.org/news-and-events/media-center/eb-awareness-campaign-images.html

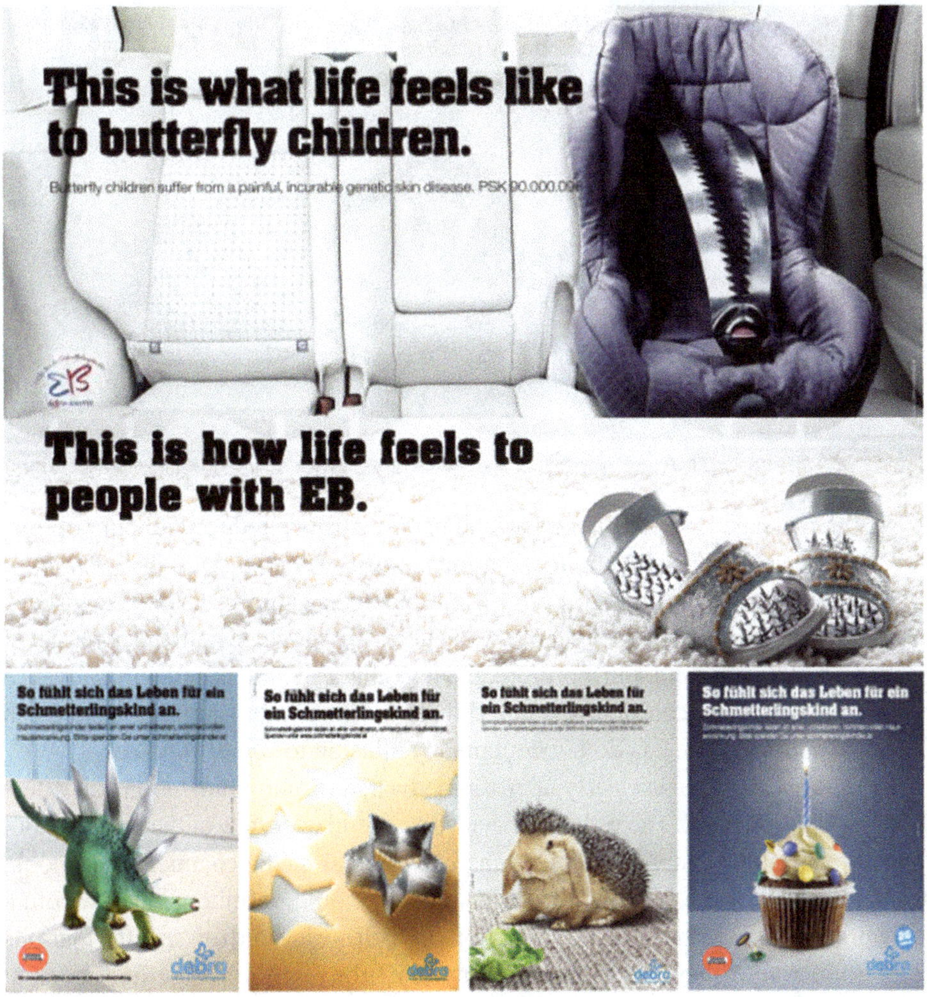

objects can be damaging for butterfly children. As such, a *negative emotional appeal* (respectively a *weakened fear appeal*) is utilized.

Following the previous examples, also this campaign targets the *general public* instead of selected audience segments. Campaign material is available in multiple languages. Therefore, instead of "targeting" sub-populations, the material is meant to raise awareness for the disease in different parts of the world.

Figure 5. Fear-evoking posters that create awareness to EB (Debra Institutional, 2016)
Source: http://www.debra-international.org/news-and-events/media-center/eb-awareness-campaign-images.html

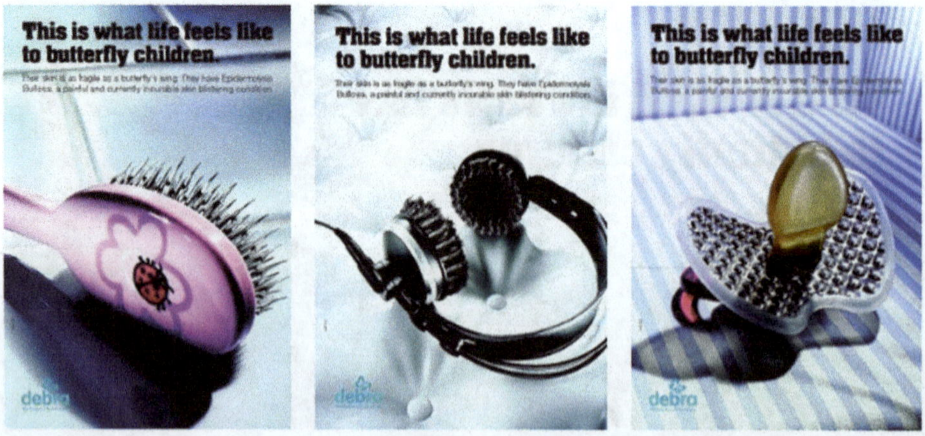

As the message is kept rather basic and benefits from a reduced amount of text, only a selective set of health communication elements are addressed. The *perceived severity* of this particular rare disease is captured in the campaign's diverse visuals, in which toys, equipment and other everyday items are shown to hold the potential of hurting a toddler or child. Furthermore, the text alludes to the necessity to advance research in this area, calling upon individuals to financially support EB research ("*cues to action*"). The ads do not contain any allusion to *social support*.

While the campaign is clearly of cross-media nature, communication still offers room for improvement. The website provides a general overview of the initiative but fails to connect the individual online channels; social media channels (Facebook, Twitter, and YouTube for the International page) would definitely benefit from a more prominent placement of switch buttons, which are located towards the margins or bottom, where they hardly receive any attention. At the same time, content preparation (in terms of currency) and posting frequency leave a lot to be desired.

DISCUSSION OF RESULTS

In response to the goal identified in the introduction, Table 2 provides an overview of the answers to each research question.

This study set out to investigate health communication campaigns for both Rare Disease Day and selected rare diseases across multiple platforms. Except for one campaign, multiple channels were used to spread the campaign message as part

Table 2. Answers to the research questions

Research Questions	Answers
RQ1: Which Channels are used to Promote Rare Diseases?	Online and Offline Channels.
RQ2: Which Message Appeals or Design Elements are used to attract Attention? Is the Reasoning rather Rational or Emotional?	Strong Visuals with Reduced Textual Elements.
RQ3: To which extent are elements of selected Health Theories integrated into these Messages and inasmuch are they used to achieve Audience Engagement?	2 Elements Featured: Cues to Action and Perceived Severity
RQ4: Do messages differ across platforms, as well as across Rare Diseases?	Messages are overall consistent. Social Media adds an "Engagement Component"
RQ5: Inasmuch are the Criteria of a "Sustainable" Health Campaign Fulfilled?	(Mostly) Fulfilled

of cross-media promotional efforts (RQ1). With regard to message design and content, visual metaphors dominated, while both negative and positive emotional appeals were used. The overarching Rare Disease Campaign used a positive appeal; individual campaigns (e.g., for Ataxia and EB) emphasized the suffering individuals had to endure when being affected by the disease; consequently, negative emotional appeals prevailed (RQ2). Depending on message purpose (awareness or persuasion), theoretical elements were integrated to varying degrees, the most common elements being perceived severity and cues to action. Social support was hardly offered by these messages, which were most commonly directed at the general public instead of specific target groups. (RQ3). Generally, messages did not differ across platforms, but, in most instances, messages provided on social media did not exploit the platform's full potential (RQ4).

With regard to each campaign's sustainable nature – according to which material is meant to provide individuals with correct and feasible information in an appealing manner and at the right time in order to bring about behavioral change – most campaigns met individuals where they searched for information (i.e. both online and offline), and used (visually-driven) emotional appeals rather than extensive and lengthy rational arguments; moreover, the fact that the disease's downsides (i.e. perceived severity) were used to draw in message recipients is more likely to positively affect individuals' intentions to donate or advance research in the field of rare diseases (i.e. cues to action) (RQ5). When compared to the Rare Disease Campaign, which emphasized the relevance of family engagement and social support, individual campaigns purposely stressed the risks of and individual's frustration with rare diseases – which can also stem from the absence of social support and help from an individual's immediate environment. Hence, the use of fear appeals in such a context might appear rather risky, for it can hold the risk to backfire; at the same time, campaign success might be grounded in this explicit risky use of fear appeals, inviting individuals to talk about the campaign (Tannenbaum et al., 2015).

Results further support that campaigns are geared towards educating individuals with regard to rare diseases, not only offering them information on health conditions they might be unfamiliar with (awareness), but also educating them as to what it is like to live with a rare condition. While Rare Disease Day utilizes a positive emotional appeal – stressing that life can still be enjoyed in spite of suffering from a rare disease -, campaigns for selected rare diseases are prone to employ a negative emotional appeal to stress the respective disease's severity. While visually driven metaphors can be used as part of print campaigns, social media extends the characteristics of traditional media by providing not only timely, but also more tailored information, thus, extending information, for instance, though personal recounts.

IMPLICATIONS FOR (HEALTH CARE) MARKETERS

By the use of three examples, this chapter intended to demonstrate how different media channels are utilized to raise awareness for rare diseases as well as how messages are positioned to appeal to the general public. Moreover, with social media being on the rise, the potential of online outlets besides traditional media channels was inquired. Even though it was found that campaigns have started to rely on social media, nonetheless, marketers do not exploit the interconnection of social networks and their interactive nature to date. The following potentials for communication about rare diseases can be pointed out:

- **Social media enables people who are affected by rare diseases to get connected:** These patients are often isolated and, owing to geographic limitations, their "offline" community might be limited. The World Health Organization (WHO, 2018) highlights that rare diseases, however, occur cross-border: "Suffering from a rare disease affects your sense of identity. [...] You start to think of yourself not as being French or English or Danish, but as a person with this particular disease. I think that is one of the reasons why the rare disease patient groups tend to be much more international and collaborative in their focus".
- **Besides enabling people who share common interests respectively health conditions to get in touch with one another, the "online crowd" is also actively looking for relevant information on a specific disease and eager to share this information amongst like-minded people.** This suggests that

reaching out goes beyond looking for people who understand what individuals are going through, but is also a way of finding out about new treatments or research that looks promising, catering to individuals' informational and affirmative beliefs.

- **Social networks might not only offer potential for engagement with content, but also might serve as a "driver to connect" with other affected individuals or groups.** Apart from the formation of new (thematic) groups, who mostly look for new information and disease experiences, the disease's visibility can be increased, resulting not only in wider reach but also in a broader awareness for the existence of selected medical conditions.
- **The interconnected and engaging nature of social media facilitates the acquisition of knowledge about the disease.** Social media can enhance communication by, for example, talking about a disease in a closed forum or group. Support can be also shown outside the borders of mostly closed groups, e.g., by adding (disease-)specific frames to one's profile picture as in the case of the PURA syndrome or the YES, WE CARE campaign by the Care-for-Rare Foundation.[5]
- **In addition to common donations, new forms of engagement emerge, too, as communication channels multiply and technology advances.** For instance, in order to "fit" the symptoms of the disease - the skins easily fractured nature when being touched - one Russian campaign took up this particular aspect, affording individuals with the opportunity to donate money in a contactless manner - or in other words: "to help without touching. [6]"
- **The advancement of the Internet has led new platforms as well as innovative forms of donation to emerge.** For example, *PledgeIt* is an online sports fundraising platform which allows users to create a custom fundraising page, which they can share with their friends and families through social media. They can select sporting events, which then serve as a reference point to their campaign. As a performance-based fundraising platform, a team's respectively an athlete's performance is used to sponsor the campaign, whereby supporters can then "pledge a donation" for every touchdown, goal, home run, point or goal in the game. Once each game is finished, pledges are automatically transferred into donations for the pre-defined (health) cause. Pages like these have already been utilized to acquire funding for rare diseases, e.g. Reps For Rare Diseases (#wetacklerare).[7]

The points made above underscore that social media and new technology offer a lot of potential to marketers when it comes to increasing awareness for rare diseases or drawing in the audience, encouraging people to share information, participate in events and advance research through donations. At the same time, social media is especially beneficial to people living with rare diseases as well as their immediate environment, as they can draw from collective knowledge provided by "the crowd" (PWC Research, 2012). Social media channels can lift communication about rare diseases to the next level. For instance, in terms of engagement, social media could be used to provide instrumental support, e.g., by organizing a charity event that is meant to assist people in living with the disease. At the same time, social media utilization also allows for emotional support (e.g. expressing sympathy for people's disease and their immediate (affected) environments), appraisal support (e.g. sharing the success-stories of people coping with the disease), and informational support (e.g., posting information on latest research findings or links for further information). The interactive nature of social media also invites contests and the collection of ideas ("calls/cues to action").

RECOMMENDATIONS: FOSTERING ENGAGEMENT AND INTERACTION

As our analysis has shown, there is still room for improvement, as campaigns fall short with regard to audience engagement, especially when it comes to reaching a younger audience segment. Messages should integrate visuals besides textual elements, as calls/cues to action including these elements have been found to be more effective when compared to plain text messages, increasing engagement by almost a quarter (note: messages do not necessarily have to be posted by a company but can even be posted by other social media users) (PWC Research, 2012). Moreover, choice of a suitable social media platform is essential. In the health context, Facebook has been found to be the most popular social media platform to be utilized amongst the plethora of social networking sites (4 Imprints, 2013). Campaigns could thus definitely benefit from putting more emphasis on social support and patient empowerment, as particularly the nature of social networking sites allows for expressing sympathy (*emotional support; affirmative support*) and offering advise (*informative support; instructional support*) (Ayme et al., 2008; Davies, 2016; Glenn, 2015). Likewise, messages could more easily appeal to individuals' willingness to financially support research on rare diseases, e.g. in form of crowdfunding campaigns (Dragojlovic & Lynd, 2014).

As acceptance rates of health content on social media are somewhat low, Weber Shandwick (2018) recommends several principles which are meant to create higher acceptance amongst message recipients:

- **Design content for discovery:** This suggests that in order to achieve the best possible goal, content needs to be provided across a multitude of platforms and prepared to fit the specific requirements of each platform. The diverse material for download – made available for Rare Disease Day 2019 - present a good example.
- **Use succinct, clear and plain language in communications.** In order to avoid confusion and misunderstandings due to the extensive use of medical jargon, it is recommended to keep information not only concise, but also short and simple, as illustrated by the EB campaign.
- **Customize approaches.** In line with "targeting" and "tailoring" communications, companies are also advised to address topics that resonate with the individual generations of health-information seekers. Rare Disease Day provided tailored content for different stakeholder groups (e.g., communities, individuals), whose information needs are very distinct from one another.
- **Use a smart channel strategy**. Companies need to realize which channel best caters to their interests: while mass media is best suited to spread information to a broad and dispersed audience, more targeted messages are best distributed through social media, where they can call upon users to participate, vote or simply entertain them. While Rare Disease Day was successful in guiding users across the multitude of channels, Ataxia was limited to one (offline) channel, leading to different engagement rates for the two campaigns.
- **Prove online credibility from the outset.** It is particularly social media which has often been doubted with regard to the quality of content. Hence, marketers have to earn consumers' trust by guaranteeing (and proving) their research results can be sustained. Therefore, transparency and supported evidence perform best. As part of Rare Disease Day, talks and interviews by experts were streamed online, enhancing both the relevance and credibility of information provided on this platform.
- **Ensure brand and content are current and portrayed accurately on medical information websites**. There is nothing worse than incomplete and outdated information, as it is the case with DEBRA's international EB campaign site (last update in 2016). For this reason, companies need to invest in and pay more attention towards more thorough reporting and an appealing design in order to enhance both message credibility and source trust. Rare Disease Day followed an elaborate strategy across multiple channels and was, thus, able to succeed.

CONCLUSION

While the Internet can never substitute face-to-face communication respectively doctor-patient encounters (Hawn, 2009), it is nevertheless a useful channel to complement traditional information offers. Especially if information is scarce and people are confronted with the challenges of connecting with like-minded people – as it is the case with people suffering from rare diseases – traditional forms and means of communication do not suffice. Instead, alternative points of reference need to be found, which are often web-based. Through social media, individuals cannot only connect over shared interests and topics, but can also retrieve information from the "crowd", who affords them access to health information without the interference of any gatekeeper ("information apomediation") (Eysenbach, 2008).

As highlighted by the changing and diverse themes of Rare Disease Day (see Table 1), it becomes obvious that both online and digital communication can help to push relevant topics above the general public's threshold, whereby offline and digital offerings can complement one another as well as extend each other. Thereby, it is especially the "crowdsourcing" nature of social media platforms that benefits individuals looking for health information (Donelle & Booth, 2012). Social networking sites allow for interaction amongst participants, inviting diverse members (patients, practitioners, family members) not only to share relevant content, but also to like, comment and spread it amongst their own network. Hence, these platforms bundle messages with diverse purposes: information, advice, and support (Eysenbach, 2008; Gray, 2011; Fox & Jones, 2009). At the same time, user-generated-content – for instance, in form of stories or collected data – becomes not only more personal, but also more relevant to the target audience (Gray, 2011; Hawn, 2009). If informational needs are satisfied, this also results in greater patient engagement and happiness (Hawn, 2009). As mentioned above, the interactive nature of social media channels offers different forms of social support and engagement, holding the potential to elevate communication about rare diseases to a next level. This engagement can also be more easily tracked, for social media offers new criteria to measure message success, including shares/retweets, likes, views, ratings and comments (Gill et al., 2007; Woerndl et al., 2008).

LIMITATIONS AND DIRECTIONS FOR FUTURE RESEARCH

There are several limitations to the study at hand. First, only a limited amount of campaigns was looked at in detail. Moreover, only message characteristics were studied, blending out consumer responses to such messages. Third, only campaigns in English or German were chosen. Hence, further research should be extended to campaigns for additional rare diseases, while also looking at both national and international campaigns in order to detect potential differences in message design and composition. It might also be interesting to look at messages' activating function in terms of design and composition, while inquiring consumers' responses to rare disease campaigns in order to generate insights into message effectiveness. Responses might also well vary with regard to consumers demographics, including sex, age and educational level.

REFERENCES

Ache, K., & Wallace, L. (2008). Human papillomavirus vaccination coverage on YouTube. American Journal of Preventive Medicine. *American Journal of Preventive Medicine*, *35*(4), 389–392. doi:10.1016/j.amepre.2008.06.029 PMID:18675530

Aetna. (2015). How consumers use social media for health care education. Retrieved from https://news.aetna.com/2015/07/how-consumers-use-social-media-for-healthcare-education/

Ahmed, O. H., Sullivan, S. J., Schneiders, A. G., & McCrory, P. (2010). iSupport: Do social networking sites have a role to play in concussion awareness? *Disability and Rehabilitation*, *32*(22), 1877–1883. doi:10.3109/09638281003734409 PMID:20367328

Ajzen, I. (1991). The theory of planned behavior. *Organizational Behavior and Human Decision Processes*, *50*(2), 179–211. doi:10.1016/0749-5978(91)90020-T

ALS. (2019). ALS Ice Bucket Challenge. Retrieved from https://www.als.net/icebucketchallenge/

Andsager, J. L., Bemker, V., Choi, H. L., & Torwel, V. (2006). Perceived similarity of exemplar traits and behavior. *Communication Research*, *33*(1), 3–18. doi:10.1177/0093650205283099

Ayme, S., Kole, A., & Groft, S. (2008). Empowerment of Patients: Lessons from the rare disease community. *Lancet*, *371*(9629), 2048–2051. doi:10.1016/S0140-6736(08)60875-2 PMID:18555918

Barnes, J. A. (1954). Class and committees in a Norwegian island parish. *Human Relations*, *7*(1), 39–58. doi:10.1177/001872675400700102

Batra, R., & Ray, M. L. (1986). Affective responses mediating acceptance of advertising. *The Journal of Consumer Research*, *13*(2), 234–249. doi:10.1086/209063

Becker, M. (1978). Compliance with a medical regimen for asthma. *Public Health Reports*, *93*, 268–277. PMID:652949

Becker, M. H. (1974). The Health Belief Model and Personal Health Behavior. *Health Education Monographs*, *2*(4), 324–508. doi:10.1177/109019817400200407

Bennett, P., & Murphy, S. (1997). *Psychology and Health Promotion*. Buckingham, UK: Open University Press.

Bernhardt, J. M. (2004). Communication at the Core of Effective Public Health. *American Journal of Public Health*, *94*(2), 2051–2053. doi:10.2105/AJPH.94.12.2051 PMID:15569948

Buntin, M. B., Jain, S. H., & Blumenthal, D. (2010). Health information technology: Laying the infrastructure for national health reform. *Health Affairs*, *29*(6), 1214–1219. doi:10.1377/hlthaff.2010.0503 PMID:20530358

Cassel, J. (1976). The contribution of the social environment to host resistance: The Fourth Wade Hampton Frost Lecture. *American Journal of Epidemiology*, *104*(2), 107–123. doi:10.1093/oxfordjournals.aje.a112281 PMID:782233

Center for Disease Control and Prevention - CDC. (2009). Social media at CDC. Retrieved from www.cdc.gov/socialmedia/campaigns/h1n1/#Microblogs

Cho, H. (2012). *Health Communication Message Design: Theory and Practice*. Thousand Oaks, CA: Sage.

Davies, W. (2016). Insights into rare diseases from social media surveys. *Orphanet Journal of Rare Diseases*, *11*(151). doi:10.118613023-016-0532-x PMID:27829465

Davis, R. E., & Resnicow, K. (2012). The Cultural Variance Framework for Tailoring Health Messages. In H. Cho (Ed.), *Health Communication Message Design: Theory and Practice* (pp. 115–135). Thousand Oaks, CA: Sage.

De la Torre-Díez, I., Díaz-Pernas, F. J., & Antón-Rodríguez, M. (2012). A content analysis of chronic diseases social groups on Facebook and Twitter. *Telemedicine Journal and e-Health*, *18*(6), 404–408. doi:10.1089/tmj.2011.0227 PMID:22650380

Debra Austria. (2013). Schmetterlingskinder. Retrieved from https://www.debra-austria.org/schmetterlingskinder/

Debra International. (2013). Epidermolysis bullosa. Retrieved from http://www.debra-international.org/what-is-eb.html

Debra International. (2016). EB awareness campaign images. Retrieved from http://www.debra-international.org/news-and-events/media-center/eb-awareness-campaign-images.html

Delbaere, M., McQuarrie, E. F., & Phillips, B. J. (2011). Personification in advertising. *Journal of Advertising*, *40*(1), 121–130. doi:10.2753/JOA0091-3367400108

Denis, A., Mergaert, L., Fostier, C., Cleemput, I., & Simoens, S. (2010). A comparative study of European rare disease and orphan drug markets. *Health Policy (Amsterdam)*, *97*(2-3), 173–179. doi:10.1016/j.healthpol.2010.05.017 PMID:20800761

Derzon, J. H., & Lipsey, M. W. (2002). A Meta-Analysis of the Effectiveness of Mass-Communication for Changing Substance-use: Knowledge, Attitudes, and Behavior. In W. D. Crano, & M. Burgoon (Eds.), *Mass Media and Drug Prevention: Classic and Contemporary Theories and Research* (pp. 231–258). London, UK: Lawrence Erlbaum Associates.

Dobrenova, F. V., Grabner-Kräuter, S., Diehl, S., & Terlutter, R. (2019). The use of advertising appeals in breast cancer detection messages: A web content analysis. *Women & Health*, *59*(8), 867–882. doi:10.1080/03630242.2019.1565904 PMID:30714487

Donelle, L., & Booth, R. G. (2012). Health Tweets: An Exploration of Health Promotion on Twitter. *Online Journal of Issues in Nursing*, *17*(3). doi:10.3912/OJIN.Vol17No03Man04 PMID:23036060

Dragojlovic, N., & Lynd, L. D. (2014). Crowdfunding drug development: The state of play in oncology and rare diseases. *Drug Discovery Today*, *19*(11), 1775–1780. doi:10.1016/j.drudis.2014.06.019 PMID:24973645

Dutta, M. J. (2008). *Communicating Health: A Culture-Centered Approach*. Malden, MA: Policy.

Eagly, A. H., & Chaiken, S. (1993). *The Psychology of Attitudes*. Orlando, FL: Harcourt Brace Jovanovich College Publishers.

Eleftheriou-Smith, L.-M. (2014). Rankin's blurred photos show what it's like to suffer from Ataxia. Retrieved from https://www.campaignlive.co.uk/article/rankins-blurred-photos-show-its-suffer-ataxia/1289566

ESB. (2019). On Thursday, February 28, 2019, The Empire State Building will be lit Green, Pink, Light Blue, and Purple in honor of Rocket Pharm & Rare Disease Day. Retrieved from https://www.esbnyc.com/tower-lighting-2019-02-28-000000

Eurodis. (2017). What is a rare disease – Fact Sheet. Retrieved from https://www.eurordis.org/sites/default/files/publications/Fact_Sheet_RD.pdf

Eysenbach, G. (2008). Medicine 2.0: Social networking, collaboration, participation, apomediation, and openness. *Journal of Medical Internet Research*, *10*(3), e22. doi:10.2196/jmir.1030 PMID:18725354

Farmer, A. D., Bruckner Holt, C. E., Cook, M. J., & Hearing, S. D. (2009). Social networking sites: A novel portal for communication. *Postgraduate Medical Journal*, *85*(1007), 455–459. doi:10.1136/pgmj.2008.074674 PMID:19734511

Fishbein, M., & Ajzen, I. (1975). *Belief, Attitude, Intention, and Behavior: An Introduction to Theory and Research*. Longman: Addison Wesley.

Fox, S., & Jones, S. (2009). The social life of health information. Retrieved from www.pewinternet.org/Reports/2009/8-The-Social-Life-of-Health-Information.aspx

Freeman, B., & Chapman, S. (2007). Is YouTube telling or selling you something? Tobacco content on the video-sharing website YouTube. *Tobacco Control*, *16*(3), 207–210. doi:10.1136/tc.2007.020024 PMID:17565142

Freimuth, V., Linnan, H. W., & Potter, P. (2000). Communicating the Threat of Emerging Infections to the Public. *Emerging Infectious Diseases*, *6*(4), 337–374. doi:10.3201/eid0604.000403 PMID:10905966

Gajaria, A., Yeung, E., Goodale, T., & Charach, A. (2011). Beliefs about attention-deficit/hyperactivity disorder and response to stereotypes: Youth postings in Facebook groups. *The Journal of Adolescent Health*, *49*(1), 15–20. doi:10.1016/j.jadohealth.2010.09.004 PMID:21700151

Gaucher Disease News. (2019). Patients, Family and Friends to Take Part in Variety of Rare Disease Day Events Worldwide. Retrieved from https://gaucherdiseasenews.com/2019/02/11/rare-disease-day-marked-by-events-worldwde/

Gill, P., Arlitt, M., Li, Z., & Mahanti, A. (2007). YouTube Traffic Characterization: A View from the Edge. IMC of the 7th ACM SIGCOMM Conference on Internet Measurement; Oct. 24–26, 2007, San Diego, CA. Retrieved from https://pages.cpsc.ucalgary.ca/~zongpeng/publications/imc07.pdf

Gkiouzepas, L., & Hogg, M. K. (2011). Articulating a new framework for visual metaphors in advertising. *Journal of Advertising*, *40*(1), 103–120. doi:10.2753/JOA0091-3367400107

Glanz, K., Rimer, B. K., & Viswanath, K. (Eds.). (2002). *Health Behavior and Health Education: Theory, Research, and Practice* (3rd ed.). San Francisco, CA: John Wiley & Sons.

Glenn, A. D. (2015). Using Online Health Communication to Manage Chronic Sorrow: Mothers of Children with rare diseases speak. *Journal of Pediatric Nursing*, *30*(1), 17–24. doi:10.1016/j.pedn.2014.09.013 PMID:25316198

Gray, C. (2011). Social media: A guide for researchers. Research Information Network. Retrieved from www.rin.ac.uk/our-work/communicating-and-disseminating-research/social-media-guide-researchers

Greene, J. A., Choudhry, N. K., Kilabuk, E., & Shrank, W. H. (2011). Online social networking by patients with diabetes: A qualitative evaluation of communication with Facebook. *Journal of General Internal Medicine*, *26*(3), 287–292. doi:10.100711606-010-1526-3 PMID:20945113

Hale, J. L., & Dillard, J. P. (1995). Fear Appeals in Health Promotion Campaigns: Too Much, Too Little, or Just Right? In E. Maibach, & R. L. Parrott (Eds.), *Designing Health Messages: Approaches from Communication Theory and Public Health Practice* (pp. 65–80). Thousand Oaks, CA: Sage. doi:10.4135/9781452233451.n4

Harwood, J., & Giles, H. (2005). *Intergroup Communication: Multiple Perspectives*. New York: Peter Lang.

Hass, B. H. (2006). Content Management – Inhalte für Neue Medien strategisch nutzen. In C. Scholz (Ed.), *Handbuch Medienmanagement* (pp. 375–391). Berlin, Germany: Springer. doi:10.1007/3-540-32879-3_18

Hawkins, J. D., Brown, E. C., Oesterle, S., Arthur, M. W., Abbott, R. D., & Catalano, R. F. (2008). Early Effects of Communities That Care on targeted risks and intention of delinquent behavior and substance use. *The Journal of Adolescent Health*, *43*(1), 15–22. doi:10.1016/j.jadohealth.2008.01.022 PMID:18565433

Hawn, C. (2009). Take two aspirin and tweet me in the morning: How Twitter, Facebook, and other social media are reshaping health care. *Health Affairs*, *28*(2), 361–368. doi:10.1377/hlthaff.28.2.361 PMID:19275991

House, J. S. (1981). *Work stress and social support*. Reading, MA: Addison-Wesley.

4. Imprints. (2013). Marketing to Baby Boomers. Retrieved from https://info.4imprint.com/wp-content/uploads/1P-19-1013-Marketing-to-Baby-Boomers2.pdf

Isles, R. (2015). Dundee Scientists on road to cure for "Butterfly Children" condition. Retrieved from http://app.dundee.ac.uk/pressreleases/prmay05/butterfly.html

Jones, S. C., & Owen, N. (2006). Using fear appeals to promote cancer screening—are we scaring the wrong people? *International Journal of Nonprofit and Voluntary Sector Marketing*, *11*(2), 93–103. doi:10.1002/nvsm.48

(•••).. . *The Journal of Consumer Research*, *21*(September), 252–273.

Simou, E. (2015). Health information sources: Trust and satisfaction. *International Journal of Healthcare*, *2*(1), 38–43. doi:10.5430/ijh.v2n1p38

Keelan, J., Pavri-Garcia, V., Tomlinson, G., & Wilson, K. (2007). YouTube as a source of information on immunization: A Content Analysis. *Journal of the American Medical Association*, *298*(21), 2482–2484. doi:10.1001/jama.298.21.2482 PMID:18056901

Kim, W., Kreps, G. L., & Shin, C. N. (2015). The role of social support and social networks in health information–seeking behavior among Korean Americans: A qualitative study. *International Journal for Equity in Health*, *14*(40). doi:10.118612939-015-0169-8 PMID:25927546

Kofinas, J. D., Varrey, A., Sapra, K. J., Kanj, R. V., Chervenak, F. A., & Asfaw, T. (2014). Adjunctive social media for more effective contraceptive counseling. *Obstetrics and Gynecology*, *123*(4), 763–770. doi:10.1097/AOG.0000000000000172 PMID:24785602

Lang, P. J. (1995). The emotion probe: Studies of motivation and attention. *The American Psychologist*, *50*(5), 372–385. doi:10.1037/0003-066X.50.5.372 PMID:7762889

Lazard, A. J., Bamgbade, B. A., Sontag, J. M., & Brown, C. (2016). Using visual metaphors in health messages: A strategy to increase effectiveness for mental illness communication. *Journal of Health Communication*, *21*(12), 1260–1268. doi:10.1080/10810730.2016.1245374 PMID:27869576

Little Black Book Online. (2014). TBWA\London Teams with Rankin to Raise Awareness of Ataxia. Retrieved from https://lbbonline.com/news/tbwalondon-teams-with-rankin-to-raise-awareness-of-ataxia/

McDivitt, J. A., Zimicki, S., & Hornik, R. C. (1997). Explaining the Impact of Communication Campaigns to Change Vaccination Knowledge and Coverage in the Philippines. *Health Communication*, *9*(2), 95–118. doi:10.120715327027hc0902_1

McNab, C. (2009). What social media offers to health professionals and citizens. Retrieved from https://www.who.int/bulletin/volumes/87/8/09-066712/en/

Messaris, P. (1997). *Visual Persuasion: The role of images in advertising*. Thousand Oaks, CA: Sage.

Moorhead, S. A., Hazlet, D. E., Harrison, L., Carroll, J. K., Irwin, A., & Hoving, C. (2013). A New Dimension of Health Care: Systematic Review of the Uses, Benefits, and Limitations of Social Media for Health Communication. *Journal of Medical Internet Research, 15*(4), e85. doi:10.2196/jmir.1933 PMID:23615206

Morris, M. E., Consolvo, S., Munson, S. A., Kramer, A. D. I., Patrick, K., & Tsai, J. (2011). Facebook for Health. Opportunities and Challenges for Driving Behavior Change. CHI'11 Extended Abstracts on Human Factors in Computing Systems. Retrieved from https://dl.acm.org/citation.cfm?id=1979489&dl=ACM&coll=DL

Mortimer, N. (2014). Ataxia UK joins forces with Rankin to launch the charity's first campaign. Retrieved from https://www.thedrum.com/news/2014/04/07/ataxia-uk-joins-forces-rankin-launch-charity-s-first-campaign

Mueller, B. (1987). Reflections of culture: An analysis of Japanese and American advertising appeals. *Journal of Advertising Research*, (August): 1–21.

Nabi, R. (2002). Anger, fear, uncertainty, and attitudes: A test of the cognitive-functional model. *Communication Monographs, 69*(3), 204–216. doi:10.1080/03637750216541

NGO CRD. (2019). Rare Disease Day Policy Event at the United Nations. Retrieved from https://www.ngocommitteerarediseases.org/rare-disease-day-policy-event-at-the-united-nations/?fbclid=IwAR0XKGVO_zukUfs7juFnb3m1PkOWQrO0cRBqH5PNN2c0148ACcmdCOBpgAA

Niebel, K., & Davidson, E. (2012). Raising the Bar for HIV Awareness. *Marketing Health Services, 32*(4), 5–7. PMID:23356034

Noar, S. M., Benac, C. N., & Harris, M. S. (2007). Does tailoring matter? Meta-analytic review of tailored print health behavior change interventions. *Psychological Bulletin, 133*(4), 673–693. doi:10.1037/0033-2909.133.4.673 PMID:17592961

O'Keefe, G. J., Boyd, H. H., & Brown, M. R. (1998). Who Learns Preventive Health Care Information From Where: Cross-Channel and Repertoire Comparisons. *Health Communication, 10*(1), 25–36. doi:10.120715327027hc1001_2 PMID:16370988

Okazaki, S., Mueller, B., & Taylor, C. R. (2010). Measuring soft-sell versus hard-sell advertising appeals. *Journal of Advertising, 39*(2), 5–20. doi:10.2753/JOA0091-3367390201

Orpha.net. (2012). About Rare Diseases. Retrieved from https://www.orpha.net/consor/cgi-bin/Education_AboutRareDiseases.php?lng=EN

Paek, H.-J., Kim, K., & Hove, T. (2010). Content analysis of anti-smoking videos on YouTube: Message sensation value, message appeals, and their relationships with viewer responses. *Health Education Research*, *25*(6), 1085–1099. doi:10.1093/her/cyq063 PMID:20923913

Paek, H.-J., Kim, K., Hove, T., & Huh, J.-Y. (2014). Reduced Harm or Another Gateway to Smoking? Source, Message, and Information Characteristics of E-Cigarette Videos on YouTube. *Journal of Health Communication*, *19*(5), 545–560. doi:10.1080/10810730.2013.821560 PMID:24117370

Pagoto, S., Schneider, K. L., Evans, M., Waring, M. E., Appelhans, B., Busch, A. M., ... Ziedonis, M. (2014). Tweeting it off: Characteristics of adults who tweet about a weight loss attempt. *Journal of the American Medical Informatics Association*, *21*(6), 1032–1037. doi:10.1136/amiajnl-2014-002652 PMID:24928175

Palmer-Wackerly, A. L., & Krieger, J. L. (2015). Dancing around infertility: The use of metaphors in a complex medical situation. *Health Communication*, *30*(6), 612–623. doi:10.1080/10410236.2014.888386 PMID:25061825

Parrott, R. (2003). Media Issues. In T. L. Thompson, A. M. Dorsey, K. I. Miller, & R. Parrott, (Eds.), Handbook of Health Communication. (pp. 445-448). London, UK: Lawrence Erlbaum Associates.

Paunio, M., Virtanen, M., Poltola, H., Cantell, K., Paunio, P., Valle, M., ... Heinonen, O. P. (1991). Increase of Vaccination Coverage by Mass Media and Individual Approach: Intensified Measles, Mumps and Rubella Prevention Program in Finland. *American Journal of Epidemiology*, *133*(11), 1152–1160. doi:10.1093/oxfordjournals.aje.a115827 PMID:2035518

PEW Internet and American Life Project. (2007). E-Patients with a Disability or Chronic Disease. Retrieved from http://www.pewinternet.org/files/old-media/Files/Reports/2007/EPatients_Chronic_Conditions_2007.pdf.pdf

Phillips, B. J. (2000). The impact of verbal anchoring on consumer response to image ads. *Journal of Advertising*, *29*(1), 15–24. doi:10.1080/00913367.2000.10673600

Piller, I. (2001). Identity constructions in multilingual advertising. *Language in Society*, *30*(2), 153–186. doi:10.1017/S0047404501002019

Porter, R. W., Steinglass, R., Kaiser, J., Olkhovsky, P., Rasmuson, M., Dzhatdoeva, F. A., ... Bragina, V. (2000). Role of Health Communication in Russia's Diphtheria Immunization. *The Journal of Infectious Diseases*, *181*(s1Supplement 1), 220–227. doi:10.1086/315566

Pricewaterhouse Cooper. (2017). Social media "likes" healthcare: From marketing to social business. Retrieved from https://www.pwc.com/us/en/industries/health-industries/library/health-care-social-media.html

Ramirez, A. G., Villarreal, R., McAlister, A., Gallion, K. J., Suarez, L., & Gomez, P. (1999). Advancing the Role of Participatory Communication in the Diffusion of Cancer Screening Among Hispanics. *Journal of Health Communication*, *4*(1), 31–36. doi:10.1080/108107399127075 PMID:10977276

Rare Disease Day. (2008). Overview of Rare Disease Day 2008. Retrieved from https://www.rarediseaseday.org/article/rare-disease-day-2008

Rare Disease Day. (2019a). What is a rare disease? Retrieved from https://www.rarediseaseday.org/article/what-is-a-rare-disease

Rare Disease Day. (2019b). What is Rare Disease Day? Retrieved from https://www.rarediseaseday.org/article/what-is-rare-disease-day

Rare Disease Day. (2019c). Rare Disease Day 2019 theme announced: Bridging health and social care. Retrieved from https://www.rarediseaseday.org/page/news/theme-2019

Rare Disease Day. (2019d). Overview of past Rare Disease Days. Retrieved from https://www.rarediseaseday.org/article/overview-of-past-rare-disease-days

Rare Disease Day. (2019e). Video out now - #ShowYourRare for Rare Disease Day 2019. Retrieved from https://www.rarediseaseday.org/page/news/video-out-now-showyourrare-for-rare-disease-day

Reinarman, C., & Levine, H. G. (1995). The Crack Attack: America's Latest Drug Scare, 1986-1992. In J. Best (Ed.), *Images of Issues. Typifying Contemporary Social Problems* (pp. 147–186). New York: Routledge.

Research, P. W. C. (2012). Social media "likes" healthcare: From marketing to social business. Retrieved from https://www.pwc.com/us/en/industries/health-industries/library/health-care-social-media.html

Rogers, E. M., & Storey, D. (1988). Communication Campaigns. In C. R. Berger, & S. H. Chaffee (Eds.), *Handbook of Communication Science* (pp. 817–847). Newbury Park, CA: Sage.

Rogers, R. W. (1975). A protection motivation theory of fear appeals and attitude change. *The Journal of Psychology*, *91*(1), 93–114. doi:10.1080/00223980.1975.9915803 PMID:28136248

Rogers, R. W. (1983). Cognitive and physiological processes in fear appeals and attitude change: A revised theory of protection motivation. In J. Cacioppo, & R. Petty (Eds.), Social Psychophysiology. (pp. 153-176). New York: Guilford Press.

Rosenstock, I. (1974). Historical Origins of the Health Belief Model. *Health Education Monographs*, *2*(4), 328–335. doi:10.1177/109019817400200403

Rossmann, C., & Ziegler, L. (2013). Gesundheitskommunikation: Medienwirkungen im Gesundheitsbereich. In W. Schweiger, & A. Fahr (Eds.), *Handbuch Medienwirkungsforschung* (pp. 385–400). Wiesbaden, Germany: Springer. doi:10.1007/978-3-531-18967-3_20

Salmon, C., & Atkin, C. K. (2003). Media campaigns for health promotion. In T. L. Thompson, A. M. Dorsey, K. I. Miller, & R. Parrott (Eds.), *Handbook of Health Communication* (pp. 449–472). Mahwah, NJ: Lawrence Erlbaum.

Sample Ward, A. (2011). Citizen tech: Social media in disaster response. Retrieved from http://amysampleward.org/2011/02/19/citizen-tech-social-media-in-disaster-response/

Sarasohn-Kahn, J. (2008). The wisdom of patients: health care meets online social media. Retrieved from https://www.chcf.org/wp-content/uploads/2017/12/PDF-HealthCareSocialMedia.pdf

Schiavo, R. (2007). *Health Communication: From Theory to Practice*. San Francisco, CA: Wiley and Sons.

Schweiger, W. (2002). Cross-Media zwischen Fernsehen und Web. Versuch einer theoretischen Fundierung des Crossmedia-Konzepts. In H. Theunert, & U. Wagner (Eds.), *Medienkonvergenz: Angebot und Nutzung* (pp. 123–136). Munich, Germany: Verlag Reinhard Fischer.

Scott, L. M. (1994). Images in Advertising: The Need for a Theory of Visual Rhetoric. *The Journal of Consumer Research*, *21*(September), 252–273. doi:10.1086/209396

Sjurts, I. (2011). *Strategien in der Medienbranche: Grundlagen und Fallbeispiele*. Wiesbaden, Germany: Springer.

Smith, D. (2013). Health care consumer's use and trust of health information sources. *Journal of Communication in Healthcare*, *4*(3), 200–210. doi:10.1179/1753807611Y.0000000010

Smith, T., Coyle, J. R., Lightfoot, E., & Scott, A. (2007). Reconsidering models of influence: The relationship between consumer social networks and word-of-mouth effectiveness. *Journal of Advertising Research, 47*(4), 387–397. doi:10.2501/S0021849907070407

Snyder, L. B. (2001). Development of Communication Campaigns. In W. B. Gudykunst, & B. Mody (Eds.), *Handbook of International and Intercultural Communication* (2nd ed., pp. 457–478). Thousand Oaks, CA: Sage.

Snyder, L. B., & Hamilton, M. A. (2002). A Meta-Analysis of U.S. Health Campaign Effects on Behavior: Emphasize Enforcement, Exposure, and New Information, and Beware the Secular Trend. In R. C. Hornik (Ed.), *Public Health Communication. Evidence for Behavior Change* (pp. 357–383). London, UK: Lawrence Erlbaum Associates.

Stellefson, M., Chaney, B., Ochipa, K., Chaney, D., Haider, Z., Hanik, B., ... Bernhardt, J. M. (2014). YouTube as a source of chronic obstructive pulmonary disease patient education: A social media content analysis. *Chronic Respiratory Disease, 11*(2), 61–71. doi:10.1177/1479972314525058 PMID:24659212

Tannenbaum, M. B., Hepler, J., Zimmerman, R. S., Saul, L., Jacobs, S., Wilson, K., & Albarracín, D. (2015). Appealing to fear: A meta-analysis of fear appeal effectiveness and theories. *Psychological Bulletin, 141*(6), 1178–1204. doi:10.1037/a0039729 PMID:26501228

Thompson, T. L. (2000). The nature and language of illness explanations. In B. B. Whaley (Ed.), *Explaining Illness: Research, Theory, and Strategies* (pp. 3–40). Mahwah, NJ: Erlbaum.

United Nations – UN. (2919). Goal 3: Ensure healthy lives and promote well-being for all at all ages. Retrieved from https://www.un.org/sustainabledevelopment/health/

U.S. Department of Health and Human Services. (2000). Healthy People 2010: Understanding and improving health and objectives for improving health. US Department of Health and Human Services. Washington, DC. Retrieved from http://www.cdc.gov/nchs/data/hpdata2010/hp2010_final_review.pdf

U.S. Department of Health and Human Services. (2005). Making Health Communication Programs Work. Retrieved from http://www.cancer.gov/publications/health-communication/pink-book.pdf

U.S. Department of Health and Human Services. (2014). What is health literacy. Retrieved from http://www.health.gov/communication/literacy/

Vance, K., Howe, W., & Dellavalle, R. P. (2009). Social Internet Sites as a source of Public Health Information. *Dermatologic Clinics*, *27*(2), 133–136. doi:10.1016/j.det.2008.11.010 PMID:19254656

Wakefield, M. A., Loken, B., & Hornik, R. C. (2010). Use of mass media campaigns to change health behaviour. *Lancet*, *376*(9748), 1261–1271. doi:10.1016/S0140-6736(10)60809-4 PMID:20933263

Weber Shandwick. (2018). The Great American Search for Healthcare Information. Retrieved from https://www.webershandwick.com/wp-content/uploads/2018/11/Healthcare-Info-Search-Report.pdf

Weiss, M. (1997). Signifying the pandemics: Metaphors of AIDS, cancer, and heart disease. *Medical Anthropology Quarterly*, *11*(4), 456–476. doi:10.1525/maq.1997.11.4.456 PMID:9408901

Winston, E. R., Dawn Medlin, B., & Adriana Romaniello, B. (2012). An e-patient's end-user community (EUCY): The value added of social network applications. *Computers in Human Behavior*, *28*(3), 951–957. doi:10.1016/j.chb.2011.12.016

Witte, K. (1992). Putting the fear back into fear appeals: The extended parallel process model. *Communication Monographs*, *59*(4), 329–349. doi:10.1080/03637759209376276

Witte, K. (1998). Fear as motivator, fear as inhibitor: Using the extended parallel process model to explain fear appeal successes and failures. In P. A. Andersen, & L. K. Guerrero (Eds.), *Handbook of communication and emotion: Research, theory, applications, and contexts* (pp. 423–450). San Diego, CA: Academic Press.

Woerndl, M., Papagiannidis, S. S., Bourlakis, M., & Li, F. (2008). Internet-induced marketing techniques: Critical factors in viral marketing campaigns. *International Journal of Business Science and Applied Management*, *3*, 33–45.

World Economic Forum. (2017). The future of treating rare diseases. Retrieved from https://www.weforum.org/agenda/2017/01/the-future-of-treating-rare-diseases/

World Health Organization - WHO. (2018). Statement for Rare Disease Day. Retrieved from https://www.who.int/mediacentre/news/statements/2018/rare-disease-day/en/

Wright, K. B., Sparks, L., & O'Hair, H. D. (2008). *Health Communication in the 21st century*. Oxford, UK: Blackwell.

Yzer, M. (2012). The integrative model of behavioral prediction as a tool for designing health messages. In H. Cho (Ed.), *Health communication message design: Theory and practice* (pp. 21–40). London, UK: Sage.

Zhao, D., & Rosson, M. B. (2009). How and why people Twitter. In *Proceedings of the ACM 2009 international conference on Supporting group work - GROUP '09* (p. 243). New York, NY: ACM Press. 10.1145/1531674.1531710

KEY TERMS AND DEFINITIONS

Cross-Media Promotion: The term refers to the distribution of content via different media channels (Sjurts, 2011).

Rare Diseases: Diseases with a low prevalence in population that often have incurable genetic conditions, being life-threatening (Orpha.net, 2012).

Sustainable Health Campaign: The term refers to all promotional material that provides individuals with the right information, at the right time, in a comprehensible, appealing, and engaging manner, in order to bring about lasting (behavioral) change.

ENDNOTES

1. Facebook Rare Disease Day, https://m.facebook.com/rarediseaseday/ (Access date: Nov. 17, 2019)
2. Twitter Rare Disease Day, https://mobile.twitter.com/rarediseaseday?lang=en (Access date: Nov. 17, 2019)
3. Twitter Rare Disease Day, https://www.youtube.com/user/rarediseaseday?app=desktop (Access date: Nov. 17, 2019)
4. DEBRA TV- Spot Cupcake. For example, see https://youtu.be/11MM4vuOF3I (Access date: Nov. 17, 2019)
5. YES, WE CARE! Photo Campaign for children with Rare Diseases. For an example, please see https://www.care-for-rare.org/en/project/yes-we-care-photo-campaign-children-rare-diseases (Access date: Nov. 17, 2019)
6. Participate in the "Help without Touching" charitable campaign at VDNH. For further information, please see https://vdnh.ru/en/news/na-vdnkh-mozhno-prinyat-uchastie-v-blagotvoritelnoy-kampanii-pomogi-ne-kasayas/ (Access date: Nov. 17, 2019)
7. 2019 REPS for Rare Diseases. For further information, please see https://pledgeit.org/for/2019-reps-for-rare-diseases (Access date: Nov. 17, 2019)

Chapter 4

Digital Media in Rare Diseases or "Knowledge Is Power": The Role of EURORDIS in Creating Awareness and Diagnosing Rare Diseases

Célia Felícia Belim Rodrigues
Instituto Superior de Ciências Sociais e Políticas, Universidade de Lisboa, Portugal

ABSTRACT

This chapter focuses on the use of digital media by EURORDIS-Rare Diseases Europe and is specifically committed to understand its contribution to the awareness and diagnosis of rare diseases. To perceive the use of digital media and role in creating awareness of rare diseases, the contents of its website and Facebook page were analyzed. In specific, a promotional video of EURORDIS and a collection of 12 videographically documented stories from 2018 and 2019. The results show the use of various types of content and inherently practices, such as information, clarification, personalization, support, appeal, and empowerment, and of several rhetorical resources. In the dimension of pathos, the author finds elements that motivate awareness and inspire the receiver. Some elements of the logos used are credibility of sender(ethos), testimony(ethos), description of disease and identification of symptoms, exemplification and personalization, factual data, statistic data, and the use of metaphors and repetition.

DOI: 10.4018/978-1-7998-2088-8.ch004

INTRODUCTION

Due to the inadequacy of the treatments, "rare disease patients have begun acting like scientists and studying themselves" (Polich, 2012, p. 167). In this context, the internet, because it addresses a large public of rare diseases, attracts patients who are internet users highly stimulated to seek information and online communities, being receptive to new interventions that respond to their needs. The internet, by providing information on rare diseases, may promote increasing competence in decoding clinical research studies and afford new insights that may be useful when the patient consults the health professional and in exploring new therapeutic modalities. This is tantamount to making tremendous progress in patient self-advocacy (Liuccio, Belotti, Comune, Zambito & Schulz, 2015, p. 5). When individuals access accurate and reliable information, they can make informed decisions. So, it can be said that "knowledge is power".

In this scenario, the author proposes to study the messages and practices of digital communication of EURORDIS-Rare Diseases Europe, concretely in its website and Facebook page, in order to understand the use of digital media and its role in creating awareness to rare diseases. EURORDIS is a unique, non-profit alliance of 837 rare disease patient organizations from 70 countries that work together to improve the lives of the 30 million people living with a rare disease in Europe.[1]

Awareness is the ability to directly know and perceive, to feel, or to be cognizant of events. In a broader sense, it is the state of being conscious of something (Korompilias, 2018, p. 71). Additionally, it has been prominent in public relations and communication campaigns. For example, Grunig and Hunt (1984) classified publics as latent, aware and active, describing the aware public as the one that recognizes that there is a problem. The emphasis on awareness in public relations and public communication circles coincided with an increase in education initiatives in the health and medical fields, because "the skills public health advocates need to amplify the voice of public health and ensure that the stories being told reflect basic public health goals and values" (Wallack, Dorfman, Jernigan & Themba-Nixon, 1993, pp. 2-3). Awareness is associated with consciousness. Anything that we are aware of at a given moment forms part of our consciousness (Velmans & Schneider, 2007, p. 1).

Furthermore, it is intended to analyze the video's potential, concretely a promotional video of EURORDIS and a collection of videographically documented stories from 2018 and 2019, present in the website, from people who share their experiences of living with a rare disease, in order to perceive how these messages can be useful in the sensitization and diagnosis of rare diseases. The defended argument is that the messages and practices of digital communication of EURORDIS contribute to awareness and diagnosis of rare diseases. Therefore, it is assumed as a starting question: *How do messages and practices of digital communication of EURORDIS contribute to create awareness and facilitate the process of diagnosis of rare diseases?* Methodologically, qualitative content analysis is used to deal with message content and rhetorical analysis to deal with form and style.

BACKGROUND

Social media, used within health care contexts for communication purposes, is increasing and becoming more acceptable (Burke-Garcia & Scally, 2014; Moorhead, 2017). Specifically, these digital tools are likely to enable: (a) Improved interactions with others; (b) More available, shared, and tailored information; (c) Increased accessibility and widening access; and (d) Increased peer/social/emotional support. These are some of numerous benefits of social media for healthcare communication (Moorhead, 2017).

Roberts, Seymour, Fish II, Robinson and Zuckerman (2017) assume that the digitally networked global public may have influenced the discourse, sentiment, and response to the Ebola epidemic originating in West Africa. The authors analyzed 109,400 English-language stories about the keyword "Ebola" published from 1 July 2014 to 17 November 2014 from the media sets U.S. mainstream media, U.S. regional media, U.S. political and popular blogs, Europe Media Monitor, and Global Voices to understand how social network theory and models of the networked global public may have contributed to health communication efforts on Ebola epidemic. The Centers for Disease Control and Prevention (CDC) and World Health Organization (WHO) were the two media sources with the most inlinks (hyperlinks directed to their sites).

In spite of recognizing that digital media have an ability to increase the reach of public health research and communication, as well as drive measurable behaviour change, Burke-Garcia and Scally (2014) identify that there is an absence of both deep and wide understanding of the opportunities within digital media, that a smart and strategic planning for its widespread use is not a common practice and that a rigorous evaluative studies of its effectiveness are few and far between.

Digital media have been contributing to the awareness of rare diseases and have even assumed diagnostic functions. Castillo-Esparcia and López-Villafranca (2016) focus on communication strategies employed by rare disease patient organizations, analyzing the media portrayal of these diseases and patient organizations in Spain between 2012 and 2014. By carrying out a descriptive analysis of the digital communication activities performed by 143 national organizations and conducting a telephone questionnaire of a representative sample of 90 organizations, the investigators explore the association between media presence, funding and public image. They observe that increased visibility of the organizations, afforded by a growth in the coverage of the topic, increments the membership - but not donations - and also increases awareness of these diseases. Most of the organizations studied do not have a specific person responsible for communication due to lack of resources and time: they are rarely able to invest in hiring a communication specialist. Generally, communication is provided by volunteers who do not receive any type of remuneration and are likely to be women between the ages of 40 and 60. It turns out that organizations develop their communication strategies mainly through the internet. More than 80% of patient organizations have active pages. It is noted a little media-oriented option, as only 21% of organizations have an online press room. However, the digital option has gained space, since more than half of organizations use online social networks for communication purposes and view these networks as their most important and effective impact tool. Davies (2016) also observes the insights of rare diseases from online surveys, a relatively new experimental method by which information can be obtained in a direct manner and can benefit affected individuals in a short timeframe. The author advocates that this approach may be especially useful for getting an overview of the wide range of phenotypes that affect patients (many of which may not be intuitive) and for gaining information on those issues which most impair affected individuals' lives.

Liuccio et al. (2015) analyze the role of communication in rare diseases through a systematic literature review, focusing on the information patients extract from (digital and traditional) media and, secondly, on interpersonal patient-physician communication. They observe that "only 56 papers" (p. 3) were found to focus on the topic and use a narrative synthesis, highlighting three specific issues:

- **The source of medication information and other information on diseases:** Patients perceive physicians and internet as credible sources of medication information. The internet offers patients with rare disease:
    - **Perceived and objective disease knowledge:** An opportunity to connect with, acquire knowledge and support from others facing identical situations (Doyle, 2015; Lasker, Sogolow & Sharim, 2005; Mursch & Behnke-Mursch, 2003; Wicks et al., 2010);
    - **Self-diagnosis and prevention:** The possibility to screen prevention, diagnosis, and treatment of the disease, and also in early identification, personalized treatment, and health management in general (e.g. Dwyer, Quinton, Morin & Pitteloud, 2014; Kowalski, Kahana, Kuhr, Ansmann & Pfaff, 2014);

- ◦ **Self-expression and communication:** It enables to express concerns that patients could hardly communicate to their doctor and to prevent disease (Hilton-Kamm, Sklansky & Chang, 2014; Jhaveri, Schrier & Mattana, 2013; Zaid et al., 2013);
- ◦ **Health-related information and education:** The access to relevant information, especially older patients with little or no education and who live without a partner.

Patients use the internet more than they ask pharmacists for medication advice, also when dealing with side effects and drug effectiveness (Carpenter, Blalock & DeVellis, 2012).

- **The patient-physician interaction:** Communication processes, in this context, are predominately affected by the role behavior of both patient and health-care provider.
- **Psycho-social support:** Families with patients with rare diseases are negatively affected by delays-in diagnosis and by the scarcity of access to peer support groups and to psychological advice.

Specifically studying the alignment of Facebook with the priorities of rare diseases associations, Subirats et al. (2018), reinforcing results from previous studies (Reguera, 2017; Reguera, Subirats & Armayones, 2017) and using computational analysis, find that photos are the type of posts with the highest number of reactions and engagement, while statuses are the type of posts with the highest number of comments, and events are the type of posts with more shares (p. 11). Among the word clouds, the authors discover that in Facebook the highlighted words are gratitude instead of help, life, people and children (more present in decalogue) and that differences among word clouds are grouped by level of engagement: the low engagement word cloud is related to spam messages, while medium/high engagement word clouds are related to treatments. It is also observed a high correlation between the polarity and the time of day. The authors recommend to users interested in rare diseases who want to maximize their engagement of their posts: (1) use photos in their posts; (2) update their status; (3) post content of common interest; and (4) post at midday or late at night.

The literature review shows that only a few studies have fully considered the communication role set in rare disease and that there is no adequate attention paid to patients' health information seeking behaviours. Bouwman, Teunissen, Wijburg & Linthorst (2010) observe that, regarding rare diseases, the use of the internet may be an important tool in the diagnostic process. The authors present two cases in which concerned parents made a correct diagnosis of a lysosomal storage disorder in their child by searching the internet after a long doctor's delay. Black and Baker (2011) also have recognized the potential of digital media. The authors consider that the IDEA League[2] is an excellent example of the impact of patient advocacy groups, the internet, and social networking on the landscape of rare diseases.

Within the studies centered on the media agenda on rare diseases, it is noted that those that approach health communication in the press have been more abundant than those involving television.

Using framing theory, Castillo Sanchez analyzed the coverage of World Rare Disease Day in the Spanish print media (2013) and the visual picture of rare diseases in these media (2012). The author suggests that these diseases require a consolidated theoretical space within the media agenda. He also points out that an image reinforces a text, particularly when it shows affected patients and families, accompanied by institutional representatives, and topics that stand out for the geographical proximity to the reader.

Meanwhile, a quantitative analysis of the Andalusian press reports on 2012 World Rare Disease Day (Urrutia, 2013) reveals that the discourse was poorly structured and error-prone, reflecting the fragility of patient organizations and the need for change of focus without resorting to morbidity and pessimism.

A study of larger audience daily television news programs (Francescutti, Martínez Nicolás & Tucho Fernández, 2012) shows that health news coverage was particularly scarce, despite the value the Spanish public attaches to these topics. Patients and family members have become key subjects in the news approach, followed by doctors, pharmacists and authorities stating the issue. Furthermore, advances in treatment are overshadowed by negligence and medical errors. The programs use mainly official sources and the health reality presented on television has little or nothing to do with reality itself. Certain diseases are overrepresented, while others and dubious medical conditions are underrepresented.

Bañón Hernández (2007) concludes that patients with rare diseases, because of their systematic exclusion from the main discussion forums, are considered a minority group with generally little capacity to exert any significant influence on political and social issues. In this line, one evidence from the studies by the Centro de Investigación Biomédica en Red de Enfermedades Raras (CIBERER) is that the training and preparation of communicators influences the quality of information, and the effectiveness of the information would increase if there was a correlation between the official sources' discourse on the what is done and what is actually accomplished (Bañón Hernández, Alcaraz, Almela & Sanchis, 2011). Therefore, there is a need for patients with rare diseases and organizations working in this field to gain an effective voice in the public sphere.

To raise awareness for rare diseases, there has to be persuasive communication. If where there is meaning there is persuasion (Burke, 1969, p. 72), all communication – which brings together meanings – is persuasive. Persuasion may attempt to influence beliefs, attitudes, intentions, motivations or behaviors (Gass & Seiter, 2010, 33). In the persuasive way, Aristotle (IV century BC/2005) points to three means of persuasion:

- ***Ethos*:** Those derived from the character of the communicator (credibility, *ethos*);
- ***Pathos*:** Those derived from emotion aroused in the public (emotion, *pathos*); and
- ***Logos*:** those based on evidence, true or probable arguments and logically extracted inferences capable of making the audience adhere to the thesis put forward (reason, the *logos*) (2005, p. 37).

Yale University studies have also shown that the characteristics of the source, the message and the receiver influence persuasion (Hovland, Janis & Kelley, 1953).

It is worth noting that there are preconditions in health communication for it to be effective, that is, to produce the expected results. It is a strategical communication made to accomplish aims and to measure. For this, it must be credible, clear, meaningful, coherent over time, based on the evidence, personalized, tailored to the user's information needs at that time, adapted to his/her cultural level and cognitive style (Teixeira 1999, p. 617), "a practice that adapts messages to individuals" (Noar, Harrington, Van Stee & Aldrich, 2011, p. 113).

The persuasion theory (e.g. Hovland, Janis & Kelley, 1953) advocates that persuasive communication, transmitting the why, is pivotal when communicating a message to ignite behavior. The Hovland group also confirmed that communicators high in expertise and trustworthiness tend to be more persuasive (Ajzen, 1992, p. 5).

Finally, Hall's concepts of "dominant-hegemonic position", which allude to the symmetry and perfect fit between the encoding (by the sender) and the decoding (by the receiver) (Hall, 1973; 1980) is a precondition to an effective communication. It means that the receiver's decoding strategies proceed along the same logic as the producer's encoding strategies. Without conflict, the meaning is secured hegemonically, i.e., correctly perceived.

METHOD AND DATA

The research question that guide the study is: How do messages and practices of digital communication of EURORDIS contribute to create awareness and facilitate the process of diagnosis of rare diseases? The specific objectives formulated are: 1. to understand the EURORDIS-Rare Diseases Europe's use of digital media (website and Facebook page) and its role on awareness to rare diseases; and 2. to perceive how the video's messages can be useful in the awareness and diagnosis of rare diseases.

To accomplish the first objective, the messages and practices of digital communication of EURORDIS-Rare Diseases Europe were analyzed, concretely in the website and Facebook page. In the Facebook, the analysis period was between January and April of 2019.

To fulfill the second one, the video's potential, concretely a promotional video of EURORDIS entitled "Rare diseases: we are 30 million in Europe. Each of us is a real person"[3], with 13855 views, was analyzed, jointly with a collection of 12 videographically documented stories from 2018 and 2019, presented in the website, in the item "Living with a Rare Disease", from people who share their experiences of living with a rare disease. In total, the corpus has 13 videos.

The techniques used are qualitative content analysis and a more formal analysis, concretely the rhetorical analysis. The qualitative content analysis is the most prevalent approach to the qualitative analysis of documents. It comprises a searching out of underlying themes in the materials being analyzed (Bryman, 2012, p. 557).

To operate the technique, the procedures suggested by Altheide (2004) were adopted:

- **Step 1:** Generate a research question (How does EURORDIS create awareness towards rare diseases?);
- **Step 2:** Become familiar with the context within which the documents were / are generated;
- **Step 3:** Become familiar with a small number of documents (contents of website and Facebook);
- **Step 4:** Generate some categories (types of content and uses) that will guide the collection of data and draft a schedule for collecting the data in terms of the generated categories.

The type of qualitative analysis is mainly thematic. This means that the data is examined to extract core themes.

The rhetorical analysis is the examination of how texts persuade their audiences of their claims (Dysart-Gale 2010, p. 29). The aim of rhetorical analysis is not simply to describe the claims and arguments advanced within the discourse, but, most importantly, to identity the specific persuasive strategies employed by the speaker to accomplish specific persuasive goals (O'Donohue, 2013). In the analysis operationalized, the rhetoric devices referred by Aristotle, specially the *pathos* and *logos*, were used.

THE POTENTIAL OF DIGITAL MEDIA FOR CREATING AWARENESS TO RARE DISEASES OR "KNOWLEDGE IS POWER": FINDINGS

The European Voice of Rare Disease Patients: The Contribution of Digital Media For Creating Awareness

Website

The EURORDIS website can be synthesized in six types of content: 1. Information; 2. Clarification; 3. Personalization; 4. Support; 5. Appeal; and 6. Empowerment. These types of content or practices are related to the uses that EURORDIS gives to website.

In the category designated "information", it can be found some notes on "who we are" (what the EURORDIS is), "what we do" (EURORDIS' mission), "international activities" (EURORDIS' vision), "membership" (list of EURORDIS member associations), "library" (e.g. publications, activity reports, fact sheets and infographics), "our funding" (financial information, health sector corporates, top five donors), "job openings", "EURORDIS events" (summer schools, workshops), EURORDIS' advocacy for incentives, "members' news and announcements", "international rare disease events", "rare diseases in the arts" (the codification and inclusion of rare diseases in diverse arts, such dance, documentaries, movies, literature, functioning as an archive of artistic material focused on rare diseases), "EURORDIS webinars" (web seminars that provide interactive training on practical skills such as how to cultivate volunteers, social media and governance), "EURORDIS press releases", "eNews" ("read past issues of our weekly newsletter").

In the "clarification" category, EURORDIS uses contents that can contribute to better understanding and demystify some conceptions on rare diseases, such as: the document "rare diseases: understanding this public health priority"[4], some deconstructive information, such as: "a disease or disorder is defined rare in Europe when it affects less than 1 in 2,000 citizens" (Orphan Drug Regulation 141/2000)[5], "no existing effective cure"[6], "there are between 6,000 and 8,000 rare diseases, 75% of rare diseases affect children, 30% of rare disease patients die before the age of 15, 80% of rare diseases have identified genetic origins"[7], "rare disease patients and their families are known to be more pro-active than patients suffering from other common illnesses"[1], the clarification of some related concepts: rare diseases, neglected diseases, orphan diseases, orphan drugs.[5]

The "personalization" is present in the item "Living with a Rare Disease"[6]. In this item, there are various videos with testimonial stories and a list from A to Z, according to disease name, of testimonial stories. The support grounds on statements, such: "useful to do"[7], "good to know"[8], "how patient groups can get involved"[9].

The appeal is anchored in some suggested behaviors, such as: "improve the safety of your medicines"[10], "get involved"[11], giving guidelines to individuals, patient groups and companies, "donate"[12], "take action"[13], "connect with others"[14].

The empowerment can be found in some titles such as: "From isolation to empowerment of patients"[1], that focuses in the context of "insufficient scientific knowledge base and human isolation"[4] and the solutions patients and parents have developed: a variety of "self-help support groups"[15], creation of associations of patients and parents whose actions have already ensured progress in healthcare and social assistance provided to the victims, development of treatments, and in raising public awareness of this type of diseases.

Facebook

The contents shared on Facebook can be organized in the categories:

- **Information**: "The gaze-controlled digital device enables people living with physical disabilities", "Intimate Audrey exhibition", "Rare Barometer survey", "The 10th World Conference on #CorneliadeLange syndrome will take place 31 July - 4 August in Germany", "EURORDIS and Rare Diseases International met Dr. Tedros, Director-General of the World Health Organization (WHO), yesterday to discuss next steps towards a future collaboration to ensure people living with a rare disease are not left behind", "EURORDIS is leading the RARE-IMPACT initiative that aims to identify challenges and solutions to patients' access to #gene and cell therapies for rare diseases with secretariat support from Dolon", "Introducing ... the recipient of the EURORDIS Photo Award 2019 DEEP DERİN", "A brand new online shop has been launched for #RareDiseaseDay where you can find t-shirts, jumpers and much more!";
- **Appeal/invitation:** "Have you heard of EyeHarp?", "Community Advisory Board in your disease area? Join a workshop to learn what's involved in starting a CAB during the EURORDIS Membership Meeting", "Ask your returning or candidate Member of the European Parliament to pledge their support for the rare disease community", "Join the first 22q11 Northern

Ireland Conference", "Would you like to contribute to shaping the next 10 years of rare disease policy? Register for a webinar on 2 May at 12.00 CET to learn more about Rare2030 - Foresight in Rare Disease Policy & how you can help shape future recommendations on rare disease policy", "Register to join an event bringing together families and experts to discuss & exchange on Cornelia de Lange syndrome", "Want to get the latest information from the #raredisease community?", "Ask your returning or candidate Member of the European Parliament to pledge their support for rare diseases ahead of the European elections taking place in May!", "Are you looking to grow your rare disease network? Register for the EURORDIS Membership Meeting 2019 Bucharest", "Live now! EURORDIS 'How to' webinar: Learn about digital health ecosystems", "Take a look at the new website for more information https://rareimpact.eu/", "Want to get the latest information from the #raredisease community? Read our eNews and share your news too!", "Get inspired to join the #ShowYourRare campaign!", "Vote for your favourite photo to win the EURORDIS Photo Award 2019!";

- **Personalization:** "Ralf is a graduate of the #EURORDISSummerSchool & #EURORDISWinterSchool and shares his experience of becoming an active patient advocate for rare vascular diseases", "Sergio and his family had a long diagnostic odyssey before getting a diagnosis of #DravetSyndrome", "On #RareDiseaseDay 2019 watch and share Lorena's story of living with Phelan-McDermid syndrome to raise awareness of rare diseases!", video of Karlo who lives with the rare disease neurofibromatosis type 1, "Anne-Dauphine Julliand is the recipient of the EURORDIS Visual and Audio Media Award in recognition of her inspiring documentary film 'Et Les Mistrals Gagnants'", "HRH Princess Maria of Romania will show her support for the rare disease community by attending the EURORDIS #BlackPearl Awards Ceremony on 12 February", "Russell is the recipient of the EURORDIS Volunteer Award in recognition of his exceptional work as a patient advocate for all rare eye conditions through LHON Society and as a patient board member of Ern-Eye and for all rare diseases in his work as one of EURORDIS' longstanding volunteers".

In Facebook, some rhetorical devices are used, such as:

- ***Logos*:**
  - The question mark as a phatic or flashy element, which establishes contact, since demands a response;
  - Repetition: some initiatives and events are remembered in an intention to optimize the reception of the message and familiarity with it;

    - The information appears as a partner of the appeal, constructing a discourse that is mainly entangled in the informational and appeal functions;
    - Exemplification and personalization by referring to people who experience illnesses, encouraging empathy and identification among subjects who deal with the same diseases and disorders, as well as the supportive and empathic spirit to those involved in the promotion of causes related to rare diseases (***pathos***);
    - Exclamation mark is used as a phatic element and, this, a magnet for the reader's attention.
- ***Ethos*:**
    - The reference to "elite figures" such as Audrey Hepburn, affected by a rare cancer, Princess Maria of Romania, Dr Tedros, Director-General of the WHO, who being public figures and credible, persuade to an active and positive behavior and leverage the causes of EURORDIS.

Video as "Knowledge is Power": Usefulness of Messages in the Awareness and Diagnosis of Rare Diseases

Video "Rare Diseases: we are 30 million in Europe. Each of us is a Real Person"

The convocation to empathy and awareness and curiosity are stimulated (*pathos*). To argue the discourse, there are: evidence / statistical data and symbology (*logos*). The Table 1 shows the main points of analysis.

Testimonial videos

In the dimension of *pathos*, we find elements that motivate awareness and inspire the recipient. As elements of the *logos*, are used: credibility of sender, testimony, description of disease and identification of symptoms, factual data, statistic data, style devices, such as metaphor. For a detailed version, see Table 2.

SOLUTIONS AND RECOMMENDATIONS

The present study attempts to give some answers to the diagnosis made by a) Burke-Garcia and Scally (2014) of that there is an absence of both deep and wide understanding of the opportunities within digital media and by b) Bañón Hernández (2007), of that patients with rare diseases are considered a minority group with

Table 1. Rhetorical analysis to the promotional video "Rare Diseases: we are 30 million in Europe. Each of us is a real person"

Pathos	*Logos*
1. **Convocation to empathy and awareness**: "Each of us is a real person", "You can see us if you try" 2. The presence in several images of hands placed on the faces of patients creates **curiosity** in the recipient.	**1. Evidence/statistical data**: "A rare disease affects less than 1 in 2000 people", "There are more than 6000 rare diseases", "Together we are 30 million in Europe", "We are 30 million real people" **2. Symbology:** a) The presence, in several images, of hands placed on the faces of subjects denotes that behind the hands is someone whose identity is hidden, suggesting that the problem of rare diseases is hidden and not visible. b) The various characters, who appear throughout the video, present diversity in terms of age, gender, ethnicity / race. This eclecticism shows that rare disease can affect any individual. It can be inferred that it is a problem that can potentially affect anyone. c) When the characters remove their hands from the face, it is symbolized that rare diseases have a face. So it is not an abstract problem: it is concrete. It can be inferred that rare diseases affect humans and are real. d) According to the Egyptian system of hieroglyphs, the hands signify manifestation, action, donating and husbandry (Cirlot, 2013). Hand (2010) refers that the hands denote deeds (p. 168). So, in the context of video, there is an intention to awaken to the action.

Source: Author's ownnership

generally little capacity to exert any significant influence on political and social issues because of their systematic exclusion from the main discussion forums. Thus, it is suggested that organizations, which act in health, specifically in rare diseases (see Table 5):

a) reinforce their presence in the digital media, thus solving what the patient with Aniridia confessed: "the internet was also no expert in this field at the time", "hardly any articles popped up and all the images I saw scared me rather than informed me of what I had";
b) use rhetorical resources in the congregated sense of raising awareness among the general public and informing patients and their families, helping them to diagnose, and guiding them.

FUTURE RESEARCH DIRECTIONS

Continuing to respond to the diagnosis by Burke-Garcia and Scally (2014) and Bañón Hernández (2007), it will be useful to study ways in which patients with rare diseases gain a more audible voice in the public sphere and ways to optimize the use of digital media that could be an effective platform for information and

Table 2. Rhetorical analysis to the testimonial videos from 2018 to 2019

Title	Disease	Aim of message	Pathos	Logos
Sergio's Story (subtitled)	Dravet syndrome	"to end the diagnostic odyssey for children with a rare disease", "avoid this situation for other children", "we [Foundation 29, "a place where you can share your pain, share your problems, and get answers"] are able to diagnose these children early and avoid the same situation that we have for Sergio, our life will have a purpose"	**Awareness**: "the problem of this gap for the proper diagnosis is that we put Sergio on a bad treatment for Dravet. One day he had 20 seizures"	**Credibility of sender**: Father tells the story of the son; **Testimony**; **Description of disease and identification of symptoms; Statistic data**: "say that the average patient with a rare disease, they need to visit 7 specialists until having diagnosis", "the average time to diagnosis is 5 years"
SoulGreg Artist – My eternal love	GM1 gangliosidosis type 1	To share "a very personal song" written for his twenty-three-month old son Viljem Julijan, "to give support to all children, in the world, with rare diseases and their families"	**Awareness**: "I ask all people of good hearts to give care and send good thoughts to Viljem Julijan and to all the children with rare diseases"	**Credibility of sender**: Father composes a song
Pensavo di essere diverso	XLPDR	To make known the journey through differences, a meeting with Alex, the only case in Italy of the rare disorder XLPDR	**Awareness**: "perfection doesn't exist, we exist with our differences"	**Credibility of sender**: Speech in the first voice – Alex; **Testimony; Description of disease and identification of symptoms**
Living in a body of open wounds with less than half his skin	Epidermolysis Bullosa	To promote the purposes of Special Books by Special Kids, "to prove no matter how you communicate or what obstacles you face you are always deserving of love and acceptance"	**Awareness and inspiration**: "John still find hope in serving as an example for others that it is possible to survive difficult times"	**Credibility of sender**: Interview to John and his family; **Testimony; Description of disease and identification of symptoms**
Short Bowel Syndrome with intestinal failure. Patient Stories: Rosie	Short Bowel Syndrome with Intestinal Failure	"Learn about how her parents managed her condition"	**Awareness**: "it is not a life for anyone basically", "our life changed completely since Rosie come home", "she is always on my mind"	**Credibility of sender**: Parents tell the story of Rosie; **Testimony; Description of disease and identification of symptoms**
Short Bowel Syndrome with intestinal failure. Patient Stories: Leo	Short Bowel Syndrome with Intestinal Failure-gastroschisis	"Learn about how his parents manage it for him here"	**Awareness**: "he loves being around people, he loves socializing, he loves doing everything that every other child love doing"	**Credibility of sender**: Parents tell the story; **Testimony; Description of disease and identification of symptoms**

Source: Author's ownership

Table 3. Rhetorical analysis to the testimonial videos from 2018 to 2019 (cont.)

Title	Disease	Aim of message	*Pathos*	*Logos*
VWM Families Foundation: Sam's story	Vanishing White Matter Disease (VWM)	To promote the VWM Families Foundation	**Awareness:** "We change our approach to life, focusing on what is important", We do not know how many years he will live, we decided to much how much time we can in family	**Credibility of sender:** Parents tell the story **Testimony; Description of disease and identification of symptoms; Statistical data:** There is no treatment or cure for VWM and there are only 250 cases worldwide
Sophie's search for a cure – Multiple system atrophy	Multiple System Atrophy (MSA)	To show and raise awareness to the Sophie's story	**Awareness:** "I feel helpless that I can't help her", "she wants as much time as she can have"	**Credibility of sender:** Diverse testimonial (e.g. Sophie, family) A medical intervention (D. M. Togasaki) **Description of disease and identification of symptoms; Factual data:** an untreatable, fatal "Parkinson's-plus" disorder; **Statistical data:** "over 50,000 people in North America are afflicted with MSA"
The last remaining light	Addison's Disease	To make known the disease: "diseased often suffer several years before receiving proper diagnosis and treatment. For some, that moment is just too late", maybe I am not just here for the story... Because this place is a pleasant sight for sore eyes and like a soothing balm for a jaded soul"	**Awareness** and **inspiration:** "The moment you think you know exactly where life is heading, it can be the moment you are losing it altogether", "I don't think even occurred to me at the time just how simple life was, when I was in good health", "never to let Addison's disease become limiting factor in my life", the hardest of feelings: that no one can see your struggle", "I feel deeper and deeper in depression", "When I ride the bike, it feels like nothing can stop me"	**Credibility of sender:** Speech in the first voice; **Testimony; Description of disease and identification of symptoms; Metaphor:** "It was like slowly dimming the light in my lamp until there was nothing but darkness", "it was like gravity", Bicycle as freedom, sights, rush of adrenaline

Source: Author's ownership

communication. As a complement and as it is noted that the rare diseases' issues have been more abundant in the press than in the television, there is a need to sensitize all media to the problems that affect patients with rare diseases and their families. And there is also a need for health communication to be more two-way.

The present study contributes to the level of the sender and the message. It is proposed to continue to study the communication of rare diseases, specifically in response to Burke-Garcia and Scally's (2014) assessment of the need for rigorous

Table 4. Rhetorical analysis to the testimonial videos from 2018 to 2019 (cont.)

Title	Disease	Aim of message	*Pathos*	*Logos*
Aniridia: My story	Aniridia		**Awareness** and **inspiration**: "to see the world as a gift and I am reminded of that every day", "the potential to become blind from aniridia is significant", "growing up as a kid with aniridia I was known as the girl who always wore sunglasses outsider", "I knew I was different"	**Credibility of sender**: Speech in the first voice; **Testimony; Description of disease and identification of symptoms; Statistical data**: "Aniridia occurs in 1 in 50,000 to 1000,000 newborns worldwide"
Butterfly children: Raed's story	Epidermolysis Bullosa	To show and raise awareness to the Raed's story and to Epidermolysis Bullosa's patients	**Awareness**: "It is not our duty to force our child to really accept this cruel and harsh society, but I feel like it is the job of every parent to make this world a less cruel place to live in", "DEBRA [which helps to support EB patients financially and emotionally] has taken three quarters of our difficulties and also built up my self-confidence", "10% per cent is what the world gives you. But 90 per cent is how you are going to react to the challenges the world throws at you"	**Credibility of sender**: Parents tell the story; Intervention of medical specialists (Dr Mark Koh, Prof E. Birgitte Lane); **Testimony; Description of disease and identification of symptoms; Factual data**: "Currently, there is no cure", "only dressing and creams can be used to help with the blistering"; **Metaphor**: "it was a skinless chicken" "the term "butterfly children" is used because the wings of a butterfly are very very fragile"
CELI4 p-/ Look at the person and not the disease	Wolf-Hirschhorn Syndrome	"Look at the person and not the disease", "Help with the investigation of Wolf-Hirschhorn Syndrome"	**Awareness** and **inspiration**: "They love her [Celia] so much and knew she could do anything", "I never give up"	**Credibility of sender**: images show the family of Celia and their experiences. The written text tells the story; **Testimony; Description of disease and identification of symptoms**

Source: Author's ownership

Table 5. Suggestions, from empirical results, to health organizations act in the digital media

<table>
<tr><th colspan="3">Types of content and uses of digital media</th></tr>
<tr><td colspan="3">1. Information: Messages that privilege objective content, such as the dissemination of events;
2. Clarification: Contents that can contribute to better understanding and demystify some conceptions;
3. Personalization: Contents that give face to the action, trying to humanize the problems, and create empathy, even though psychological mechanisms of projection and identification, inspire and motivate;
4. Support: Contents that guide action, suggesting useful behaviors;
5. Appeal: Contents that are, in essence, motivators of action, stimulating, convincing, making happen;
6. Empowerment: Contents that allow to give more power to the receiver, providing him with self-efficacy.</td></tr>
<tr><td colspan="3">Rhetorical devices</td></tr>
<tr><td>Ethos</td><td>Pathos</td><td>Logos</td></tr>
<tr><td>1. Reference to "elite figures" (e.g. medical specialists)
2. Credibility of sender</td><td>1. Awareness
2. Inspiration
3. Convocation to empathy
4. Curiosity</td><td>1. Use of the question mark as a phatic or flashy element, to stablish contact;
2. Repetition, in order to assist in the memorization;
3. Mix of information and appeal;
4. Exemplification and personalization, in order to show that the problems are real, concrete and human;
5. Use of the exclamation point a phatic element and, thus, a magnet for the reader's attention
6. Factual data;
7. Statistical data;
8. Symbology;
9. Style figures (e.g. metaphor);
10. Credibility of sender;
11. Testimony;
12. Description of disease and enumeration of symptoms.</td></tr>
</table>

Source: Author's ownership

evaluative studies of effectiveness of the message among recipients, including patients, are few and far between. It may also be a future research direction, in methodological terms, to use computational analysis tools in order to complement the qualitative dimension of the given analysis.

Therefore, studies on communication with the commitment to raise awareness among the general public, studies evaluating communication based on digital media or a multimedia dimension, and studies that focus on the potential of communication to sustain diagnoses are welcome.

CONCLUSION

EURORDIS uses digital media to raise awareness of its causes, corresponding to the idea that social media, used within health care contexts for communication purposes, are increasing and becoming more acceptable (Burke-Garcia & Scally, 2014; Moorhead, 2017). EURORDIS uses social media to inform, clarify, personalize, support, appeal, and empower, benefiting from the uses of social media for healthcare communication (Moorhead, 2017), such as: improved interactions with others; more available, shared, and tailored information; increased accessibility and widening access; and increased peer/social/emotional support are some of numerous benefits of social media for healthcare communication (Moorhead, 2017).

Although Burke-Garcia and Scally (2014) ascertain that there is an absence of both deep and wide understanding of the opportunities within digital media and that the smart and strategic planning for its widespread use is not the common practice, it seems that EURORDIS has been able to leverage its communication through digital means and that has perceived the digital potential for the dissemination of information, which helps in the diagnosis, and awareness of the causes in which it is involved.

The results coincide with the topics found by Liuccio et al. (2015): (a) the source of information on diseases: it is notorious the effort that EURORDIS makes to be multidimensional (information, clarification, personalization, support, appeal and empowerment) in the contents that it offers; b) psycho social support: families with patients with rare diseases are negatively affected by delays-in diagnosis and by the scarcity of access to peer support groups and to psychological advice. Sergio's father, in their testimonial video, refers to the difficulty in correctly diagnosing Sergio and has created a foundation to help the correct diagnosis in a timely manner.

The results can confirm that the internet offers patients with rare disease: 1. an opportunity to connect with, acquire knowledge and support from others facing identical situations (Doyle, 2015; Lasker, Sogolow & Sharim, 2005; Mursch & Behnke-Mursch, 2003; Wicks et al., 2010); 2. the possibility to screen prevention, diagnosis, and treatment of the disease, and also in early identification, personalized treatment, and health management in general (e.g. Dwyer, Quinton, Morin, & Pitteloud, 2014; Kowalski, Kahana, Kuhr, Ansmann & Pfaff, 2014); 3. permits to express concerns that patients could hardly communicate to their doctor (Hilton-Kamm, Sklansky & Chang, 2014; Jhaveri, Schrier & Mattana, 2013; Zaid et al., 2013); 4. the access to relevant information. Patients use the internet more than they ask pharmacists for medication advice, also when dealing with side effects and drug effectiveness (Carpenter, Blalock & DeVellis, 2012).

By sharing information and testimonies listing disease symptoms and experiences with rare diseases, EURORDIS, through its online resources, can help with diagnosis. Bouwman et al. (2010), also, observe that, for rare diseases, the use of the internet may be an important tool in the diagnostic process.

In the testimonial videos, the patient tends to be accompanied by his/her families, and their difficulties to deal with the disease can be visually and verbally observed by publics. The visual complement that allows viewing tends to have a sharper effect on empathy and awareness. Castillo Sanchez (2012; 2013), also, on the visual picture of rare diseases in media, highlight that an image reinforces the text, particularly when it shows affected patients and families, accompanied by institutional representatives, and topics that stand out for the geographical proximity to the viewer.

The rhetorical devices used in Facebook's messages, to communicate with patients and members, make them more attractive and motivate for persuasion: a) the question as a phatic or flashy element, which establishes contact, since demands a response; b) repetition: some initiatives and events are remembered in order to optimize the reception of the message and familiarity with the message; c) the information appears as a partner of the appeal, constructing and improving the potential of a discourse that is mainly entangled in the informational and appeal functions; d) exemplification and personalization by referring to people who experience illnesses, encouraging empathy and identification of people who deal and not deal with same diseases and disorders, and to those involved in the promotion of causes related to rare diseases, as stimulating a supportive and empathic spirit (*pathos*); e) the exclamation point is used as a phatic element and, thus, a magnet for the reader's attention; f) the reference to "elite figures" makes the speech credible. The credibility of the sender is also present in all testimonial videos, through the presence of the patient and his/her family and also through the presence of medical specialists. The construction of personal stories of suffering helps individuals to understand certain situations (Sharf & Vanderford, 2003, p. 29). Hovland group confirmed that communicators high in expertise and trustworthiness (such as medical specialists) tend to be more persuasive (Ajzen, 1992, p. 5); g) the description of disease and enumeration of symptoms contribute to a potential diagnosis of the receiver. The factual and statistical data and style resources help to persuade. For Aristotle (IV century/2005), proof and demonstration are fundamental in oratory discourse (p. 49). Style figures concretize and clarify the sender's speech (Corbett, 2004, 143). The use of examples gives a better illustration of the speaker's statement (Petric, 2007, p. 263).

Given the conclusion by Bañón Hernández (2007) that patients with rare diseases, owing to their systematic exclusion from the main discussion forums, are considered a minority group with generally little capacity to exert any significant influence on political and social issues, all means and resources will be welcome to give voice to patients with rare diseases. Subirats et al. (2018), previously, made some recommendations regarding the Facebook. Overall, digital media can give voice and knowledge, and both are power.

REFERENCES

Ajzen, I. (1992). *Persuasive communication theory in social psychology: A historical perspective* (pp. 1–16). Amherst, MA: University of Massachusetts.

Altheide, D. L. (2004). Ethnographic content analysis. In M. S. Lewis-Beck, A. Bryman, & T. F. Liao. (Eds.), The Sage encyclopedia of social science research methods, 3 vols. (pp. 325-326). Thousand Oaks, CA: Sage.

Aristotle. (IV century BC/2005). Retórica. Lisboa, Portugal: Imprensa Nacional-Casa da Moeda.

Bañón Hernández, A. M. (2007). Las enfermedades raras y su representación discursiva. Propuestas para un análisis crítico. *Discurso & Sociedad*, *2*(1), 188–229.

Bañón Hernández, A. M., Alcaraz, J. F., Almela, J. S., & Sanchis, I. R. (2011). *Desafíos y estrategias comunicativas de las enfermedades raras: La investigación médica como referente: Estudio cuantitativo-discursivo de la prensa escrita impresa y digital española (2009-2010).* Valencia, Spain: CIBERER.

Black, A. P., & Baker, M. (2011). The impact of parent advocacy groups, the Internet, and social networking on rare diseases: The IDEA League and IDEA League United Kingdom example. *Epilepsia*, *52*(Suppl 2), 102–104. doi:10.1111/j.1528-1167.2011.03013.x PMID:21463291

Bouwman, M. G., Teunissen, Q. G. A., Wijburg, F. A., & Linthorst, G. E. (2010). 'Doctor Google' ending the diagnostic odyssey in lysosomal storage disorders: Parents using internet search engines as an efficient diagnostic strategy in rare diseases. *Archives of Disease in Childhood*, *95*(8), 642–U96. doi:10.1136/adc.2009.171827 PMID:20418338

Bryman, A. (2012). *Social records methods.* New York: Oxford University Press.

Burke, K. (1969). *A rhetoric of motives.* Berkeley, CA: University of California Press.

Burke-Garcia, A., & Scally, G. (2014). Trending now: Future directions in digital media for the public health sector. *J. Public Health*, *36*(4), 527–534. doi:10.1093/pubmed/fdt125 PMID:24468840

Carpenter, D. M., Blalock, S. J., & DeVellis, R. F. (2012). Patients with rare diseases using pharmacists for medication information. *Journal of the American Pharmaceutical Association*, *52*(6), e175–e182. doi:10.1331/JAPhA.2012.12047 PMID:23942759

Castillo-Esparcia, A., & López-Villafranca, P. (2016). Communication strategies employed by rare disease patient organizations in Spain. *Ciência & Saúde Coletiva, 21*(8). Retrieved from http://www.scielo.br/scielo.php?pid=S1413-81232016000802423&script=sci_arttext&tlng=en (Access date: August 25, 2019)

Castillo Sánchez, S. (2012). Representación social de las enfermedades raras en la prensa española. Aposta. *Revista de Ciencias Sociales*, *54*, 1.

Castillo Sánchez, S. (2013). Las enfermedades raras en la prensa española: una aproximación empírica desde la teoría del framing. *Ambitos: Revista internacional de comunicación,* 22, 71-80.

Cirlot, J. E. (2013). *A dictionary of symbols*. New York: Philosophical Library.

Corbett, E. (2004). Classical Rhetoric. In J. Rivkin, & M. Ryan (Eds.), Literary theory, an anthology (pp. 142-161). Malden, MA: Blackwell Publishing.

Davies, W. (2016). Insights into rare diseases from social media surveys. *Orphanet Journal of Rare Diseases*, *11*(1), 151. doi:10.118613023-016-0532-x PMID:27829465

Doyle, M. (2015). Peer Support and Mentorship in a US Rare Disease Community: Findings from the Cystinosis in Emerging Adulthood Study. *Patient*, *8*(1), 65–73. doi:10.100740271-014-0085-9 PMID:25231828

Dwyer, A. A., Quinton, R., Morin, D., & Pitteloud, N. (2014). Identifying the unmet health needs of patients with congenital hypogonadotropic hypogonadism using a web-based needs assessment: Implications for online interventions and peer-to-peer support. *Orphanet Journal of Rare Diseases*, *9*(1), 83. doi:10.1186/1750-1172-9-83 PMID:24915927

Dysart-Gale, D. (2010). Techne, technology, and disenchantment in the wind in The Wind in the Willows. In J. C. Horne, & D. R. White (Eds.), *Kenneth Grahame's the wind in the willows: A children's classic at 100*. Lanham, MD: Scarecrow Press.

Francescutti, L. P., Martínez Nicolás, M., & Tucho Fernández, F. (2012). *La información sanitaria en los telediarios*. Madrid, Spain: Almud Ediciones.

Gass, R. H., & Seiter, J. S. (2010). *Persuasion, social influence, and compliance gaining*. Boston, MA: Allyn & Bacon.

Grunig, J., & Hunt, T. (1984). *Managing public relations*. New York, NY: CBS College Publishing.

Hall, S. (1973). *Encoding and decoding in the media discourse. Stencilled Paper 7*. Birmingham: CCCS.

Hall, S. (1980). Encoding/decoding. In D. Hobson, A. Lowe, & P. Willis (Eds.), *Culture, media, language* (pp. 128–138). London, UK: Hutchinson.

Hand, S. S. (2010). *Finishing the mysteries of gods and symbols* (Vol. 0, p. II). Lawrence, W.

Hilton-Kamm, D., Sklansky, M., & Chang, R. K. (2014). How not to tell parents about their child's new diagnosis of congenital heart disease: An Internet survey of 841 parents. *Pediatric Cardiology, 35*(2), 239–252. doi:10.100700246-013-0765-6 PMID:23925415

Hovland, C. I., Janis, I. L., & Kelley, H. H. (1953). *Communication and Persuasion: Psychological studies of opinion change. Yale*. Yale University Press.

Jhaveri K. D., Schrier P. B., Mattana J. (2013). Paging Doctor Google!. *Heuristics vs. technology, 2*, 90. doi:10.12688/f1000research.2-90.v2

Korompilias, V. (2018). *Relational awareness: Experience architecture manuals*. Copyrighted material.

Kowalski, C., Kahana, E., Kuhr, K., Ansmann, L., & Pfaff, H. (2014). Changes over time in the utilization of disease-related internet information in newly diagnosed breast cancer patients 2007 to 2013. *Journal of Medical Internet Research, 16*(8), e195. doi:10.2196/jmir.3289 PMID:25158744

Lasker, J. N., Sogolow, E. D., & Sharim, R. R. (2005). The role of an online community for people with a rare disease: Content analysis of messages posted on a primary biliary cirrhosis mailing list. *Journal of Medical Internet Research, 7*(1), e10. doi:10.2196/jmir.7.1.e10 PMID:15829472

Liuccio, M., Belotti, R., Comune, A., Zambito, V., & Schulz, P. J. (2015). Communication in rare diseases: A literature review. *Journal of Communication Research, 7*(3), 2–10.

Moorhead, S. A. (2017). Social media for healthcare communication. *Oxford Research Encyclopedias*. Retrieved from https://oxfordre.com/communication/view/10.1093/acrefore/9780190228613.001.0001/acrefore-9780190228613-e-335 (Access date: August 25, 2019)

Mursch, K., & Behnke-Mursch, J. (2003). Internet-based interaction among brain tumour patients. Analysis of a medical mailing list. *Zentralblatt fur Neurochirurgie*, *64*(2), 71–75. doi:10.1055-2003-40375 PMID:12838475

Noar, S. M., Harrington, N. G., Van Stee, S. V., & Aldrich, R. S. (2011). Tailored health communication to change lifestyle behaviours. *American Journal of Lifestyle Medicine*, *5*(5), 112–122. doi:10.1177/1559827610387255

O'Donohue, W. (2013). *Clinical psychology and the philosophy of science*. Switzerland: Springer. doi:10.1007/978-3-319-00185-2

Petric, B. (2007). Rhetorical functions of citations in high- and low-rated master's theses. *Journal of English for Academic Purposes*, *6*(3), 238–253. doi:10.1016/j.jeap.2007.09.002

Polich, G. R. (2012). Rare disease patient groups as clinical researchers. *Drug Discovery Today*, *17*(3-4), 167–172. doi:10.1016/j.drudis.2011.09.020 PMID:22016088

Reguera, N. (2017). *Las enfermedades raras en grupos de Facebook: Evaluación de la línea de actuación de FEDER mediante minería de textos* (Master's thesis), Universitat Oberta de Catalunya, Barcelona, Spain.

Reguera, N., Subirats, L., & Armayones, M. (2017, June 22–24). Mining Facebook data of people with rare diseases. In *Proceedings of 2017 IEEE 30th International Symposium on Computer-Based Medical Systems (CBMS)* (pp. 588-593). Thessaloniki, Greece: CBMS. 10.1109/CBMS.2017.124

Roberts, H., Seymour, B., Fish II, S. A., Robinson, E., & Zuckerman, E. (2017). Digital health communication and global public influence: A study of the ebola epidemic. *J. Health Communication, 22*(sup1), 51-58. doi:10.1080/10810730.2016.1209598

Schneider, S., & Velmans, M. (2007). *The Blackwell Companion to Consciousness*. Victoria, Australia: Blackwell Publishing Asia.

Sharf, B., & Vanderford, M. (2003). Illness narratives and the social construction of health. In T. Thompson, A. Dorsey, K. Miller, & R. Parrott (Eds.), *Handbook of health communication* (pp. 9–34). New Jersey: Lawrence Erlbaum Associates.

Subirats, L., Reguera, N., Bañón, A., Gómez-Zúñiga, B., Minguillón, J., & Armayones, M. (2018). Mining Facebook data of people with rare diseases: A content-based and temporal analysis. *International Journal of Environmental Research and Public Health, 15*(9), 1877. doi:10.3390/ijerph15091877 PMID:30200209

Urrutia, J. M. (2013). El Día Mundial de las Enfermedades Raras en las noticias de prensa. El ejemplo de Andalucía. *Discurso & Sociedad, 1*(7), 224–247.

Wallack, L., Dorfman, L., Jernigan, D., & Themba-Nixon, M. (1993). *Media advocacy and public health: Power for prevention*. Newbury Park, CA: Sage.

Wicks, P., Massagli, M., Frost, J., Brownstein, C., Okun, S., Vaughan, T., ... Heywood, J. (2010). Sharing health data for better outcomes on PatientsLikeMe. *Journal of Medical Internet Research, 12*(2), e19. doi:10.2196/jmir.1549 PMID:20542858

Zaid, T., Burzawa, J., Basen-Engquist, K., Bodurka, D. C., Ramondetta, L. M., Brown, J., & Frumovitz, M. (2014). Use of social media to conduct a cross-sectional epidemiologic and quality of life survey of patients with neuroendocrine carcinoma of the cervix: A feasibility study. *Gynecologic Oncology, 132*(1), 149–153. doi:10.1016/j.ygyno.2013.10.015 PMID:24145111

KEY TERMS AND DEFINITIONS

Awareness: Ability to directly know and perceive, to feel, or to be cognizant of events.

Dominant-Hegemonic Position: When the receiver takes the connoted meaning from the media content, full and straight, and decodes the message in terms of the reference code in which it has been encoded. It can be said that the receiver is operating inside the dominant code, being this case an ideal-typical case of "perfectly transparent communication."

Ethos: Credibility derived from the character of the communicator.

EURORDIS: A non-profit alliance of 837 rare disease patient organizations from 70 countries that work together to improve the lives of the 30 million people living with a rare disease in Europe.

Inlinks: Hyperlinks directed to own websites.

Logos: Based on evidence, true or probable arguments and logically extracted inferences capable of making the audience adhere to the thesis put forward (reason).

Online Press Room: A section of the website for media's use, containing all news releases (archived by date, typically), photos, videos, brochures, catalogs.

Pathos: Those derived from emotion aroused in the public (emotion).

ENDNOTES

1 Further information can be obtained in the following link: https://www.eurordis.org/who-we-are (Access date: September 4, 2019)

2 The International Dravet syndrome Epilepsy Action League (IDEA League), founded by parents of children with Dravet syndrome in October 2005 and officially designated a tax-exempt public charity in the United States of America in November 2006, is the leading patient advocacy organization for Dravet syndrome and related genetic ion-channel epilepsy disorders. The organization spurred the creation of regional affiliates, becoming international. The IDEA League's mission encompasses international support and outreach for patients and families, as well as collaboration with physicians, medical education, health care coordination, and research

3 Rare Diseases: We are 30 million in Europe. Each of us is a real person. Available in https://www.youtube.com/watch?time_continue=1&v=-N8zbmMONSc (Access date: September 4, 2019)

4 Rare Diseases: Understanding this Public Health Priority. Available in https://www.eurordis.org/IMG/pdf/princeps_document-EN.pdf (Access date: September 4, 2019)

5 What is a Rare Disease? Available in https://www.eurordis.org/IMG/pdf/Fact_Sheet_RD.pdf (Access date: September, 4, 2019)

6 Living with a Rare Disease, Available in https://www.eurordis.org/living-with-a-rare-disease (Access date: September, 4, 2019)

7 EURORDIS - Useful to do, Available in https://www.eurordis.org/pharmacovigilance-useful-to-do (Access date: September, 4, 2019)

8 EURORDIS – Good to Know, Available in https://www.eurordis.org/pharmacovigilance-good-to-know (Access date: September, 4, 2019)

9 EURORDIS – How Patients can get involved, Available in https://www.eurordis.org/get-involved/patient-groups (Access date: September, 4, 2019)

10 EURORDIS – Pharmacovigilance: Improve the safety of your medicines, Available in https://www.eurordis.org/pharmacovigilance (Access date: September, 4, 2019)

11 EURORDIS – Get Involved, Available in https://www.eurordis.org/get-involved (Access date: September, 4, 2019)

12 EURORDIS – Donation, Available in https://donation.eurordis.org/ (Access date: September, 4, 2019)

13 EURORDIS – Get involved, Available in https://www.eurordis.org/get-involved-individuals-take-action (Access date: September, 4, 2019)

14 EURORDIS – Connect with others, Available in https://www.eurordis.org/get-involved-individuals-connect-with-others (Access date: September, 4, 2019)

15 Code of Practice Between Patients' Organisations and the Healthcare Industry, Available in https://www.eurordis.org/sites/default/files/thumbnails/0904-PO-Code%20of%20practice.pdf (Access date: September, 4, 2019)

Chapter 5
Public Media Coverage of Rare Diseases and Disorders:
The Case of Spanish Public Broadcasting Corporation

Yolanda Berdasco-Gancedo
https://orcid.org/0000-0003-0291-0617
Universidad a Distancia de Madrid, Spain

ABSTRACT

Rare diseases and disorders are, as the names suggest, a strange or unusual health condition, and so the coverage given by the media is not as extensive as it could be. However, researchers point out that this situation is changing little by little, and there is now more information about those who suffer from these conditions, and their experience. It is quite interesting to see how the public media, especially in the case of Spain, are making a great effort to give a voice and space to people affected by such diseases. In the case of public media, there are many other aspects to be considered. Firstly, the Spanish Broadcasting Corporation, Radio Televisión Española (RTVE) is not tied to private finance. Secondly, these channels are expected to be more independent and, subsequently, there may be no additional pressure to reach high audience share or obtain external funding from private media companies. This is especially interesting in the case of radio broadcasting, as it tends to be a medium with a high level of credibility, and closeness to the audience.

DOI: 10.4018/978-1-7998-2088-8.ch005

INTRODUCTION

Public media services are committed to improving people's quality of life and serving the public interest by contributing to an informed society and having a great impact on individual's daily living (*e.g.* voting, behaviour change, protesting) (Perse, Kubey, & Csikszentmihalyi, 1991; Wright, 1960). Indeed, a number of organizations, such as United Nations Educational, Scientific and Cultural Organization (UNESCO) have attempted to clarify the role of Public Service Broadcasting (PSB) and explain what would be expected from those media. One of the most obvious tasks of PSB is covering issues that are out of the scope of commercial media but meet the citizens' general interest. RTVE follows United Nations Public Service Broadcasting (PSB) recommendations[1] and as such, it aims to give a voice and a space to a general audience.

This chapter focuses on media coverage of rare diseases in Spanish public media. RTVE has a wide coverage of this area, using all the available channels: TV, radio, web services and social media profiles.

The investigation takes the form of a case-study in which RTVE broadcasts dealing with information about rare diseases are analysed, focusing on the content, data sources and the way information is included and presented.

The main aim of this chapter is to understand the way health-related information about rare diseases is covered in Spanish Public Broadcasting Corporation, namely, its conditions and treatments. Furthermore, it discusses the role of RTVE in satisfying Public Broadcasting Service (PBS) duties in spreading health-related information. Comparisons between public and commercial media are also made.

The author makes a distinction between programmes which deal with global and general information about these conditions, and those in which the individual situation of a person affected by a rare disease is presented. Likewise, the difference is noted between those programmes in which the disease and illness-related topics are the focus and those in which the interrelationships between different actors, such as doctors, organization spokespersons are in the spotlight.

The rationale for spreading health-related information about rare diseases is twofold: (a) underline that a rare disease exists; and (b) inform about the diagnostics and effects, in order to obtain some funding or research investment. Nonetheless, health-related journalism is still in need of accuracy, reliability and depth stories (Holtzman, et al., 2005; Smith, 2006).

By analysing information and communication in mass media, it is important to take into account polarization, frequency, or campaign initiatives, e.g. World Day of Rare Disease. Another significant aspect is also the relevancy to know whether they are using only traditional channels, i.e. television and radio to spread this information, or if they are including other platforms, such as a multimedia page (rtve.es) and social media channels (i.e. Twitter, Facebook).

Finally, the way in which this information is presented also shows the strength of commitment of a chosen media source (in this case, RTVE) to people affected by rare diseases and disorders. Whether this content is presented only as part of a longer informative programme as a one-minute-piece, or is given more attention, with a documentary or with a more thorough treatment.

BACKGROUND

Public Broadcasting Service (PBS) in Europe: A Brief Overview

Public Broadcasting Service (PSB) has existed in Europe for more than eighty years now and has evolved and faced many challenges, such as financial problems or commercial channels creation. However, it is not accurate to speak broadly of public media in Europe considering that there are several models of public service broadcasting, depending on their place in the national media system, the way they are funded or the relationship between public authorities and public media.

David Hendy (2013: 26) overstates the importance of content in comparison with profit-seeking media services. In his words:

Whereas in a commercial system, programmes would be made to acquire money, in this public system money was henceforth acquired to make programmes (Hendy, 2013:26).

Furthermore, PBS may support democracy (Harrison, & Woods, 2001) or, as Hendy puts it, 'nourishing democracy' and as d'Haenens and colleagues (2011:197) state, these media have the mission to ensure content provision regardless of its interest to audience share and popularity, fostering education and cultural programmes.

Focusing on thematic patterns, the study carried out by d'Haenens and colleagues (2011:197) unravels the following:

Public broadcasting time mainly goes to fiction, information, news, and to a lesser degree, to arts, humanities and sciences (d'Haenens et al., 2011:197)

In terms of the global ecosystem in the Spanish media, Spain was classified by Hallin and Mancini (2004: 3) as a country with a 'polarized pluralist model' 'with considerable levels of politicisation, state intervention and clientelism'. This applies not only to PSB but also to the media in general.

Papatheodorou and Machin (2003: 31-54) delve into Spanish public broadcasting peculiarities and they note:

The Press made a pact with the political forces in the first years of the transition to strengthen the brand-new democracy, but this agreement lasted too long, preventing the press from evolving towards a more mature and less partisan media system.

This evolution does not seem to be easy, either in Spain or in other European countries with an important tradition of public radio broadcasting, as the Dutch public broadcaster Nederlandse Omroepprogramma Stichting (NOS, 1999) recognizes:

Public broadcasting is associated with effort, commercial broadcasting with relaxation. Young people in particular are turning away from the public broadcaster.... A public broadcasting system that wishes to play a significant role in society must have a significant audience' (Nos, 1999:2).

As it will be later described, audience gathering is one of the main difficulties of public service broadcasting, and it seems that a process of adaptation is needed to achieve this aim, something that has been acknowledged by several authors since the beginning of the new century:

It is not easy to be a successful public service broadcaster now, particularly because the yardstick against which public broadcasters are often measured is one formulated when competition and choice were very much less developed than they now are. But the conclusion that if circumstances have changed, so must public service broadcasting, seems inescapable (Collins et. Al., 2001: 6).

Spanish Public Media Corporation: RTVE

In such a highly decentralized country as Spain, two public broadcasting systems coexist: a national television broadcaster, RTVE, that can be accessed all around the Spain; and many autonomic TV channels, which only broadcast within their respective Autonomous Community.

The Spanish public media corporation, RTVE Corporation, is a state-owned company, known as RTVE Public Entity until 2006. It is the largest Spanish-speaking broadcasting group and it is entirely funded by public subsidies. Within the company umbrella, there are three main divisions: Spanish National (Radio RNE), Spanish Television (TVE) and Interactive media (RTVE.es). An orchestra and a formative institute are also part of the Public Media Corporation.

In terms of the RTVE funding, legal changes in TV commercials have occurred after the 2006, but some sponsorship information is still present in television programmes. In the case of radio broadcasting, however, commercials have never been broadcast. Although it is not privately owned and there is no pressure from commercial firms, some groups argue that this media corporation suffers from political interference and that its independence is not complete.

Based on its operation and aims, RTVE can be considered a complete public service media corporation (Fernández-Alonso, & Fernaández-Viso, 2012; León, 2010) as it follows public service general requirements, informing, educating and entertaining citizens, guaranteeing pluralism, programming diversity, editorial independence, appropriate funding, accountability and transparency.

RTVE Corporation is a clear example of public broadcasting because a wide range of their programmes, not only on television but also on it radio channels, try to cover the gaps existing in the commercial media, such as educational and formative reports; health, social and environmental problems are also extensively covered, and time is devoted to cultural and religious matters with a respectful view that provides a clear example of public service.

In a broader sense, it is necessary to focus on radio broadcasting, as it is an important space chosen to broadcast a great deal of information related to health issues (Skuse, Butler, Power, Woods, & 2004; Smith, Menn, & McKyer, 2011; Turner, Dewnckhahn, & Bates, 1935) and this chapter will cover the case the Spanish National Radio (RNE) and Radio 5 All-News.

Radio: Credibility and Intimacy

From the early days, Spanish radio has revealed itself as a highly respected medium with great influence among its listeners. Nowadays, despite the broad range of existing media, there are still loyal radio listeners. This is due to the intrinsic characteristics of the medium, including its versatility, which allows us to listen while people are driving, cooking or doing sport, for example.

In general terms, according to the last audience data gathered, through the Estudio General de Medios, 23 million people listen to the radio in Spain every day, which is approximately half the population, including people from 0 to 110 years of age. However, there is a much more important consideration than the listener numbers, and that is the listener loyalty, and the reliability of the medium.

One of the most recent surveys on Public Relations in Spain (PR Noticias, 2015) included some questions about media credibility, and the results are clear. When people are asked to choose which medium is more impartial and more credible, they choose radio as their answer, before other options such as the Internet or TV. In addition, not only do traditional listeners consider radio as the most credible and impartial source of information, but also journalists and communication professionals, as the study suggests.

Radio is an "intimate medium" (Orfanella, 1998) that as such, is very likely to not be the most widely used (European Commission, 2011). Listeners can reach radio broadcasting from traditional devices or the latest applications designed to be heard through mobiles, tablets, among others. Furthermore, by using mobile networks, radio can promote its unique sense of intimacy and group belonging, which have been always seen distinctive features of the medium (Piñeiro-Otero and Ribeiro 2015: 291).

When referring to radio as an intimate medium, one should understand the relationship established between listeners and presenters. In fact, most of the listeners follow their favourite presenter and change from one station to another to continue listening to his or her programme, and many fan clubs have been created to support them.

Another aspect that characterize it as an intimate medium is because it can be heard in a series of situations that imply some kind of intimacy; such as when going to sleep or having a shower, or in your car, on your own, singing along shamelessly. Rodero and Sánchez (2007) point out that in its eighty years of existence; radio broadcasting had to adapt to social, cultural and technological changes. Indeed, these mentioned aspects need to be taken into account when planning to spread information and to reach an audience who will have more difficulty in accessing culture or knowledge in other ways and doing it with a credibility and closeness that other media are not able to reach.

Research in radio broadcasting is not so common as would be desirable, at least in the Spanish and European context in general. However, as Rodero and Sánchez (2007) overstate, radio continues to be part of the sound of people lives, and it will depend on the work of everyone: companies, advertisers, media professionals, students, researchers and listeners.

Bearing in mind these research goals, health issues and media intimacy can be easily linked, as explained by Díezhandino (1994: 89). She defines Public Service Journalism as:

It must contain information which gives the audience the effective possibility to act and react; be offered accurately; present personal interest; with the requirement of being useful information for individuals, materially and psychologically (Díezhandino, 1994:89)

Similarly, Casasús and Ladèveze (1991: 25) state that public radio must be a 'utility service', devoted to 'offer[ing] a kind of information that makes listeners' decision making easier and improves their daily life, in any of its facets: housing, health services, education and other financial aspects, work or entrepreneurial problems, etc.' as they consider that 'these issues are part of an individual's daily life' and 'should be addressed by public media'.

Spanish National Radio (RNE) and Radio 5 All-News

Spanish National Radio was created in 1937, in Salamanca, and it was the only official source of information until the end of the dictatorship (Balsebre, 2001). It includes six channels: the original Radio 1, Classical Radio devoted to classical music, Radio 3 with a cultural and more modern approach; Radio 4 for the Catalan public; Radio 5 All-News and REE, which produce international multi-language broadcasting.

Radio 5, the station this research is interested in, is a thematic channel, based on an All-News formula. This means that most of the time it broadcasts informative programmes. The format followed by Radio 5 is the traditional All-News with some adaptations and the main informative slots are broadcast twice an hour: on the hour and a half past the hour. These news bulletins last five minutes and include international, national, financial, sporting, and other information. The prevailing criterion for news selection is, apart from news relevance, immediacy. Also, every fifteen minutes, they outline the main headlines of the moment. It shares some slots with the main channel, Radio 1, and every day, it offers some sections that differ by region, with local and regional information.

Apart from these purely informative bulletins and headlines, to complete the rest of the schedule, small pieces from a broad range of fields are broadcast. They never last more than five minutes, and they are a great example of public service information because they are not only intended, like traditional radio programmes, to gain an audience or to improve commercial results, but also to improve the audience's knowledge and to fulfil a social function of presenting social problems and realities, a culture far removed from mainstream and formative content.

Spanish National Radio is included in the Estudio General de Medios[2] (EGM) system for measuring listenership, although it has not always been measured through this system. The EGM is an audience study in three stages, with results published in April, July and December. EGM depicts a rich and complete scenario of media consumption at both local and regional levels.

It may seem strange that public radio broadcasting follows the same measurement system as commercial stations because, as it does not follow the same funding system. In addition, it does not have to fight for commercials, having very different duties that need to be fulfilled, even if this compromises audience numbers. However, it can be useful as illustrative data as to how the situation varies, since there is a quite spread assumption that if public media only pay attention to public service duties and they mostly rely on the audience's need to get informed instead of only displaying information accordingly with their preferences, they will become minority media and they will not be able to satisfy their function of reaching as many people as possible. This latter view is held by many researchers and executives, especially when dealing with US Public media.

To sum up the discussion of audiences, and according to the EGM study, 275,000 different listeners heard Radio 5 every day in April 2019. This data is not comparable with audience attraction relative to general interest radio stations, such as Radio 1 or the most listened to, COPE, Onda Cero and SER, which have more than a million daily listeners. The difference between specialized and general interest stations must, therefore, be considered, as well as the fact that Radio 5 has a high level of credibility among the general public and be also considered as a trustworthy source among journalists.

When dealing with absolute data, the estimated audience of Radio 5 must be seen in its context. Spain has a large number of radio stations and audience is not the strongest point of public media. There are several reasons for this.

RTVE does not receive income from advertisements and so they present a mixed form of funding with income from the public budget and a smaller part coming from sponsorships, which supports specific television programmes. In the case of radio (RNE), there is no other form of funding than from the public budget. This implies that in the case of radio especially, they cannot afford to pay large amounts to their presenters, and therefore well-known presenters are hired by commercial stations.

Most of the audience thus goes to these stations, following these presenters. The audience of national public radio stations is not, therefore, as high as it could be. However, RNE has never, in 80 years, used advertisements as a way of funding itself, and this is said to guarantee some independence for the medium.

As it has been previously mentioned, Radio 5 is only one of the five channels of the national public radio (RNE), being the all-news channel. It only broadcasts information, every fifteen minutes, and Public Service Information.

Finally, it is needed to think of a very decentralised country, with seventeen regions, all of them with their own public media, so gathering an audience for such a small and specialised channel is not easy. It should be also highlighted that Radio 5 is the youngest of the RNE channels, with just 28 years on the air, and it is the only all-news channel in Spain, despite which, it has increased its audience from year to year.

COMMUNICATION OF RARE DISEASES

The Situation in Spain

Nearly 3 million Spanish people are affected by chronic rare diseases or disorders (FEDER, 2018).[3] Nevertheless, the media does not always pay as much attention to these issues as might be expected. The commercial media devote their efforts to products with a high level of market acceptance, and thus with high audience numbers.

Some authors like Villa et al. (2014: 2) also ascertain that when this kind of illness is represented in the media, it may not be fully and individually covered by those broadcasting the final result. They suggest the media are merely acting as an 'echo', because they repeat press agency releases, without going more deeply into real cases.

According to López-Villafranca and Castillo-Esparcia (2018: 142), more than half the pieces related to this issue are broadcast by TVE, in both the first and the second channel of public television, while commercial television channels broadcast only 5 to 15% of total television coverage. Similarly, there has been some radio coverage of rare diseases, as the same authors mention that 42% of radio slots related to rare illnesses and disorders are broadcast on RNE, including Radio 1 and Radio 5. They believe that this is, in part, due to the agreement between the health authorities and the public media corporation (RTVE), which states that the latter must broadcast a series of radio and television programmes with an informative and educational purpose, so that they become better known in society.

They also note a significant increase in this news coverage year by year, and in February there is a greater presence of these issues in the media, because Rare Disease Day takes place on the last day of February each year. December is also a very important month, as solidarity programmes tend to be run close to Christmas.

Spanish Public Television Coverage

In the case of public television, López-Villafranca and Castillo-Esparcia (2018: 144) state that 44% of slots devoted to rare diseases run from 1 to 5 minutes, 28% vary from 5 to 30 minutes and 6% lasts more than 30 minutes. One in two pieces has an informative purpose, 3% are part of an advertisement, and the rest, 48%, are part of programmes.

Television channels tend to change the focus and they pay more attention to 'human interest' issues rather than commemorative events. More attention is paid to individual situations, in which a person suffers from this kind of illness, and they frequently demand a stronger commitment of the authorities towards these people.

As there are too many examples that could be studied independently, this research does not aim to be a quantitative representation of what is being broadcast, but a summary and initial classification of programmes which include information about rare diseases and disorders.

Example 1. Broadcast of an Event of the Spanish Federation of Rare Diseases (FEDER)

This programme was completely given over to a broadcast of the annual event created by FEDER, the national federation of rare diseases, which takes place on the last day of February, established as Rare Diseases Day.

This public event was broadcast live by Televisión Española (TVE). It lasted 45 minutes and included several speeches, given by FEDER members, and finally, an address by the Spanish Queen, Dña. Letizia Ortiz Rocasolano. Her commitment to social causes is well known, and events in which she plays an important role are widely followed and broadcast all over the country.

The main aim of this event is to raise people's awareness of rare diseases and disorders, research necessities and the progress of medical treatments.

Example 2. Information Given on the Main News Bulletin of TVE

The information, entitled 'More than 90% of the 3 million Spanish people affected by rare diseases have no specific treatment for their illness.'[4]

This piece lasted 1 minute and 23 seconds and was broadcast on Rare Diseases Day. It was part of the main news bulletin on Spanish public television. It focused on Rett syndrome, one of the more common illnesses among rare disorders in Spain. The piece was based on the experience of a four-year-old child, who is attending equine therapy as part of her treatment. It has an important emotional element, as it talks about a child and there are other people involved, the child's mother and a psychologist, trying to explain how they feel.

This way of telling things attempts to touch people's hearts and make them more sensitive to this kind of problem. The use of a child and her mother is also part of the strategy of increased sensitivity, and to make people aware of these diseases among people of different ages.

Example 3. Diagnosis: Rare disease. Documentary (Second channel).[5]

The documentary called 'Diagnosis: rare disease' was broadcast on the second channel of Spanish public television (TVE). It lasted 32 minutes and it was based on the description and diagnosis of an illness. The programme was also aimed at explaining the lack of research investment in this area.

The main characters involved in this documentary are people who work as researchers, doctors, and association spokespeople. They all make clear that, as well as making people aware of rare diseases, an efficient system for funding research and diagnosis would be needed.

This documentary goes deeper into this kind of disorder than short pieces of information, but it was broadcasted on the second television channel. This is because longer programmes with a deeper perspective cannot find a place on the main channel, which pays more attention to daily news and entertainment formats.

Spanish Public Radio Coverage

López-Villafranca and Castillo-Esparcia (2018: 144) conclude that on radio, more than half of pieces devoted to this issue have a length of more than 5 minutes and less than 30, whereas only 2% of them last more than 30 minutes, and 25% last between 1 and 5 minutes. This explains why the coverage on radio is wider, as it includes not only short informative pieces, but also longer stories and documentaries. There is a high presence of interviews embedded in longer pieces, and they give a deeper and closer view of these diseases.

The most common items dealing with this issue are events organized around important dates, such as Rare Disease Day, as well as interviews and reports centred on people suffering from different diseases. For RNE, scientific awareness in society plays an important role, as it is one of the goals of the public corporation. This consists of explaining pathology, diagnosis, symptomatology and available or future therapies.

Huertas and Gutiérrez have conducted general research about radio and health coverage, and they argue that there are some problems involving the people at whom the information is aimed.

It is clear information directed towards the sick person, with little attention to caregivers and family members. This implies that information about the most immediate news (conferences, scientific discoveries, work problems in the health sector, etc.) is in the hands, almost exclusively, of the merely informative programmes (Huertas and Gutiérrez, 2014:60)

On the same lines, it is important to note that there are some differences between commercial and public radio stations, and there are even internal differences between the different channels which constitute public radio, in the way of addressing this kind of subject. Furthermore, the fact that RNE has several channels makes a difference with respect to commercial stations.

Radio 5 All News, the channel previously described, plays a crucial role in dealing with health, diseases, research and other issues, considered less relevant by the main channels.

Given that there are many examples of content related to rare diseases, this study offers only three different examples of the treatment that the subject receives in public radio and its various channels.

Example 1. Information and Interview in an Informative Programme (RNE 1)[6]

In this case, an interview took place during the morning news programme of the main radio station, Radio 1. It included a brief introduction by the presenter, who subsequently asked a series of relevant questions to the vice president of the Spanish Federation of Associations of Rare Diseases.

The introduction was very brief, serving to justify the interview and only very general data were offered. Subsequently, the interview was quite generic, and the conclusions reached were the lack of knowledge of these pathologies and the need to continue researching them. In total, the item lasted just over three and a half minutes. This is not a very long time for a radio programme, and it was also an interview that took place as part of the awareness activities for the World Day of Rare Diseases.

Example 2. Rare Diseases: The Challenge. Radio Programme. (RNE1)[7]

In the week in which the World Day of Rare Diseases was celebrated, the programme 'Memory of Dolphin' was dedicated to this subject. It was a two-hour programme, so that almost all journalistic genres were represented: reports, chronicles, interviews, among others. It includes many testimonies, some focusing on research, others on the patients themselves and their families or the associations that represent them.

The best thing about this programme was the depth with which it was allowed to deal with the subject matter. The opportunity to have two hours to address multiple perspectives made it a very complete programme enriched by a variety of contributions.

The programme was broadcast at the weekend and from two to four o'clock in the morning, so a priori, the expected audience was not very large. Fortunately, RTVE has an important online platform from which the programme can be heard on demand.

Example 3. (Cómo lo ves) So You Can See! Short Radio Programme (Radio 5)[8]

This programme, which is broadcast weekly on Radio 5 All News is a clear example of the commitment to public service of Spanish public radio. It is a programme of very short duration, just 5 minutes, broadcast on the all-news channel, not the main one, of public radio.

The slot arose from a collaboration between the public media corporation and the Spanish federation of associations of rare diseases. A negative point to highlight is its brevity, and it is also broadcast on a channel with a lower audience share.

However, a weekly slot dedicated to these 'less frequent' diseases is a good opportunity to make information about this type of disease more than a matter just for February.

Issues, Controversies, Problems

Rare diseases and disorders are increasingly 'less rare' because the number of people affected in Spain for example, already exceeds three million and there are some issues that may be relevant not only for the information treatment of them.

There are a number of issues that, although they are relevant for the population as a whole, do not have the expected representation in the media. In this sense, it can be stated that there is a lack of understanding between media and audience.

Previous research in this area shows not only the lack of time devoted to this kind of disease, but also the concentration this content in scarcely one week a year. It could be added that this content is commonly presented as elements conceived to move spectators to tears, and other interesting perspectives are left out.

In general, the case of Spanish public media presents similarities with other European media. They are expected to cover the gap left by commercial media and to fulfil their public service commitments, and in the case of Spain, there are some particularities. Radio Televisión Española (RTVE) suffers from a high level of political interference, and so everything related to it, including funding and programming, is not only linked to its public service function, but to a variety of other interests. That is reflected in the broadcasting of subjects like rare diseases and disorders, which do not find a home on the first channel, as they are not considered attractive enough to gain a large audience. The constant battle between quality and relevant content and audience figures is still present in the public media.

SOLUTIONS AND RECOMMENDATIONS

Firstly, there is a question of language to be clarified, as people still continue to talk about 'rare diseases' when, just in Spain, one out of every fifteen people suffers from one of these diseases.[9] The language that helps to shape reality is important and perhaps the nomenclature used to refer to them should be revised. Maybe, it would be much more accurate talking about 'less prevalent diseases' or similar.

Associations also have a very important role in the task of making this reality known. While it is true that their spokespersons and several experts are always willing to help the media, they may have to look for a more consistent and lasting strategy over time. So far, the fact is that information about rare diseases is only broadcast for a few weeks every year, so the strategy should be modified so that there is real awareness of rare diseases and so people can receive information more frequently.

In this same sense, authorities have the responsibility to go further and offer not only financial aid but also institutional coverage to people suffering from rare diseases and disorders. The Spanish Ministry, as an example, devotes large sums of money to advertising campaigns, for instance to encourage people to avoid tobacco or to be careful when choosing alternative therapies. These campaigns have a considerable cost that cannot be afforded by individual institutions or private associations for the sick, but they are very effective at reaching public opinion.

This is not the only role that public authorities can play. They are responsible for distributing budget items to facilitate the welfare of citizens, and for choosing which issues deserve greater attention. Therefore, in addition to awareness campaigns, they are also responsible for allocating more resources to centres dedicated to researching this type of disease.

Governments and politicians also have a role to play, which is also usually direct, in the content made available and in its promotion by means of public funding. If it is considered that there are numerous commercial media that already occupy their programming with issues such as politics, the economy, events, etc. day after day, the public media must make a difference. They do not meet purely economic criteria, since their funding is guaranteed from other sources, and they must therefore maintain quality standards that are not available to commercial media.

This is why it does not make much sense for citizens to receive the same information via the public and private media every day. The commitment to public service has to be noticed, even more than it currently is, when dealing with this kind of content.

Thus, these media should include content as specific as this, but so necessary for the awareness of the audience, in more predominant places in programming schedules.

FUTURE RESEARCH DIRECTIONS

So far, all the research carried out in this field has looked at the national media, in the case of Spain, and it is likely that a deep and serious comparison with foreign media will allow accurate conclusions to be drawn about what is being done in surrounding countries, and what can be improved in the Spanish case.

It would likewise be interesting to know what motives cause some health or research topics to keep their place among the most habitual contents addressed by the media, in order to try to apply those same methods to the awareness of rare diseases.

CONCLUSION

As might have been expected, the Spanish Public Television and Radio Corporation (RTVE) is the most outstanding example of the attention given to rare diseases in Spain. Both television and radio give a voice and an outlet to patients, associations and researchers, while the commercial media are still far from offering the quantity and quality of information that is possible in this field.

In general terms, the focus is on events to raise awareness of rare diseases among the population and, to a lesser extent, to deepen knowledge of the scientific reality of these diseases.

The use of personal stories, the daily situation of sufferers, works as a way to give visibility and voice to the disease and to reach the public emotionally. There is also a significant tendency to use relevant opinions by professionals from the associations of patients, researchers and doctors. This is especially interesting in longer slots, such as documentary programmes.

Focusing on the case of Televisión Española (TVE) the highest level of coverage is given in approximately, one month, between February and March. This is because the day devoted to making these diseases visible is the last day of February.

Most bulletins last from 1 to five minutes, and they are broadcast as part of longer programmes. That are very often broadcast on the first channel (which has the highest level of audience). They tend to deal with research breakthroughs or with individual cases in which a sick person's needs are expressed.

In the case of longer programmes, from thirty to sixty minutes, they are broadcast on lower audience channels, such as the second or the 24-hour channels. However, these latter do have the opportunity to go further into the subject, and to provide much more information.

In the case of radio, the general framework is similar. Informative programmes tend to include shorter slots, in which little content can be offered beyond the latest discovery or a specific event. The most complete pieces, which include the most relevant content and provide personal experience and expert voices, do not easily find a place, and are relegated to a secondary channel, such as Radio 5, All News.

In the case of radio, the fact that it conveys a greater sense of intimacy and closeness allows journalists to create very personal spaces, in which this type of information is better received and better accepted by the listener.

As a general conclusion, and bearing in mind research initial approach, the Spanish radio and television corporation offers adequate coverage of rare diseases, research in the field, and the personal situations that occur as a result of them. This is easily plausible if readers take into account the other media that currently broadcast in Spain, and that have commercial interests that do not allow them to pay attention, or at least as much as they should, to content that does not directly attract an audience.

REFERENCES

Asociación para la investigación en medios de comunicación. (2015). 'Datos EGM. Resumen General – AIMC'. Retrieved from http://www.aimc.es/-Datos-EGM-Resumen-General-.html. [Access date: 18 May 2016].

Balsebre, A. (2001). *Historia de la radio en España*. Madrid, Spain: Cátedra.

Casasús, J. M., & Núñez Ladèvèze, L. (1991). Estilo y géneros periodísticos. Barcelona, Spain: Ed. Ariel.

Collins, R., Finn, A., McFadyen, S., & Hoskins, C. (2001). Public service broadcasting beyond 2000: Is there a future for public service broadcasting? *Canadian Journal of Communication*, *26*(1). doi:10.22230/cjc.2001v26n1a1192

D'haeneens, L., Sousa, H., & Hultén, O. (2011). From Public Service Broadcasting to Public Service Media, In T. Josef, M. Werner, & D. Leen (Eds.), Media in Europe today, Bristol, UK: Intellect, pp. 187-197.

Diezhandino, M. P. (2002). Periodismo de Servicio. Madrid, Spain: Bosch Ed.

European Commission. (2011). Media Use in The European Union [Report]. Standard Eurobarometer 76/Autumn 2011. Retrieved from https://ec.europa.eu/commfrontoffice/publicopinion/archives/eb/eb76/eb76_media_en.pdf [Access date: Aug 20th, 2019]

FEDER – Federacíon Española de Enfermedades Raras. (2018). ¿Qué son las enfermedades raras o poco frecuentes? Retrieved from https://enfermedades-raras.org/index.php/enfermedades-raras (Access date: August 13, 2019)

Fernández-Alonso, I., & Fernández-Viso, A. (2012). Internal pluralism in the governance of public service broadcasters in Spain and the role of social groups and professionals. The case of RTVE. Vol XXV, Nr. 2, 203-230.

Hallin, D., & Mancini, P. (2004). *Comparing media systems: Three models of media and politics*. Cambridge, UK: Cambridge University Press. doi:10.1017/CBO9780511790867

Harrison, J., & Woods, L. M. (2001). Defining European public service broadcasting. *European Journal of Communication*, *16*(4), 477–504. doi:10.1177/0267323101016004003

Hendy, D. (2013). *Public service broadcasting*. Hampshire: Andrew Crisell. doi:10.1007/978-1-137-32898-4

Holtzman, N. A., Bernhardt, B. A., Mountcastle-Shah, E., Rodgers, J. E., Tambor, E., & Geller, G. (2005). The quality of media reports on discoveries related to human genetic diseases. *Public Health Genomics*, *8*(3), 133–144. doi:10.1159/000086756 PMID:16113530

León, B. (2010). Spanish public service media on the verge of a new era. In P. Iosifidis (Ed.), *Reinventing Public Service Communication* (pp. 197–208). London, UK: Palgrave Macmillan; doi:10.1057/9780230277113_16

López-Villafranca, P., & Castillo-Esparcia, A. (2018). El encuadre de las enfermedades raras en los medios de comunicación españoles. *Observatorio (OBS*), 12*(2), 136-155. doi:10.15847/obsOBS12220181074

Nederlandse Omroepprogramma Stichting (NOS). (1999). *Hilversummary. Broadcasting news from the Netherlands*. Hilversum, The Netherlands: NOS.

Noticias, P. R. (2015). Prnoticias y TyC presentan el estudio 'Prospectiva del sector de las RRPP', Retrieved from http://prnoticias.com/comunicacion/20141311-relaciones-publicas-estudio-prospectiva?jjj=1489486462614. [Access date: 28 Jun. 2019]

Orfanella, L. (1998). Radio: The intimate medium. *English Journal*, *87*(1), 53–55. doi:10.2307/822022

Papatheodorou, F., & Machin, D. (2003). The Umbilical Cord That Was Never Cut: The Post-Dictatorial Intimacy between the Political Elite and the Mass Media in Greece and Spain. *European Journal of Communication*, *18*(1), 31–54. doi:10.1177/0267323103018001225

Perse, E. M., Kubey, R., & Csikszentmihalyi, M. (1991). Television and the Quality of Life: How Viewing Shapes Everyday Experience. *Contemporary Sociology*, *20*(2), 284. doi:10.2307/2072983

Piñeiro-Otero, T., & Ribeiro, F. (2015). Radio mobility in the digital era: Interactivity, participation and content share possibilities in Iberian broadcasters. *Comunicação e Sociedade*, *28*, 291–308. doi:10.17231/comsoc.28(2015).2282

Poon, G. P. (2003). 'Making Money and Serving the Public Interest. Public Broadcasting Can and Should do Both', In M. P. McCaulay, E. E. Peterson, B. L. Artz, & D. Halleck (Eds.), Public Broadcasting and the Public Interest.

Rodero, E., & Sánchez, C. (2007). 'Radiografía de la radio en España', Revista Latina de Comunicación Social, 62, Retrieved from http://www.ull.es/publicaciones/latina/200714RoderoySanchez.htm. [Access date: 19 June 2019]

Skuse, A. J., Butler, N., Power, F., & Woods, N. (2004). *Radio broadcasting for health: A decision maker's guide* (pp. 1–50). London, UK: Department for International Development.

Smith, M. L., Menn, M., & McKyer, E. L. J. (2011). Effectiveness of the radio as a health information source. *Journal of Radio & Audio Media*, *18*(2), 196–211. doi:10.1080/19376529.2011.615776

Smith, R. (2006). Medical journals and the mass media: Moving from love and hate to love. *Journal of the Royal Society of Medicine*, *99*(7), 347–352. doi:10.1177/014107680609900717 PMID:16816264

Turner, C. E., Drenckhahn, V. V., & Bates, M. W. (1935). Effectiveness of radio in health education. *American Journal of Public Health and the Nation's Health*, *25*(5), 589–594. doi:10.2105/AJPH.25.5.589 PMID:18014216

Villa, À. À., Llombart, B. E., Solanillo, C. F., Queralt, A. R. & Castillo, S. S. (2014). *Las Enfermedades Raras en los Medios*. Madrid: Observatorio de Enfermedades Raras, OBSER.

Wright, C. R. (1960). Functional analysis and mass communication. *Public Opinion Quarterly*, *24*(4), 605–620. doi:10.1086/266976

ADDITIONAL READING

Dentzer, S. (2009). Communicating Medical News— Pitfalls of Health Care Journalism. *The New England Journal of Medicine*, *360*(1), 1–3. doi:10.1056/NEJMp0805753 PMID:19118299

Donders, K. (2014). *Public service media and policy in europe*. UK: Palgrave Macmillan.

Harrison, J., & Wessels, B. (2005). A new public service communication environment? Public service broadcasting values in the reconfiguring media. *New Media & Society*, *7*(6), 834–853. doi:10.1177/1461444805058172

Holtzman, N., Bernhardt, B., Mountcastle-Shah, E., Rodgers, J., Tambor, E., & Geller, G. (2005). The Quality of Media Reports on Discoveries Related to Human Genetic Diseases. *Public Health Genomics*, *8*(3), 133–144. doi:10.1159/000086756 PMID:16113530

Jivkova Semova, D. (2011). RTVE sin publicidad: Un modelo de financiación en estado de emergencia. *Vivat Academia*, *0*(116), 75. doi:10.15178/va.2011.116.75-91

Kostic, Z. (2008). Review: From Public Service Broadcasting to Public Service Media. *Media International Australia*, *129*(1), 159–160. doi:10.1177/1329878X0812900123

Nutbeam, D. (2000). Health literacy as a public health goal: A challenge for contemporary health education and communication strategies into the 21st century. *Health Promotion International*, *15*(3), 259–267. doi:10.1093/heapro/15.3.259

Seale, C. (2004). *Health and the media*. Oxford: Blackwell.

Young, M., Norman, G., & Humphreys, K. (2008). Medicine in the Popular Press: The Influence of the Media on Perceptions of Disease. *PLoS One*, *3*(10), e3552. doi:10.1371/journal.pone.0003552 PMID:18958167

KEY TERMS AND DEFINITIONS

Commercial Media: Media that do not rely, directly and only, on public funding. Those media have to get their money from private investors and commercials, but they do not have a public commitment. They do not pay so much attention to issues which are not attractive for many people, as they need high audience levels to obtain more commercials and finance themselves.

Documentary: A documentary is an audio-visual genre that can vary greatly from one medium to another. In principle, it is conceived to give a more complete view of a specific subject. Its duration and the manner in which its content is presented, with greater depth, a greater variety of actors, etc. make it the ideal format to raise awareness of unusual issues in traditional media.

Informative Programme: Content and informative slots are based on recent and relevant news for all citizens, or at least for the potential audience of the medium that produces them. In general, these programmes act as the backbone of the programming schedule.

Programme: Each of the spaces that are broadcast, on television or radio. They are collected in a programming schedule. It is important to know the length of these spaces, as well as the place they occupy in the schedule, to determine the importance that is given to each one.

Public Media/Public Broadcasting: Those media that have a vocation for public service and are therefore intended to cover gaps in programming that other media, for commercial purposes, cannot cover. In general, they have specific forms of funding that include public money and their return to society should respond to that investment.

Radio Nacional de España (RNE): The Spanish public radio receives this name collectively. It is made up of several radio stations devoted to information (such as Radio 5 All News), music (such as Classical Radio) or culture in general (such as Radio 3).

Radio Televisión Española (RTVE): Public audio-visual media corporation in Spain. It includes several television channels, radio stations and a platform for digital and interactive media.

Televisión Española (TVE): This is the name given to Spanish public television, collectively. It comprises several channels, among which are the first and second channel, 24-hour channel and international channel.

ENDNOTES

1 Public Service Broadcasting, http://www.unesco.org/new/en/communication-and-information/media-development/public-service-broadcasting/ (Access date: November 4, 2019)

2 Asociación para la Investigación de Medios de Comunicación – Audiencia General de Medios, http://reporting.aimc.es/index.html#/main/cockpit (Access date: November 4, 2019)

3 FEDER – Federation of Rare Diseases, https://enfermedades-raras.org (Access date: November 4, 2019)

4 RTVE – TeleDiário, http://www.rtve.es/alacarta/videos/telediario/ (Access date: November 4, 2019)

5 RTVE – News: Diagnosing rare diseases, http://www.rtve.es/television/20170912/diagnostico-enfermedad-rara-noche-tematica/1613300.shtml (Access date: November 4, 2019)

5 RTVE – News: Diagnosing rare diseases, http://www.rtve.es/television/20170912/diagnostico-enfermedad-rara-noche-tematica/1613300.shtml (Access date: November 4, 2019)

6 News – Todo Noticias, http://www.rtve.es/alacarta/audios/todo-noticias-manana/problemas-quienes-padecen-enfermedades-raras/5021439/ (Access date: November 4, 2019)

7 News – RTVE, http://www.rtve.es/alacarta/audios/todo-noticias-manana/problemas-quienes-padecen-enfermedades-raras/5021439/ (Access date: November 4, 2019)

8 News – RTVE, http://www.rtve.es/alacarta/audios/para-que-veas/para-veas-enfermedades-raras-05-12-18/4876152/ (Access date: November 4, 2019)

9 ABC España, https://www.abc.es/espana/abci-mas-tres-millones-personas-sufren-espana-alguna-enfermedad-rara-201902280748_video.html (Access date: November 4, 2019)

Chapter 6
Representation of Patients With Rare Diseases in Spanish Media

Paloma López Villafranca
https://orcid.org/0000-0003-4193-1365
University of Málaga, Spain

ABSTRACT

There are more than 360 associations of patients with rare diseases in Spain that strive for visibility to obtain funding and encourage clinical pathologies. The Spanish Year of Rare Diseases has been a considerable effort to be part of media agenda since 2013 and a "collective voice" throughout the media has been encouraged with the international initiatives devoted to the cause. Over the past years, representation of patients with rare diseases in Spanish media has been very superficial, despite the renewed interest during the Spanish Year of Rare Diseases. Certain cases as "Paco Sanz" or "Los Padres de la Pequeña Nadia" have negatively affected this representation by using the disease to pursue economic benefit. This chapter reports on the representation of rare diseases through Spanish media and the way it evolved in the last 6 years. The findings highlight the effort that has been made by patient advocacy groups with rare diseases and their relatives and caregivers, who have been recognized and proactive to get the treatment and medication needed.

DOI: 10.4018/978-1-7998-2088-8.ch006

INTRODUCTION

Rare diseases are characterized by a low prevalence in general population, but they are often chronic, life-threatening and a high rate of people with such diseases are very likely to experience a deterioration in quality of life (Avellaneda, Izquierdo, Torrent-Farnell, & Rámon, 2007; Aymé & Schmidtke, 2007; Cohen & Biesecher, 2010; López-Bastida, Oliva-Moreno, Linertová, & Serrano-Aguilar, 2016; López-Bastida, Perestelo-Pérez, Mónton-Alvarez, Serrano-Aguilar, 2008; Pasculli, Resta, Guastamacchia, Suppressa, & Sabbà, 2004). According to the World Health Organizations (WHO, 2012), rare diseases are those who affect less than 100.000 patients, and they may stem from both a genetic condition and/or environmental cause or bacterial infection (Hunter, 2005).

These diseases often affect the individual's longevity, being incurable and a threat to life. It was not until 1980s that policymakers and general community considered rare diseases worthy of scholarly attention. Avellaneda and colleagues (2007, p.178) claim that this interest has been a result of improving health conditions, increase in life expectancy and wellbeing in population (Aymé, Kole, & Groft, 2008). Commenting on these recent developments in society, Carretón and López (2016) draw our attention to the fact that these "orphan patients" (Kontoghiorghe, Andreou, Constantinou, & Kontoghiorghes, 2014) with rare diseases may have suffered from disease heritage and still face an 'unrecognized risk' (Trujillano, et al., 2017).

The Spanish Federation of Rare Diseases, FEDER (2018)[1] points out that there are more than 6000 rare diseases affecting 300 million people worldwide (cf. ASHUA, 2018) and more than 3 million patients in Spain (FEDER, 2018a). In terms of disease diagnosis and treatment, an average of five years is the estimated time that patients take to be diagnosed with the disease and, in 20% of the cases, it can exceed 10 years to have a proper diagnosis. Almost half of the patients do not receive any treatment and the same proportion show no improvements and get worse in their disease (FEDER, 2018b). Escobar (2018) argues that the major problem that patients and caregivers are facing is the lack of access to reliable information, physicians and experts in the field. As a result, they face a delay in disease diagnosis and, therefore, treatment (Knight, & Senior, 2006; Zurynski et al., 2017).

In Spain, there have been some attempts to raise awareness to rare diseases and its importance. For example, the Council of Ministers declared 2013 as the The Spanish Year of Rare Diseases with the purpose of uniting citizens and foster knowledge towards these diseases. The strategy adopted by the Ministry of Health (Ministerio de Sanidad y Política Social, 2009) fall under three courses of action: (a) sanitary (*i.e.* prevention and detection); (b) scientific (research promotion); and (c) social (through information and sensitization campaigns). In 2016, the International Year of Rare Diseases was celebrated and following the action approved by the Spanish

State in March 2015, the health, social and economic consequences of rare diseases were analyzed. Subsequently, the Ministry of Health, Social Services and Equality of Spain addressed the following priorities: improving medical and psychosocial care of patients and their families; advancing research; and raising awareness to rare diseases among general population (Ministerio de Sanidad y Política Social, 2016).

In this chapter, a follow-up of a previous research undertaken by the author in 2013 in the field of communication and rare diseases is discussed and updated. In specific, it covers: (a) the courses of action carried out by patient organizations; (b) identify the patients' problems in coping with the disease; and (c) strategies adopted by public and private organizations to raise awareness towards rare diseases in the community. Whilst there has been a lack of information and resources in this field (Simoens, Cassiman, Dooms, & Picavet, 2012; Stakišaitis, Špokienė, Juškevičius, Valuckas, & Baiardi, 2007; Zurynski, Frith, Leonard, & Elliott, 2008) and the initiatives rely too much on volunteerism, health communication has become a central issue for patient organizations (Huyard, 2009; Pinto, Martin, & Chenhall, 2016; Rajasimha et al., 2014).

Furthermore, media has been important to disseminate health communication (Moorhead, Hazlett, Harrison, Carrol, Irwin, & Hoving, 2013; McMullan, 2006) and media professionals have a prominent role in communicating current advances in science and medicine (Nelkin, 1996; Petersen, 2001).

A PORTRAIT OF PATIENTS WITH RARE DISEASES IN THE SPANISH PRESS

Much of the literature (*e.g.* Castillo, 2012a, 2012b, 2013; Hernández et al., 2011; Holtzman et al., 2005; Lupton, 1993; Revuelta, & Semir, n.d.) on representation of patients in media have taken into account their portrayal by the press. "El Informe Quiral 10 Años, Medicina y Salud" published by Observatorio de la Comunicación de la Universidad Pompeu Fabra is a good illustration of the coverage of health in media between 1997 and 2006 (Revuelta, & Semir, n.d.).

Relative to rare diseases, the publication entitled "Desafíos y estrategias comunicativas de las enfermedades raras: la investigación médica como referente" (Hernández et al., 2011) compile the work and efforts carried out by CIEBER (Centro de Investigación Biomédica en Red de las Enfermedades Raras)[2], ECCO (Research Group at Universidad de Almería) [3] and GIDYC (Universidad de CEU Cardenal Herrera).[4] In this latter publication, a total of 2455 pieces of information and photos were analyzed, in which 335 different rare diseases were identified. In addition, a set courses of action were proposed in order to create awareness towards rare diseases and overcome the lack of information validated by official political sources or/and a patient spokesperson.

In 2014, the Spanish "Observatorio sobre Enfermedades Raras" (OBSER, 2019)[5] is also an example of an entity that analyzes information and communication practices about rare diseases and reach medical professionals and experts on the field, aiming at ensuring the most accurate and credible information.

Prior work on the visual representation of patients with rare diseases in the Spanish Press was undertaken by Castillo (2012a). Following a framing theory, it covers cognitive perception of the general public about rare diseases. In 2013, the same author (Castillo, 2013) performed a content analysis of the coverage of International Day of Rare Diseases in press from 2010 to 2012. A total of 214 articles from popular newspapers (i.e. El País[6], El Mundo[7], ABC[8], Qué! [9], 20 Minutos y ADN[10], other medical journals, regional and local newspapers, sports press and other general newspapers) have been collected, re-read and analyzed. Findings indicated that patients were represented as discouraged people, who seek visibility and obtain financial resourced for their needs.

As such, Sánchez Castillo (2013, p.75) advocates the need for strengthening the connection between health institutions and information professionals. Castillo and Mercado (2014) also report that news press and information on rare diseases are usually disseminated for Human interest and, therefore there is a request for responsibilities that affect patients, physicians and scientific community as a whole.

In the same vein, other authors (*e.g.* Arcos, 2013; Urrutia, 2013) have also analyzed the way this 2013 International Day of Rare Diseases has been covered in the media. This latter is a mixed-method analysis in the Spanish autonomous community Andalucía and, according to Urrutia (2013), the discourse that appeared in the media was poorly elaborated, leading to misleading information, incredibility of patient associations and a message of pessimism and morbidity.

Bañón and Requena (2014, p.216) argue that the patients' discourse and the interrelationship between patients and patients' representatives may lead to metonymy and self-discrimination, based on the disease portrayal in the press.

In a study investigating the role of health communication in the news press (López-Villafranca, 2016), a low percentage of communication professionals qualified to divulgate health-related information about rare diseases has been revealed. The major challenges found were: (a) lack of information, resources and time; (b) co-operation with patient organizations; and (c) few journalists specialized in health (López-Villafranca & Castillo-Esparcia, 2018). As a result, poorly elaborated and interpreted data is likely to be published by communication agencies owing to the lack of time or/and specialization in the field. Furthermore, Santos and Pérez (2019) affirm that rare diseases should have the same coverage as other diseases, with a general focus on these pathologies.

Figure 1. Coverage of patients with Rare Diseases - El Mundo
Source: https://www.elmundo.es/comunidad-valenciana/alicante/2017/02/27/58ad8695e5fdea4d408b45f2.html

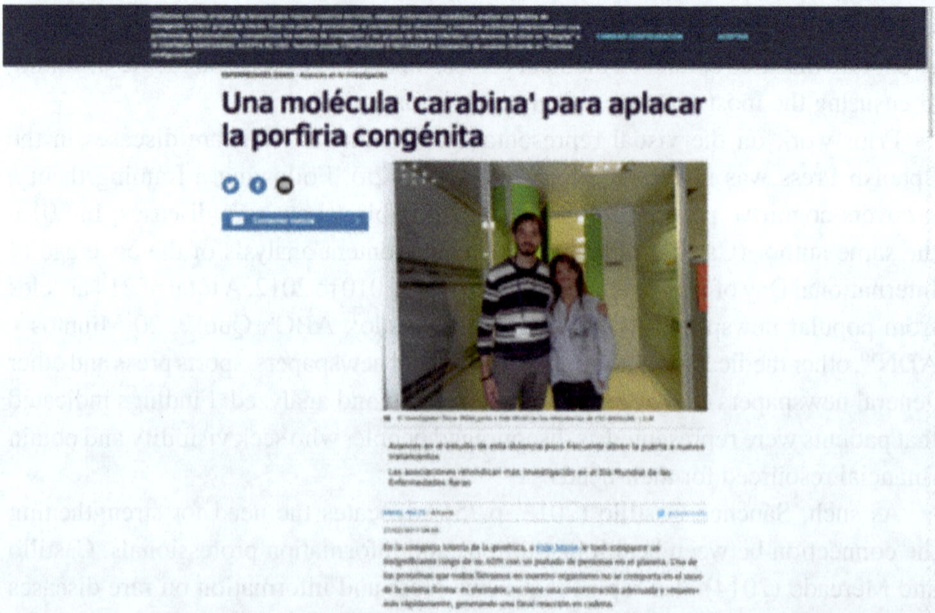

Figure 1 shows the coverage of patients with rare diseases in the Spanish newspaper El Mundo.

As shown in Figure 1, the interconnection between the scientific research community and the patients is evident. Nevertheless, patients with rare diseases tend to have serious doubts about their appearance in media because of the lack of rigor and possible association of media coverage to some biases and previous cases that have negatively affected the representation of these patients by using the disease to pursue economic benefit. Some examples of cases that have negatively affected the representation of these patients are:

- **Los Padres de la Pequeña Nadia:** Nadia is a girl with trichothiodystrophy (TTD), whose parents asked for compassion and money from celebrities and citizens to fund treatments that were not carried out.
- **Paco Sanz:** A patient with 2000 tumors exaggerated the syndrome in order to raise 100 000 euros for a treatment that did not exist.

In an analysis of these two cases, López-Villafranca (2018) concludes that these damaged the representation of patients with rare diseases in the media, being negative in terms of the patients' actions and family history scams. By contrast, these are isolated cases of so many others, in which misleading information and messages of pessimism and incredibility of patient associations need to be demystified.

THE ROLE OF AUDIOVISUAL MEDIA IN RARE DISEASE AWARENESS

Radio and television are two means of communication that can "give voice" to the voiceless and vulnerable people and, therefore, improve their visibility and demystify some stereotypes. Indeed, the way patients are represented in the media may affect the perception of general community towards the severity of the diseases, characteristics and challenges faced on a daily basis. For that, the following obstacles need to be overpassed: (a) avoid sensationalism during a sweeps period (Cooper, Roter, 2000); (b) clarify some bias in news coverage (Tanner, 2004) and (c) lack of journalists specialized in health (Leask, Hooker, & King, 2010) and involvement of the patient in news production (Aledo, 2007).

Aledo (2007, p.95) highlights that the radio has the potential of informing the listeners about illness prevention, rehabilitation, technical advances, research, guides on existing services and aids, self-help associations, books and publications, and health professionals.

A number of Spanish radio stations cover these rare diseases. For example, the private radio station "Onda Cero" [11], the health programme "En buenas manos" [12] addresses these diseases. Another radio station "Cope" [13], a programme "Los Decanos" targeted at older adults, has covered health issues since 1992. In the public broadcaster, "A su Salud" [14], "Alimento y Salud" [15] and "Entre probetas"[16] are scientific dissemination programmes that treat these diseases. Nevertheless, it was not until 2013 that public or private television and radio stations considered rare diseases worthy of exclusive coverage.

Detailed examination of discursive and audiovisual strategies of news relative to the World Rare Disease Day 2012 by Cruz and Requena (2013) suggested some improvements for covering health information through the use of these media: inform society about the concept of rare diseases and social and health problems that are faced; present data relative to the investment needed in terms of research and treatment; and offer data, images that support these pieces of information.

Meanwhile, the coverage of Rare Diseases in the Spanish Public Radio Broadcasting RTVE[17] was analyzed (López-Villafranca 2015a). It was found that patient organizations appeared on TVE during a series of specialized programmes (*e.g.*

Figure 2. Telemaratón - RTVE
Source: https://www.rtve.es

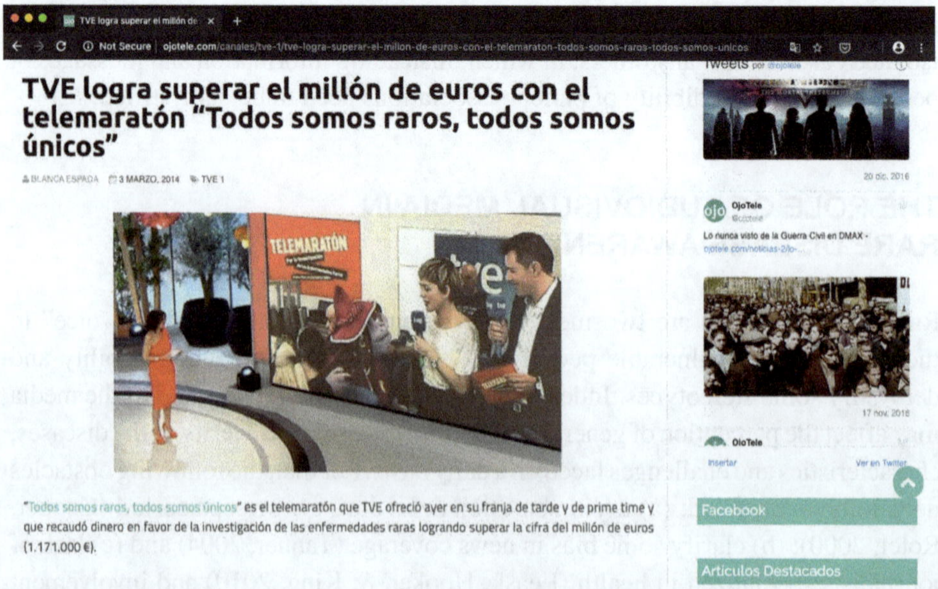
TVE logra superar el millón de euros con el telemaratón "Todos somos raros, todos somos únicos"
3 MARZO, 2014
TVE 1
TELEMARATÓN
"Todos somos raros, todos somos únicos" es el telemaratón que TVE ofreció ayer en su franja de tarde y de prime time y que recaudó dinero en favor de la investigación de las enfermedades raras logrando superar la cifra del millón de euros (1.171.000 €).
OjoTele
Facebook
Articulos Destacados

Telemaratón) (Figure 2). In fact, the author considers that patient organizations have gained some visibility and increased news coverage in both TVE and representatives of radio associations – RNE.[18]

Patient organizations also created their own space in the media to disseminate information and their experiences. The Internet Television Minoritaria TV[19] is an example of a medium that is used to inform and create awareness to rare diseases and get resources for patients' treatments. The Non-Governmental Alliance of Organizations of Patients with Rare Diseases, EURORDIS, also has a television channel entitled EURORDIS TV.[20] This channel aims to spread news and events and vital experiences associated to rare diseases, while informing about orphan drugs[21] or health policies and strengthen the interactions between scientific community, physicians, patients and general citizens.

In the USA TV series "Doctor House" [22], rare diseases are also addressed (*e.g.* Dawson Disease, Rabies, Bubonic Wilson Disease) (Valenzuela-Rodríguez, 2012), in which the characters face with ethical dilemmas and difficulties in diagnosis (Francescutti, Nicolás y Fernández, 2011). These diseases have also been portrayed in cinema. According to Sánchez, Sánchez and Marcos (2008), cinema is also a medium that can guide citizens in their knowledge about rare diseases and create awareness to the stigmatization of such diseases as Tourette's or Treacher Collins

Figure 3. 'Campeones', la película Española más taquillera de 2018
Source: http://www.solidaridaddigital.es/noticias/cultura/campeones-la-pelicula-espanola-mas-taquillera-de-2018

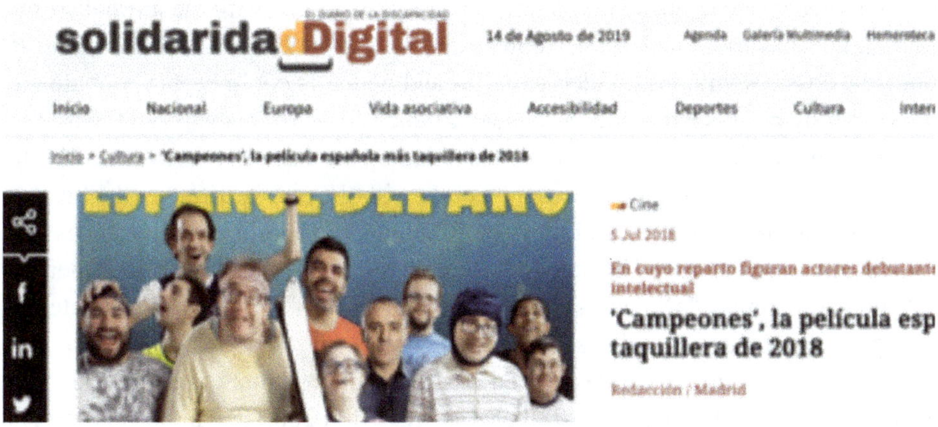

syndromes. This latter was covered in the American commercial movie Wonder[23], released in 2018.

The movie Campeones [Champions] [24], which won the el Goya Spanish movie award in 2019, has also raised awareness to people with disabilities and some of them with rare diseases.

Collectively, these coverage in audiovisual media pave the way into such values as diversity and inclusion, ensuring patients' visibility.

WEB-BASED INFORMATION AND SOCIAL NETWORKS IN RARE DISEASES

For Fornieles and Bañon (2011) [25], web enabled the dissemination of health information and patient support. Social networks, web pages and blogs are part of the services that patients can use in order to share their experiences and information (Kamel Boulos, & Wheeler, 2007). For the authors, social networks are ideal in order to spread the messages and create interest in citizens. Similarly, Torrente and colleagues (2010) stress the role of virtual spaces, which offer patients the possibility to share their experiences and exchange information (Nambisan, 2011), advices and emotional support (Antheunis, Tates, & Nieber, 2013; Hackworth, & Kunz, 2011; Kuehn, 2011). These virtual health communities and online support groups (Wright et al., 2013) usually depend on such variables as membership, shared activities, vision, social norms, among others.

In a comprehensive analysis of communication management in the social networks of 143 patient's organizations relative to rare diseases in Spain, Castillo-Esparcia and López-Villafranca (2016) found that their dissemination strategy is not oriented to a target audience and a close interconnection could be forged with the journalists by, for example, having a virtual press room on the web, in which such materials as press releases, dossiers, graphics, video galleries and podcasts could be easily obtained.

The study by Basagoiti and Fernández Luque (2011, p.77) analyzed the role of Social Network Sites in patient initiatives, including the case 'El Diario de Pedro.' In this mentioned initiative, the parents of a child with the rare syndrome - the Sturge-Weber syndrome, use the social network Facebook to share their experiences and fight against the disease. The authors use such terms as "ePacientes" (ePatients), "ePadres" (eParents), "eMenores" (eChild) and "eFamilias" (eFamily) to characterize the agents involved in rare disease management.

There are a number of specialized networks that address rare diseases. An example is Patientslikeme[26] (2019) that was created in 2005 by Heywood brothers after Stephen Heywood was diagnosed with Amyotrophic Lateral Sclerosis (Gupta & Riis, 2011), becoming a digital tool for sharing information on the disease (Wicks et al., 2010). Another specialized network is RareConnect[27] (Tommasetti, Toisi, & Cosimato, 2014), run by the organizations EURORDIS and NORD[28] in order to exchange accurate information about each rare disease in different languages (e.g. French, Spanish, English, Italian, German).

In Spain, the website FEDER brings together 360 patient organizations and the "Share4Rare"[29] is a community that aims to unite patients, relatives and researchers towards rare diseases (Athanasiou, Nafría, Vroom, 2018). In addition, the #LoweResearchProject [30] (Subirats et al., 2018) is run by UOC, CIBERER, Universitat Oberta de Calalunya and Centro de Investigación Biomédica en Red de Enfermedades Raras, which purpose is to advance biomedical research and foster quality of life in people suffering from Lowe Syndrome through the use of the general Social Network Sites Facebook and Twitter.

Health blogs also play a very important role for patient groups, in that these enable patients to share their experiences and reinforce the interconnection with health professionals. The following are known examples of these blogs: PsyBlog[31], The Patient Experience[32], Maternity Matters[33], Bad Medicine[34], Disabled People Against Cuts (DPAC)[35], Dr. Grumble[36], Aspie in the family[37], and Frontier Psychiatrist[38] (González Pacanowski, & Medina Aguerrebere, 2014).

Overall, such digital tools as social network sites, websites, blogs and online videos tend to be relevant to educate, unite, create awareness towards diseases and strengthen the interconnection between patients, relatives and health professionals (López-Villafranca & Castillo-Esparcia, 2014).

DEVELOPING RARE DISEASE COMMUNICATION CAMPAIGNS

According to Estevez and Terrón Blanco (2011), health campaigns have the purpose of giving visibility to a certain disease. In the case of rare diseases, these aim to create awareness, provide further information and raise funds for research.

In Spain, these health communication campaigns are mainly performed through the use of digital media, mainly, social networks and closed groups in order to disseminate information, encourage fundraising, and ensure visibility (López-Villafranca, 2015b). The Federación Española de Enfermedades Raras, FEDER, is usually the entity that fosters these campaigns in both the traditional media and Web. One of the campaigns launched in 2014, entitled "Enfermedades Raras, Pacientes Únicos. Si no las conoces no las reconoces" ["Rare diseases, Unique patients. If you don't know them, you don't recognize them."] was created by the agency Ilusionlabs[39], being awarded with the prize 'Aspid de oro 2014'. Figure 4 shows the poster for the campaign.

Health video campaigns are also used in such video channels as Youtube. The challenge of the ice cube was a viral campaign to create awareness to Amyotrophic Lateral Sclerosis, in which celebrities from sports, film and entertainment industry adhered to the challenge and 'gave voice' to the cause (Hrastej, & Robertson, 2016; Koohy & Koohy, 2014).

Among the most striking campaigns created by both patients and caregivers was Ignasi Serrahima relative to the rare disease Ectodermal Dysplasia, which affects 1 in 5000-10000 newborns and there is no treatment or cure (Killic et al., 2017).[40] This disease affects the ectoderm structures or derivatives (Priolo, 2009), e.g. skin, teeth, nail, eyes, nose. Patients with this disease lack sweat glands, which may lead to serious symptoms of hyperthermia (Mortier, & Wackens, 2004). The campaign raised more than 14,800 eur through crowdfunding and enabled to fund a research project of the Spanish Association of Ectodermal Dysplasia, carried out jointly with the Medical Genetics Unit of the Hospital Pediatrics service at the Hospital Virgen de la Arrixaca de Murcia.

Celebrities have also an important role in these campaigns, as it is the case of the Asosiación Síndrome Poland[42] in which Spanish celebrities embraced the cause (Figure 5). Likewise, other foundations adopted the same strategy – *e.g.* Fundación Isabel Gemio[43] or Fundación Menudos Corazones.[44]

Collectively, these initiatives are essential to the motte launched by the TVE Telemarathon "Todos Somos Raros, Todos Somos Únicos" [We Are All Rare, We Are All Unique]. In Spain, radio and television programmes are still the prior media in which messages of solidarity and research relative to rare diseases are disseminated. In terms of fundraising, the means have also evolved to embody short messages – SMS or platforms of crowdsourcing. In addition, Spanish celebrities

Figure 4. Poster for the Day of Rare Diseases in 2014
Source: Federación Española de Enfermedades Raras, FEDER

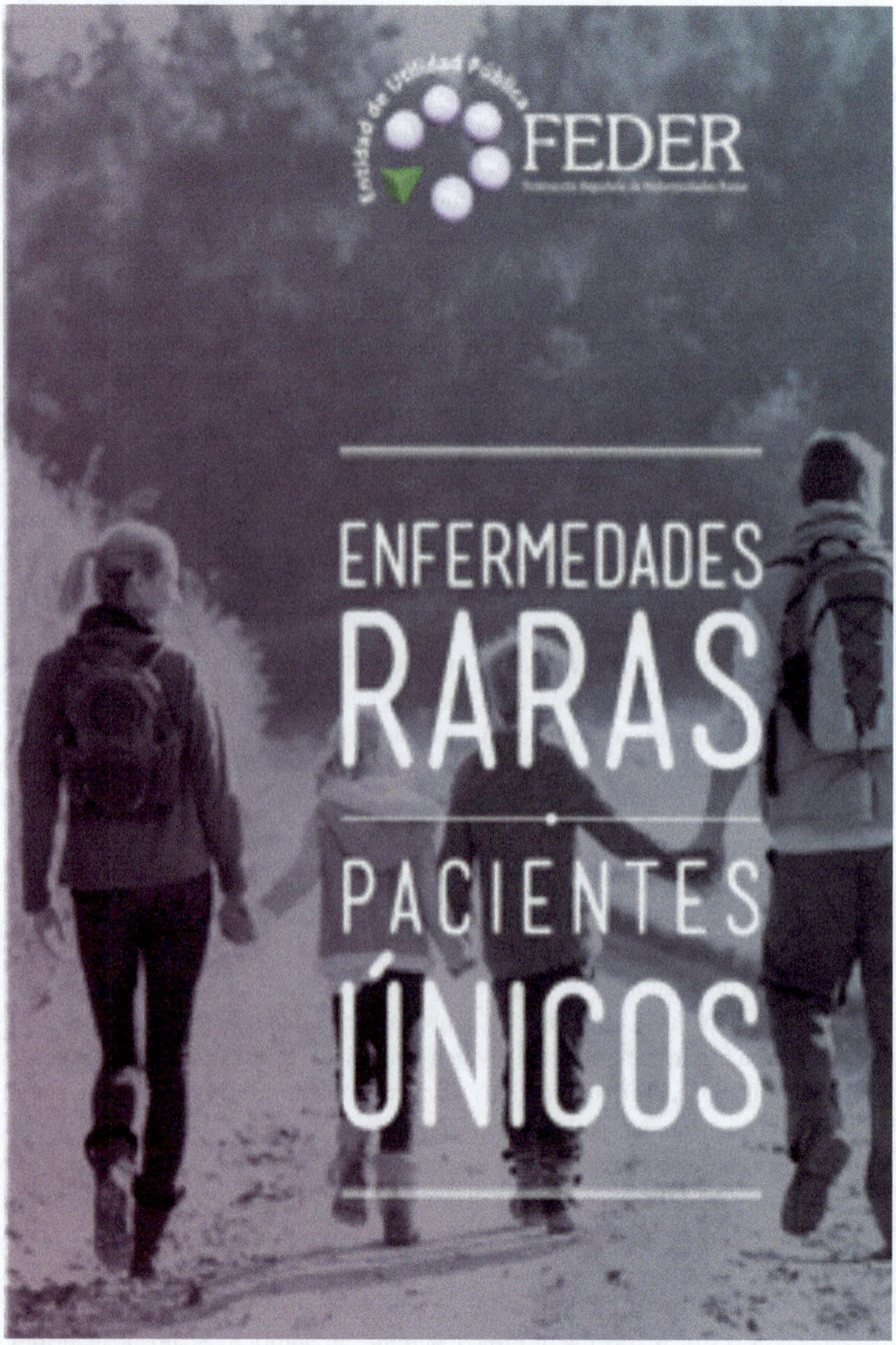

Figure 5. Campaign – Poland Syndrome on Facebook
Source: https://www.facebook.com/asociacionespanoladesindromedepoland?fref=ts

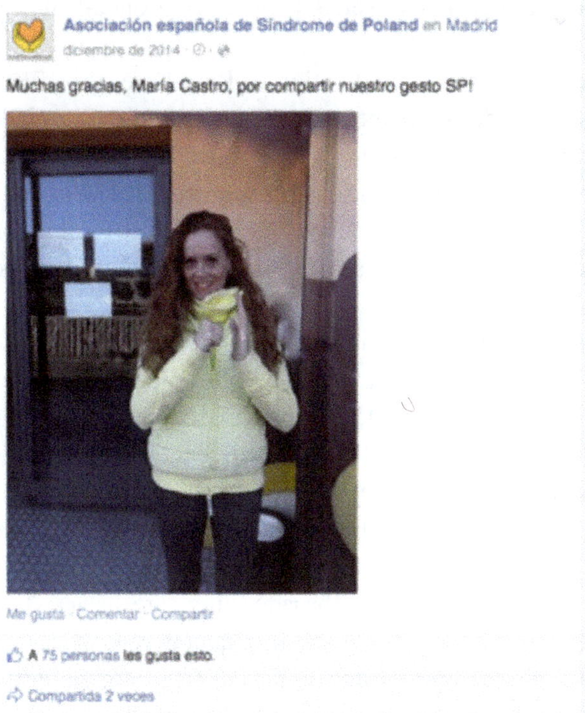
Asociación española de Síndrome de Poland en Madrid
diciembre de 2014
Muchas gracias, María Castro, por compartir nuestro gesto SP!
Me gusta · Comentar · Compartir
A 75 personas les gusta esto.
Compartida 2 veces

from different fields, who embrace this causes, function as models to follow in the community (Wadhera, 2016). Lastly, such support of Spanish enterprises as Telefónica, La Caixa, Inditex or Mercadona have also contributed to the success of the rare disease campaigns in Spain.

CONCLUSION

This chapter reported on the representation of rare diseases through Spanish media and the way it evolved during the last 6 years. It was observed that although patients with rare diseases have managed to be on the media agenda, their exposure have also been compromised.

Since the 2013 Spanish Year of Rare Diseases, the patient organizations have increased their impact on both the traditional media and social networks. It is worth noting, however, that these organizations often lack of economic and Human resources to carry out communication actions or hire professionals. Furthermore, there is a lack of journalists specialized in health and, as consequence, data that is published by communication agencies tend to be poorly elaborated and interpreted in a short-time period (Leask, Hooker, & King, 2010; López-Villafranca & Castillo-Esparcia, 2018).

The creation of the Spanish Federation of Rare Diseases - FEDER was also a landmark in the spread of positive messages (Castillo & Mercado, 2014), information and support towards the diseases, demystifying some bias.

Two important dates marked the visibility of these patients in the media: the aforementioned 2013 Spanish Year of Rare Diseases and 2016 -that corresponds to the International year devoted to rare diseases (Castillo-Esparcia & López- Villafranca, 2016; Cruz, & Requena, 2013).

In recent years, rare disease patients have gained some visibility in press, radio and press, outgrowing its interest in media and communication research (Bañón, & Requena, 2014; Castillo, 2012, 2013; Urrutia, 2013; López-Villafranca & Castillo-Esparcia, 2018; Santos & Pérez, 2019). Alongside these advancements in the field, there has also been a change in the way rare disease patients were regarded – *i.e,* victims, unprotected or with no authority and its portrayal evolvement to people who have a role in the community and are constantly challenged in their daily lives.

In the specific case of Spanish radio broadcasting, rare diseases have been covered with the use of in-depth interviews (Castillo-Esparcia & López-Villafranca, 2016), whereas, in television, such programmes as the RTVE Telemarathon or the movement "Todos somos raros.Todos somos únicos." ["We are all rare. We are all unique"] are limited to a short time agenda. To overcome this limitation towards television, other media formats were also effective to transmit the message – *e.g.* scientific debates on the radio, health-related issues in magazines and 24h updated pieces of web-based information (Díaz, 2004). Patients and caregivers also use direct contacts and events to raise public awareness to the disease and, in turn, these are likely to have an impact on traditional media, i.e. press, radio, and television. Celebrities have also an important role in campaigns in order to help patient organizations to gain visibility in the media.

Audio-visual strategies have also been adopted to fight against stereotypes that often affect these patients, e.g. the movie Campeones [Champions]. Indeed, the coverage of rare diseases in audiovisual media seem to pave the way into such values as diversity and inclusion.

While comparing the Spanish case with other countries, similarities can be observed in the investigations of Emerich and colleagues (2017) in Brazil that highlight the negative aspects of news in press about these diseases. In social networks, the same conclusions are reached by Jacobs et al (2016), who confirm that there is a need for the participation of patients and families in Facebook groups about these diseases. Finally, the study by Liuccio et al. (2015) concludes that it is important to promote more studies on communication and on patients' health information and on the way to spread correct information, not alarmist and easy to decode in rare diseases.

To sum up, the findings highlight the effort that has been made by patient advocacy groups with rare diseases and their relatives and caregivers, who have been recognized and proactive in order to get the treatment and medication needed.

REFERENCES

Aledo, L. D. (2007). La representación de la discapacidad en los medios de comunicación. *Comunicación e cidadanía: revista internacional de xornalismo social= Social Journalism International Review*, (1), 289-306.

Antheunis, M. L., Tates, K., & Nieboer, T. E. (2013). Patients' and health professionals' use of social media in health care: Motives, barriers and expectations. *Patient Education and Counseling*, *92*(3), 426–431. doi:10.1016/j.pec.2013.06.020 PMID:23899831

Arcos, J. M. (2013). El Día Mundial de las enfermedades raras en las noticias de prensa: el ejemplo de Andalucía. *Discurso y Sociedad*, 7(1), 224-247. Recuperado de http://www.dissoc.org/ediciones/v07n01/DS7(1)

ASHUA – Associación Síndrome Hemolítico Urémico Atípico España. (2018, February). *ASHUA reivindica el papel de los pacientes em la investigación sobre el diagnóstico del SHUa em el Día Mundial de las Enfermedades Raras*. Retrieved from https://www.ashua.es/blog/55

Athanasiou, D., Nafría, B., Vroom, E. (2018). Share4Rare: Social media platform dedicated to rare diseases, using collective intelligence for the generation of awareness and knowledge. *Orphanet Journal of Rare Diseases 2018, 13*(Suppl 2):P2, 167. doi:10.118613023-018-0895-2

Avellaneda, A., Izquierdo, M., Torrent-Farnell, J., & Ramón, J. R. (2007). Enfermedades raras: Enfermedades crónicas que requieren un nuevo enfoque sociosanitario. *Anales del Sistema Sanitario de Navarra*, *30*(2), 177–190. doi:10.4321/S1137-66272007000300002 PMID:17898813

Aymé, S., Kole, A., & Groft, S. (2008). Empowerment of patients: Lessons from the rare diseases community. *Lancet*, *371*(9629), 2048–2051. doi:10.1016/S0140-6736(08)60875-2 PMID:18555918

Aymé, S., & Schmidtke, J. (2007). Networking for rare diseases: A necessity for Europe. *Bundesgesundheitsblatt, Gesundheitsforschung, Gesundheitsschutz, 50*(12), 1477–1483. doi:10.100700103-007-0381-9 PMID:18026888

Bañón Hernandezy, A. M., & Requena Romero, S. (2014). La representación de las enfermedades poco frecuentes en el discurso periodístico español. Propuestas para el análisis. *Pragmática Sociocultural/Sociocultural Pragmatics, 8*(2), 180-222. doi:10.1515oprag-2014-0023

Basagoiti, I., & Fernández-Luque, L. (2011). Compartir información sanitaria: ePacientes: comunicación e interacción. In V. *Traver Salcedo, & L. Fernández Luque (Coords.), El ePaciente y las redes sociales.* Valencia, Spain: Publidisa.

Carretón Ballester, M. C., & López Villafranca, P. (2016). The impact of the Ebola Virus and rare diseases in the media and the perception of risk in Spain. *Catalan Journal of Communication & Cultural Studies, 8*(2), 245–263. doi:10.1386/cjcs.8.2.245_1

Castillo, S. (2012b). *Discurso visual de las enfermedades raras: encuadres latentes.* Tonos digital: Revista electrónica de estudios filológicos, 23, 1-24.

Castillo S. (2013) . Las enfermedades raras en la prensa española: una aproximación empírica desde la teoría del framing. Ambitos: *Revista internacional de comunicación*, (22), 71-80.

Castillo, S. S. (2012a). Representación social de las enfermedades raras en la prensa española. Aposta. *Revista de Ciencias Sociales*, (54): 1–31.

Castillo, S. S., & Mercado Sáez, M. T. (2014). El encuadre de las enfermedades raras en la prensa española. *Anuario Electrônico de Estudios en Comunicación Social, 7*(1), 104-128. Recuperado de https:// dialnet.unirioja.es/servlet/articulo?codigo=4800928 (Access date: August 13, 2019)

Castillo-Esparcia, A., & López-Villafranca, P. (2016). Las estrategias de comunicación de las organizaciones de pacientes con enfermedades raras (ER) en España. *Ciencia & Saude Coletiva, 21*(8), 2423–2436. doi:10.1590/1413-81232015218.19852015 PMID:27557016

Cohen, J. S., & Biesecker, B. B. (2010). Quality of life in rare genetic conditions: A systematic review of the literature. *American Journal of Medical Genetics. Part A, 152*(5), 1136–1156. doi:10.1002/ajmg.a.33380 PMID:20425818

Cooper, C. P., & Roter, D. L. (2000). If it bleeds it leads"? Attributes of TV health news stories that drive viewer attention. *Public Health Reports*, *115*(4), 331–338. doi:10.1093/phr/115.4.331 PMID:11059426

Cruz Moya, O., & Requena Romero, S. (2013). El día de las enfermedades raras en las noticias televisivas. análisis crítico de su representación audiovisual. *Discurso & Sociedad*, *7*(1), 200–223.

Díaz, E. J. (2004). La radio y el multimedia, dos alternativas para la divulgación científica. *Quark: Ciencia, medicina, comunicación y cultura*, 34, 40-49.

Emerich, T. B., Cavaca, A. G., Santos-Neto, E. T., Gentilli, V. I., & Oliveira, A. E. (2017). Media valuations of health journalism and health dynamics in brazilian print media. *International Journal of Social Science Studies*, *5*(1), 31–42. doi:10.11114/ijsss.v5i1.1997

Escobar Pérez, L., Ávalos Sandoval, P., & Medeiros, M. (2018). Espacios digitales y enfermedades raras. *Revista Digital Universitaria*, 19(5).

Estevez Jimenez, P., & Terrón Blanco, J. L. (2011). El diseño de campañas sobre el ictus y su evaluación. Una revisión de 10 años de literatura científica (1999-2009). *Observatorio (OBS*)*, *5*(1), 123- 156. doi:10.15847/obsOBS512011410

FEDER – Federacíon Española de Enfermedades Raras. (2018, March). *ASHUA se suma al Día Mundual de las ER*. Retrieved from https://enfermedades-raras.org/index.php?option=com_content&view=article&id=10200 (Access date: August 13, 2019)

FEDER – Federacíon Española de Enfermedades Raras. (2018a). *¿Qué son las enfermedades raras o poco frecuentes?* Retrieved from https://enfermedades-raras.org/index.php/enfermedades-raras (Access date: August 13, 2019)

FEDER – Federacíon Española de Enfermedades Raras. (2018b). *Las Enfermedades Raras em cifras*. Retrieved from https://enfermedades-raras.org/index.php/enfermedades-raras/enfermedades-raras-en-cifras (Access date: August 13, 2019)

Fornieles, J., & Bañón, A. M. (2011). Análisis del discurso multimodal: las fotografías en la información sobre Enfermedades Raras. In A. M. Bañón & ... (Eds.), *Desafíos y estrategias comunicativas de las enfermedades raras: la investigación médica como referente* (pp. 189–200). Valencia, Spain: CIBERER.

Francescutti, L. P., Nicolás, M. M., & Fernández, F. T. (2011). *La información sanitaria en los telediarios*. Toledo: Almud Ediciones.

González-Pacanowski, T., & Medina-Aguerrebere, P. (2011). Blogs para pacientes como nueva fuente de información de salud. *El Profesional de la Información*, *20*(6), 652–658. doi:10.3145/epi.2011.nov.08

Gupta, S., & Riis, J. (2011). *Patientslikeme: An online community of patients*. Harvard Business School Marketing Unit Case, (511-093).

Hackworth, B. A., & Kunz, M. B. (2011). Health care and social media: Building relationships via social networks. *Academy of Health Care Management Journal*, *7*(2), 1.

Hernández, A. M., Fornieles Alcaraz, J., Solves Almela, J. A., & Rius Sanchis, I. (2012). (Coords.) Desafíos y estrategias comunicativas de las enfermedades raras: la investigación médica como referente: estudio cuantitativo-discursivo de la prensa escrita impresa y digital española (2009-2010). Valencia, Spain: Centro de Investigación Biomédica em Red de Enfermedades Raras (CIBERER).

Holtzman, N. A., Bernhardt, B. A., Mountcastle-Shah, E., Rodgers, J. E., Tambor, E., & Geller, G. (2005). The quality of media reports on discoveries related to human genetic diseases. *Public Health Genomics*, *8*(3), 133–144. doi:10.1159/000086756 PMID:16113530

Hrastelj, J., & Robertson, N. P. (2016). Ice bucket challenge bears fruit for amyotrophic lateral sclerosis. *Journal of Neurology*, *263*(11), 2355–2357. doi:10.100700415-016-8297-7 PMID:27734164

Hunter, D. J. (2005). Gene–environment interactions in human diseases. *Nature Reviews. Genetics*, *6*(4), 287–298. doi:10.1038/nrg1578 PMID:15803198

Huyard, C. (2009). Who rules rare disease associations? A framework to understand their action. *Sociology of Health & Illness*, *31*(7), 979–993. doi:10.1111/j.1467-9566.2009.01177.x PMID:19619152

Jacobs, R., Boyd, L., Brennan, K., Sinha, C. K., & Giuliani, S. (2016). The importance of social media for patients and families affected by congenital anomalies: A Facebook cross-sectional analysis and user survey. *Journal of Pediatric Surgery*, *51*(11), 1766–1771. doi:10.1016/j.jpedsurg.2016.07.008 PMID:27522307

Kamel Boulos, M. N., & Wheeler, S. (2007). The emerging Web 2.0 social software: An enabling suite of sociable technologies in health and health care education 1. *Health Information and Libraries Journal*, *24*(1), 2–23. doi:10.1111/j.1471-1842.2007.00701.x PMID:17331140

Katz, M. S., Utengen, A., Anderson, P. F., Thompson, M. A., Attai, D. J., Johnston, C., & Dizon, D. S. (2016). Disease-specific hashtags for online communication about cancer care. *JAMA Oncology*, *2*(3), 392–394. doi:10.1001/jamaoncol.2015.3960 PMID:26539640

Kilic, S., Altintas, S. H., Yilmaz Altintas, N., Ozkaynak, O., Bayram, M., Kusgoz, A., & Taskesen, F. (2017). Six-Year Survival of a Mini Dental Implant-Retained Overdenture in a Child with Ectodermal Dysplasia. *Journal of Prosthodontics*, *26*(1), 70–74. doi:10.1111/jopr.12366 PMID:26418841

Knight, A. W., & Senior, T. P. (2006). The common problem of rare disease in general practice. *The Medical Journal of Australia*, *185*(2), 82–83. doi:10.5694/j.1326-5377.2006.tb00477.x PMID:16842062

Kontoghiorghe, C. N., Andreou, N., Constantinou, K., & Kontoghiorghes, G. J. (2014). World health dilemmas: Orphan and rare diseases, orphan drugs and orphan patients. *World Journal of Methodology*, *4*(3), 163. doi:10.5662/wjm.v4.i3.163 PMID:25332915

Koohy, H., & Koohy, B. (2014). A lesson from the ice bucket challenge: Using social networks to publicize science. *Frontiers in Genetics*, *5*, 430. doi:10.3389/fgene.2014.00430 PMID:25566317

Kuehn, B. M. (2011). Patients go online seeking support, practical advice on health conditions. *Journal of the American Medical Association*, *305*(16), 1644–1645. doi:10.1001/jama.2011.509 PMID:21521841

Leask, J., Hooker, C., & King, C. (2010). Media coverage of health issues and how to work more effectively with journalists: a qualitative study. *BMC public health*, *10*(1), 535, 1-7. doi:10.1186/1471-2458-10-535

López-Bastida, J., Oliva-Moreno, J., Linertová, R., & Serrano-Aguilar, P. (2016). Social/economic costs and health-related quality of life in patients with rare diseases in Europe. *The European Journal of Health Economics*, *17*(S1), 1–5. doi:10.100710198-016-0780-7 PMID:27023708

López-Bastida, J., Perestelo-Pérez, L., Montón-álvarez, F., & Serrano-Aguilar, P. (2008). Social economic costs and health-related quality of life in patients with degenerative cerebellar ataxia in Spain. *Movement Disorders*, *23*(2), 212–217. doi:10.1002/mds.21798 PMID:17999424

López Villafranca, P. (2015a). "La representación de las asociaciones de pacientes en el ente público RTVE. El caso de las Enfermedades Raras". En Peñafiel, C y Echegaray, L. (2015). Estudios de Comunicación y Salud: innovaciones e información científica para el progreso social. Cuadernos Artesanos de Latina, 84. Tenerife: Sociedad Latina de Comunicación Social, 157- 174.

López Villafranca, P. (2015b). Análisis de las campañas de comunicación de pacientes con enfermedades raras en España. *Opción*, *31*(1), 1039–1055.

López Villafranca, P. (2016). Estudio de la presencia de los gabinetes de comunicación en las organizaciones de pacientes con enfermedades raras en España. *Revista Internacional de Relaciones Públicas*, *11*(6), 27–46. doi:10.5783/RIRP-11-2016-03-27-46

López Villafranca, P. (2018). Análisis de estafas de pacientes en la prensa española. El caso de Paco Sanz, el hombre de los 2.000 tumores y el caso de Nadia, la niña con tricodistrofia. *Revista Española de Comunicación en Salud*, *9*(1), 5–13. doi:10.20318/recs.2018.4256

López Villafranca, P., & Castillo Esparcia, A. (2014). El papel del vídeo online en la promoción y difusión de las Enfermedades Raras. In *González, J. E., y Valderrama, M. (2014). Comunicación actual: Redes sociales y lo 2.0 y 3.0* (pp. 127–137). Madrid, Spain: Editorial McGraw Hill.

López Villafranca, P., & Castillo-Esparcia, A. (2018). El encuadre de las enfermedades raras en los medios de comunicación españoles. *Observatorio (OBS*)*, *12*(2), 136-155. doi:10.15847/obsOBS12220181074

Lupton, D. (1993). The construction of patienthood in medical advertising. *International Journal of Health Services*, *23*(4), 805–819. doi:10.2190/FPDH-CXKD-RJH3-8REJ PMID:7506237

McMullan, M. (2006). Patients using the Internet to obtain health information: How this affects the patient–health professional relationship. *Patient Education and Counseling*, *63*(1-2), 24–28. doi:10.1016/j.pec.2005.10.006 PMID:16406474

Meseguer, J. A. P. (2011). La realidad en un# hashtag. Ponencia presentada en Congreso Aecpa, Sevilla, España.

Ministerio de Sanidad y Política Social. (2009). *Estrategia em Enfermedades Raras del Sistema de Salud*, Valencia, SP: CIBER de Enfermedades Raras (CIBERER). Instituto de Salud Carlos III w Instituto de Biomedicina de Valencia, CSIC. Ministerio de Sanidad y Política Social (03/032016). *La investigación y la atención sociosanitaria, claves de la estrategia de Sanidad frente a las enfermedades raras* [Press release], Retrieved from https://www.mscbs.gob.es/gabinete/notasPrensa.do?id=3916

Moorhead, S. A., Hazlett, D. E., Harrison, L., Carroll, J. K., Irwin, A., & Hoving, C. (2013). A new dimension of health care: Systematic review of the uses, benefits, and limitations of social media for health communication. *Journal of Medical Internet Research, 15*(4), e85. doi:10.2196/jmir.1933 PMID:23615206

Mortier, K., & Wackens, G. (2004). Ectodermal dysplasia anhidrotic. *Orphanet Encyclopedia, 3*, 1–6.

Nambisan, P. (2011). Information seeking and social support in online health communities: Impact on patients' perceived empathy. *Journal of the American Medical Informatics Association, 18*(3), 298–304. doi:10.1136/amiajnl-2010-000058 PMID:21486888

Nelkin, D. (1996). An uneasy relationship: The tensions between medicine and the media. *Lancet (London, England), 347*(9015), 1600–1603. doi:10.1016/S0140-6736(96)91081-8 PMID:8667872

OBSER. (2019). *Observatorio Sobre Enfermedades Raras.* Retrieved from https://obser.enfermedades-raras.org (Access date: August 13, 2019)

Pasculli, G., Resta, F., Guastamacchia, E., Suppressa, P., & Sabbà, C. (2004). Health-related quality of life in a rare disease: Hereditary hemorrhagic telangiectasia (HHT) or Rendu–Osler–Weber Disease. *Quality of Life Research: An International Journal of Quality of Life Aspects of Treatment, Care and Rehabilitation, 13*(10), 1715–1723. doi:10.100711136-004-7865-y PMID:15651542

Patientslikeme. (2019). *About us.* Retrieved from https://www.patientslikeme.com/about (Access date: August 13, 2019)

Petersen, A. (2001). Biofantasies: Genetics and medicine in the print news media. *Social Science & Medicine, 52*(8), 1255–1268. doi:10.1016/S0277-9536(00)00229-X PMID:11281408

Pinto, D., Martin, D., & Chenhall, R. (2016). The involvement of patient organisations in rare disease research: A mixed methods study in Australia. *Orphanet Journal of Rare Diseases, 11*(1), 2. doi:10.118613023-016-0382-6 PMID:26754025

Priolo, M. (2009). Ectodermal dysplasias: An overview and update of clinical and molecular-functional mechanisms. *American Journal of Medical Genetics. Part A*, *149*(9), 2003–2013. doi:10.1002/ajmg.a.32804 PMID:19504607

Rajasimha, H. K., Shirol, P. B., Ramamoorthy, P., Hegde, M., Barde, S., Chandru, V., ... Babar, I. A. (2014). Organization for rare diseases India (ORDI)–Addressing the challenges and opportunities for the Indian rare diseases' community. *Genetical Research*, *96*, e009. doi:10.1017/S0016672314000111 PMID:25579084

Revuelta, G., & Semir, V. (n.d.). Medicina y salud em la prensa diária, Informe Quiral 1997-2006, *Análisis de 10 años de información sanitária em El País, El Mundo, ABC, La Vanguardia Y El Periódico de Catalunya*. Barcelona, Spain: Observatorio de la Comunicación Científica. *Universitat Pompeu Fabra.*

Santos, M. T., & Pérez, J. A. (2019). Las enfermedades raras y su representación en la prensa española. *Palabra Clave (La Plata)*, *22*(1), 254–287. doi:10.5294/pacla.2019.22.1.10

Saxton, G. D., Niyirora, J., Guo, C., & Waters, R. (2015). # AdvocatingForChange: The strategic use of hashtags in social media advocacy. *Advances in Social Work*, *16*(1), 154–169. doi:10.18060/17952

Simoens, S., Cassiman, D., Dooms, M., & Picavet, E. (2012). Orphan Drugs for Rare Diseases. *Drugs*, *72*(11), 1437–1443. doi:10.2165/11635320-000000000-00000 PMID:22747423

Stakišaitis, D., Špokienė, I., Juškevičius, J., Valuckas, K., & Baiardi, P. (2007). Access to information supporting availability of medicines for patients suffering from rare diseases looking for possible treatments: The EuOrphan Service. *Medicina*, *43*(6), 441. doi:10.3390/medicina43060054 PMID:17637514

Subirats, L., Reguera, N., Bañón, A., Gómez-Zúñiga, B., Minguillón, J., & Armayones, M. (2018). Mining Facebook Data of People with Rare Diseases: A Content-Based and Temporal Analysis. *International Journal of Environmental Research and Public Health*, *15*(9), 1877. doi:10.3390/ijerph15091877 PMID:30200209

Tanner, A. H. (2004). Agenda building, source selection, and health news at local television stations: A nationwide survey of local television health reporters. *Science Communication*, *25*(4), 350–363. doi:10.1177/1075547004265127

Tommasetti, A., Troisi, O., & Cosimato, S. (2014). Patient empowerment and health online community: two ways to give the new viability doctor-patient relationship= Cooperación y intercambio de conocimiento en la era de Internet: dos maneras de dar nueva viabilidad a la relación médico-paciente. Comunitania. *Revista Internacional de Trabajo Social y Ciencias Sociales*, (8), 9-23. doi:10.5944/comunitania.8.1

Torrente, E., Escarrabill, J., & Martí, T. (2010). Impacto de las redes sociales de pacientes en la práctica asistencial. *Revista de Innovación Sanitaria y Atención Integrada*, *2*(1), 1.

Trujillano, D., Oprea, G. E., Schmitz, Y., Bertoli-Avella, A. M., Abou Jamra, R., & Rolfs, A. (2017). A comprehensive global genotype–phenotype database for rare diseases. *Molecular genetics & genomic medicine, 5*(1), 66-75. doi: . eCollection 2017 Jan. doi:10.1002/mgg3.262

Urrutia, J. M. (2013). El Día Mundial de las Enfermedades Raras en las noticias de prensa. *El ejemplo de Andalucía, Discurso, & Sociedad*, *7*(1), 224–247.

Valenzuela-Rodríguez, G. (2012). Análisis de los casos clínicos presentados en la serie médica televisiva Dr. House. *Rev Soc Peru Med Interna*, *25*(2), 65.

Wadhera, R. (2016). Celebrities and social cause–detailed analysis of importance of choosing a celebrity followed by pulse polio advertisement. *International Journal of Advance Research, Ideas. Innovations in Technology*, *2*(6), 1–9.

WHO -World Health Organization. (2012, June). *Coming together to combat rare diseases.* Bulletin of the World Health Organization, 90(6), June 2012, 401-476. Retrieved from https://www.who.int/bulletin/volumes/90/6/12-020612/en/ (Access date: August 13, 2019)

Wicks, P., Massagli, M., Frost, J., Brownstein, C., Okun, S., Vaughan, T., ... Heywood, J. (2010). Sharing health data for better outcomes on PatientsLikeMe. *Journal of Medical Internet Research*, *12*(2), e19. doi:10.2196/jmir.1549 PMID:20542858

Wright, K. B., Bell, S. B., Wright, K. B., & Bell, S. B. (2003). Health-related support groups on the Internet: Linking empirical findings to social support and computer-mediated communication theory. *Journal of Health Psychology*, *8*(1), 39–54. doi:10.1177/1359105303008001429 PMID:22113899

Xu, W. W., Chiu, I. H., Chen, Y., & Mukherjee, T. (2015). Twitter hashtags for health: Applying network and content analyses to understand the health knowledge sharing in a Twitter-based community of practice. *Quality & Quantity*, *49*(4), 1361–1380. doi:10.100711135-014-0051-6

Zurynski, Y., Deverell, M., Dalkeith, T., Johnson, S., Christodoulou, J., Leonard, H., & Elliott, E. J. (2017). Australian children living with rare diseases: Experiences of diagnosis and perceived consequences of diagnostic delays. *Orphanet Journal of Rare Diseases*, *12*(1), 68. doi:10.118613023-017-0622-4 PMID:28399928

Zurynski, Y., Frith, K., Leonard, H., & Elliott, E. (2008). Rare childhood diseases: How should we respond? *Archives of Disease in Childhood*, *93*(12), 1071–1074. doi:10.1136/adc.2007.134940 PMID:18684747

KEY TERMS AND DEFINITIONS

Amyotrophic Lateral Sclerosis (ALS): A progressive motor neuron degeneration disease. This disease affects muscle control and movement, leading to a number of difficulties as muscle twitching, slurred speech, stiffness, respiratory failure, among others.

Audio Podcasts: Episodic series of digital audio files, usually recorded about a certain theme, available on the Web and that can be downloaded.

Ectodermal Dysplasia (ED): This disease affects the ectoderm structures or derivatives (Priolo, 2009), e.g. skin, teeth, nail, eyes, nose. Patients with this disease lack sweat glands, which may lead to serious symptoms of hyperthermia.

FEDER (Federación de Enfermedades Raras): Spanish Federation of Rare Diseases that support more than 360 associations of patients with rare diseases in Spain.

Framing Theory: A theory that overstates that media devotes more time and attention to certain events rather than others, depending on the information meaning they convey.

Health Campaigns: A media campaign that addresses health interventions.

Lowe Syndrome: A multisystem X-linked recessive disorder that is often characterized by anomalies in the eye, nervous system and kidney problems.

Patient Organizations: Organizations that aim to support patients in policymaking, representation in such basic rights as access to health, drugs and treatments and ease the communication among patients, physicians, caregivers and other stakeholders.

Poland Syndrome: Rare congenital disease that is often characterized by the absence of muscle development on one side of the body, mainly observable through the lack of chest wall muscles and webbed fingers.

Press Releases: Official statements delivered by the organizations to the media.

Sturge-Weber: Rare congenital disease that is often characterized by a port-wine stain birthmark and neurological and eye abnormalities.

Sweeps Period: Rating time periods in which media companies reach a larger audience through a broadcast programming that meets the viewers' likes and interests and may, subsequently, increase advertisement time, promotions and some TV show cancellations.

Treacher Collins Syndrome (TCS): Genetic disorder that is often characterized by an abnormal gene that affect bone and tissue development relative to the face. There are usually deformities of the ears, eyes, cheekbones and chin.

TVE: National television broadcaster in Spain.

ENDNOTES

1 Federación Española de Enfermedades Raras (FEDER), https://enfermedades-raras.org
2 CIEBER (Centro de Investigación Biomédica en Red de las Enfermedades Raras), https://www.ciberer.es/en
3 ECCO (Research Group at Universidad de Almería), http://cvirtual.ual.es/webual/jsp/investigacion/nuevo/pInicio.jsp?id_grupo=HUM852&idioma=en
4 GIDYC (Universidad de CEU Cardenal Herrera), https://www.uchceu.es/grupos-lineas-investigacion/gidyc-grupo-de-investigacion-en-discapacidad-y-comunicacion
5 OBSER (Obervatorio sobre Enfermedades Raras), https://obser.enfermedades-raras.org
6 El País, https://elpais.com
7 El Mundo, https://www.elmundo.es
8 ABC, https://www.abc.es
9 Qué, https://www.que.es/
10 20 Minutos y ADN, https://www.20minutos.es/minuteca/adn/
11 Onda Cero, https://www.ondacero.es
12 En buenas Manos, https://www.enbuenasmanos.com
13 Radio COPE, https://www.cope.es
14 A su salud, http://www.rtve.es/alacarta/audios/a-su-salud/
15 Alimento y salud, http://www.rtve.es/alacarta/audios/alimento-y-salud/
16 Entre probetas, http://www.rtve.es/alacarta/audios/entre-probetas/
17 Spanish Public Radio Broadcasting RTVE, http://www.rtve.es
18 Radio Nacional en Directo– RNE, http://www.rtve.es/radio/radio-nacional/directo/
19 Internet Television Minoritaria TV, http://www.minoritaria.tv
20 EURORDIS TV, https://www.eurordis.org/tv

21 According to EURORDIS, "The orphan drugs" are medicinal products that serve to diagnose, prevent and treat life-threatening disorders are serious and rare. These drugs are entitled "orphan" because they have been overlooked by the pharmaceutical industry and, thus, non-profitable to the market owing to its low prevalence.

22 Doctor House, https://www.imdb.com/title/tt0412142/

23 Movie Wonder. https://www.imdb.com/title/tt2543472/

24 Campeones, https://www.imdb.com/title/tt6793580/

25 See Book "Desafíos y estrategias comunicativa de las enfermidades raras: la investigación médica como referente" edited by CIBERER, in collaboration with Universidad de Almería and Universidad Ceu-Cardenal Herrera de Valencia, which analyze the press relative to rare diseases from 2009 to 2010

26 Patientslikeme, https://www.patientslikeme.com

27 RareConnect, https://www.rareconnect.org

28 NORD-National Organization for Rare Disorders, https://rarediseases.org

29 "Share4Rare", https://www.share4rare.org/diseases

30 "#LoweResearchProject", https://www.facebook.com/LoweResearchProject/

31 PsyBlog, https://www.spring.org.uk/about-this-blog

32 The patient experience blog, http://blog.theberylinstitute.org

33 Maternity Matters, https://blogs.psychcentral.com/maternity-matters/

34 Bad Medicine, http://badmedicine.org

35 Disabled People Against Cuts, https://dpac.uk.net

36 Dr. Grumble, http://drgrumble.blogspot.com

37 Aspie in the family, http://www.aspieinthefamily.com

38 Frontier Psychiatrist, http://frontierpsychiatrist.co.uk

39 Further information on the campaign can be found at: https://enfermedades-raras.org/index.php/actualidad/2911-la-campana-enfermedades-raras-pacientes-unicos-galardonada-con-un-premio-aspid-de-oro

40 "Quiero sudar porque mis hijos no pueden", https://enfermedades-raras.org/index.php/fundacion-feder/2-feder/3560-quiero-sudar-porque-mis-hijos-no-pueden

41 "Asociación Española de Esclerodermia – ELA", https://esclerodermia.com

42 "Asociación Española SindromePoland – AESIP", http://www.aesip.es

43 "Fundación Isabel Gemio", http://www.fundacionisabelgemio.com

44 "Fundación Menudos Corazones", https://www.menudoscorazones.org

Chapter 7
Networks in Rare Diseases:
Identities, Partnership, and Advocacy in Brazil

Maria Angelica de Faria Domingues de Lima
Hospital Universitário Gaffrée e Guinle, Brazil

Ana Cristina B. Gilbert
https://orcid.org/0000-0001-9695-3946
Independent Researcher, Brazil

Dafne D. G. Horovitz
Instituto Fernandes Figueira, Brazil

ABSTRACT

Rare diseases are characterized by their low prevalence in a population, and since 1980 a social movement has gathered around this cause in many countries. In Brazil, the category of rare diseases emerged in 2000, culminating with the enactment of a National Policy geared at rare diseases. Rare disease patient organizations are the main actors of this social movement and since this is very recent in Brazil, this research was conducted to explore the topic. Using netnography as method, a content analysis of the Social Media Network Facebook was performed, aiming at understanding the way social movements have assembled around rare diseases and its role in portraying this type of diseases in Brazil. This chapter offers important insights into the way patient organizations are using social media to convey ideas and discourses, and to foster lay expertise on rare diseases.

DOI: 10.4018/978-1-7998-2088-8.ch007

INTRODUCTION

Rare diseases are defined by their low prevalence in population, and in the past years they have only been described in the biomedical literature as a way to classify a disease (Wilson, 2013). Then, the term 'rare diseases' has evolved in order to become a category, a way to classify people who share the experience of living with a rare disease. Actors of a social movement in health began to use this term in consequence of a series of events that took place – *e.g.* development in surgery treatments, gather disease information in a database (*e.g.* Orphanet), emergence of networks and associations, and media coverage (Dooms, 2016; Huyard, 2009a).

The legislation on pharmaceutical products has changed in the United States of America (USA) over the years, and it also became required to demonstrate the effectiveness and safety of those substances in order for them to be commercialized. This made pharmaceutical products safer, but also raised the cost of drug development. Therefore, the industry focused only on the development of drugs for common diseases, which could be profitable.

Before the early 80s, diseases which were not contemplated by research of new treatments and were considered 'orphan diseases.' By contrast, in the following decades, people with 'orphan/rare diseases' and their families had begun to claim access to treatment and a way to solve those inequities was a new law – the Orphan Drug Act, which included several incentives for the development of drugs for orphan/rare diseases (Greene & Podolsky, 2012).

The Orphan Drug Act, enacted in 1984 had two criteria to define what was meant by an orphan drug (Huyard, 2009a): (1) the drug would be used to treat diseases with a prevalence of lower than 200.000 patients in the United States of America; or (2) although the disease prevalence would exceed 200.000 patients, the drug would not be profitable in the American market. The incentives granted by this law focused on the industry's profitability and not on its innovation capacities. Therefore, people with rare diseases tended to be overlooked as health consumers and, as such, they began to make political demands for access to specific treatments.

In Europe, the social movement of rare diseases has emerged in the 1990s. The French government, alongside rare diseases patient organizations, founded a non-governmental organization (NGO) dedicated to rare diseases, EURORDIS – Rare Diseases Europe (EURORDIS, 2018). The policy geared at rare diseases in the European Union (EU) also included incentives for the pharmaceutical industry.

It is worth noting that the European policy makes a clear distinction between orphan diseases and rare diseases. Orphan diseases are the ones that mainly affect people living in the underdeveloped world, which makes them an unprofitable market due to economic restrictions and rare diseases are the ones that mainly affect few people living in the developed world, which makes them unprofitable due to a very small market (Huyard, 2011a).

The social movement aimed at rare diseases has emerged in Brazil almost 30 years later than the Orphan Drug Act. The cornerstone of 'rare diseases' in Brazil was in 2009 with the I Brazilian Congress on Rare Diseases, promoted by Fundación Gêiser (Oliveira, Guimarães & Machado, 2012; Sergent, Cagliari & Teixeira, 2010). Since then, Brazil joined the 'Rare Disease Day' movement, and patient organizations alongside with health professionals and delegates of the State assembled to develop a National Policy for Rare Diseases (Santos, Cagliari &Teixeira, 2010; Tejada, 2010). Unlike the USA and the EU, Brazilian's National Policy, enacted in 2014, has not introduced financial aids for the pharmaceutical industry. It is mainly focused on the development and financing of rare diseases reference centers in order to grant the population access to diagnosis and treatment of those patients (Fonseca, 2014).

The aim of this chapter is to understand the way social movements have assembled around rare diseases and its role in portraying this type of diseases in Brazil. Hence, this chapter proceeds with the research background, purpose and introduction to netnography. Then, the rare disease patient organizations are presented and both group identities and individual's subjectivity are addressed. Finally, it summarizes the relevant events that are part of social movements relative to rare diseases in Brazil.

BACKGROUND

The idea that people with different diseases could be represented under a single group was what made possible the emergence of a social movement in health geared at rare diseases. Patients and their families realized that even though diseases were different, they shared the experience of living with a rare disease and that they had similar needs. Soon the identity of 'rare' was shaped and rare diseases became a category with political use (Forman et al., 2012; Giugliani, Vairo, Riegel, de Souza, Schwartz, & Pena, 2016; Melo, et al., 2015; Williams, 2011).

A category is a way to classify someone or something. Classifications promote a structure and, as such, it aids with assimilation of people and the society. However, this has consequences, owing to the fact that certain designations are likely to exclude individual features. Therefore, equalizing people inside a social matrix generates a certain way to act and think. Discourses and practices shape the social construction of an idea, or a category. In turn, it frames the experience of living under a certain classification (Hacking, 1999).

Patient organizations are main actors in the generation of health policies, as they serve as spokesperson for a whole group. They have a major role in the advancement of democracy in a society as they collaborate with individual development, represent certain groups in political domains and build public opinion. In general, they are frequently part of a social movement (Lüchmann, 2014). Indeed, a social movement can be defined as "collective actions of socio-political-cultural nature that make feasible the organization of a population to express its demands" (Gohn, 2011, p.335).

Since this is a recent phenomenon in Brazil, it is not well understood. Furthermore, a National Policy geared at genetic diseases exists in the country since 2009. However, this policy was never embodied beyond its theory. It is worth noting that the liberal democracies of the North have different cultural and historical backgrounds when compared to democracies of the South (Frossard & Dias, 2016; Rose, 2007). So, how exactly social movements in health assemble around 'rare diseases' in the country and what means to 'be rare' in Brazil have been a subject of interest during the past few years in the country.

In this chapter, the researchers analyze how the identity of 'rare' is shaped by patient organizations in Brazil. The study was undertaken in the Social Network Site – Facebook, owing to the fact that very recently virtual communities have enabled new forms of relationships and patient organizations use the cyberspace like many other companies to propagate ideas and publish their accomplishments in order to gather more followers, consolidating a social movement (Armayones, Requena, Gómez-Zuñiga, Pousada & Bañón, 2015).

METHOD

For this research, sources were all pages created and maintained by patient organizations that represented people with rare diseases of genetic etiology in Brazil. The definition of rare diseases in this study was the same employed by the National Policy on rare diseases in Brazil, which states that a disease is rare when it affects less than 65/100.000 individuals (Ministério da Saúde, 2014). After consulting the Orphanet document on the frequency of rare disorders (Rath, Wakap, Demarest & Lanneau, 2016), the researchers defined which diseases would be included in this study. A total of 65 diseases are represented by patient organizations in the country, which added to a total of 191 organizations. One organization was excluded because it was not active. The authors, then, searched for patient organizations on the social network and found 102 Facebook pages. All items published by the organizations on the pages between 2010 (the year the first post appeared) and 2016 were analyzed using netnography as a method. In order to preserve individual's identities, the authors did not report names of people who published on the social network. In addition, patient organizations were identified only by the disease they represent and not by their full names.

In regard to the method used, netnography is a qualitative research method that uses data gathered from the Internet. It is an adaptation of ethnography to digital media because in cyberspace we need to analyze not only language, but also images, videos, sounds, among other digital files. Netnography considers that participant-observation involves an immersion of the researcher in the theme. Kozinets (2005) proposes that data should be analyzed in seven steps:

Step 1 **Imaging**: The researcher collects data and makes conscious observations, taking note of all reactions;
Step 2 **Re-memorying:** The researcher thinks about the data that was previously collected and writes down everything he/she can remember;
Step 3 **Abduction:** The researcher tries to identify theories that might explain the data;
Step 4 **Visual abstraction:** It is the expansion of local observations to universal data;
Step 5 **Ratifying:** The researcher analyzes data using artistic expression in such a way that it may help to evoke metaphors. It is also a visual tool to connect all data;
Step 6 **Cultural decoding:** Cultural framing of data, which requires the recognition of patterns from the evaluation of each part;

Step 7 **Tournament play**: *The researcher tests as many ideas as possible that might explain the data and choose the one that fits the best.*

In the following sections, the authors will discuss the main functions of a group identity; how patient organizations craft this identity; what is the identity of 'rare diseases' in Brazil, and critics to the models established so far in the country.

RARE DISEASE PATIENT ORGANIZATIONS IN BRAZIL

Patient organizations have many roles. They help to disseminate information about disease symptoms, diagnosis and treatment; create a place where individuals may share the experience of living with a rare disease without the feeling of being judged; articulate in political sphere to guarantee access to the health system, treatment and social security benefits, among other roles (Ingelfinger & Drazen, 2011). Simultaneously, those actions demand and help setting up a group identity, which is crucial to social movements (Lüchmann, 2014).

Caroline Huyard (2009b) in her research about rare diseases patient organizations in France, she identified two main kinds of associations: (a) 'pluralistic' organizations, and (b) 'monistic' organizations. This division is based on the associations' actions, vision and mission defined by its members. These organizations differ in the following ways:

- **Pluralistic associations:** In pluralistic associations, patients, families and health professionals share decisions and activities, focusing mainly on patient care. Therefore, their actions are aimed at emotional support, guidance to patients and health professionals and social and political recognition. These organizations do not expect major breakthroughs that will change the natural history of the disease they represent unlike the monistic associations, which are focused on the cure.
- **Monistic associations:** Monistic associations are managed by one single actor (either patients, families or health professionals) and their tasks are directed either to disease recognition, through advertisement, hoping that treatment breakthroughs arise in the future, or to the development of a cure.

It is well known that patient organizations use cyberspace to divulgate their activities and information about diseases regarding diagnostics and treatment, to convey social, psychological and medical support, to promote scientific research and to raise money for the cause (Armayones et al., 2009). On Facebook, each association may have a profile or a page. Usually organizations use pages to spread their message, and it is through images, audios, videos and written text that discourses are built. It is important to mention that discourses represent a set of propositions created in accordance to social rules shared in a specific historical moment. As such, they are meaningful, relational and circumstantial. They are cultural practices that relate to an individual who speaks of something, in a certain way, for someone in a certain time/space.

Through discourses, collective identity is built and acknowledged by patient organizations (Osakabe, 2002). According to Goodwin, Jasper and Polletta (2001, p.285), collective identity is defined as:

An individual's cognitive, moral, and emotional connection with a broader community, category, practice, or institution. It is a perception of a shared status or relation, which may be imagined rather than experienced directly, and it is distinct from personal identities, although it may form part of a personal identity (Goodwin, Jasper, & Polletta, 2011, p.285)

The elaboration of such an identity is not only cognitive but also an emotional process. It is an important mechanism in social movements as it promotes the group union, the maintenance and commitment of individuals to the group and to the cause, the integration of new members and constitute persuasive strategies employed by the group (Goodwin, Jasper & Polletta, 2001).

Patient organizations also provide guidance to patients, their families and health professionals through social network posting live or online lectures. The main themes are the diagnosis, treatment, health care and some other practices they consider beneficial. Those actions represent the circulation of knowledge outside the traditional sphere and are understood as redistribution of power between patients and specialists (Rabeharisoa, 2008, p13).

Mutual-help groups are the pioneers to experience the distribution of knowledge outside biomedical institutions, during the 1940s. Throughout the 20th century, the knowledge produced by non-specialists gained validity in the society, especially because of a legitimacy crisis of specialists (Prior, 2003; Rabeharisoa, 2008). In the 1990s, Arksey (1994), in a research with patients suffering from repetitive strain injury and Epstein (1995), in his study with AIDS patient groups and social movement noted that lay people have a major role in the construction of knowledge, what is regarded as lay expertise.

Lay experts acquire knowledge by experience and defy biomedical hegemony (Prior, 2003). However, in the context of rare diseases, when patient organizations establish partnership with experts, their knowledge help to advance science (Rabeharisoa, 2008). The following posts serve as examples on how patient organizations appear as lay experts:

People, when you undergo an ECO (echocardiogram), ask the doctor to pay attention to this detail which is the presence or absence of left ventricular noncompactation - Posted by a Muscular Dystrophy Patient Organization on January 2013.

Attention, doctors! Diagnostics delay and inadequate treatment are the worst enemies of patients with porphyria. Access our content and inform yourself about this rare disease - Posted by a Porphyria Patient Organization on August 2016.

Rare diseases are characterized not only by its low prevalence but also by physicians' lack of knowledge about the disease, what influences the patient-physician relationship (Budych, Helms, & Schultz, 2012), as patients no longer expect physicians to respond to all their needs. When facing a physician, who does not have all the answers or meets the patient or his/her family demands, patients and families set out to gain information about the disease (Budych, Helms & Schultz, 2012; Engel, Bagal, Broback & Boice, 2013) through contact with other families, patient organizations and they may even do the research on their own.

While general practitioners regard their self-knowledge about rare diseases as insufficient, experts do not share the same opinion (Engel, Bagal, Broback & Boice, 2013). Considering that most rare diseases are of genetic etiology this imposes another problem in Brazil, as medical genetics is the specialty with the least number of physicians in the country (Scheffer, Biancarelli & Cassenote, 2018) and the majority of them is based on seven of the 27 states of Brazil (Passos-Bueno, Bertola, Horovitz, Ferraz & Brito, 2014), which makes access to proper health care even harder.

The lack of knowledge about rare diseases results in diagnostic delay, which may be of several years, holds back the initiation of proper treatment, and provokes the onset of irreversible complications and psychological stress in patients and their families. Another common consequence of diagnostic delay is income decrease in families affected by rare diseases. Since the majority of rare diseases are chronic conditions, the quest to understand all symptoms someone presents leads to work withdrawal, from the patient or family member (Aghamohammadi et al., 2010; Barataud, 2001; Bruni, Lavery & Broomfield, 2016; Streinraths, Vallance & Davidson, 2008; Vieira et al., 2008).

In this setting, patient organizations may even take on diagnosis, as it is shown in the following statement:

More and more I believe that my son has Williams syndrome for [his] many physical and mental characteristics, and based on all the information available on this syndrome - A woman comments on a post by the Williams syndrome's association that presents the characteristics of the syndrome

[..] and gets a reply from another woman: Send his photos to us... look at my Williams granddaughter. The first woman then shares her son's picture and the second states: From what I saw on the pictures... it's not.

The process of diagnosis is supported by biomedical classifications and is associated to the existing power of medical profession (Dew & Jutel, 2014). While avoiding the dichotomy of expert x layperson, Epstein (1996) argues that patient organizations become professionalized within social movements and develop *credibility tactics* (Epstein, 1995, p.417). Credibility tactics are strategies that patient organizations use in order to be accepted as equals by health professionals, society and the State while defending their cause and, in order for this to happen, they have to learn the language and culture of Medicine (Epstein, 1995).

In Brazil, becoming a 'lay expert' not only gives patient organizations the authority to turn into true representatives of patients in the political sphere, but also they are almost imposed by the biomedical institution in the country as there are many gaps in the health system that impair the proper care of people with rare diseases. There is still a debate on scientific literature (Héon-Klin, 2017; Polich, 2012; Prior, 2003) about the means of being a lay expert. Prior (2003) points that, since lay expert acquire knowledge mainly by experience, this may not be valid, as the experience will not show them the full amplitude of knowledge (Prior, 2003). In turn, Rabeharisoa understands that since the concept of lay expert emerged amidst uncommon and lethal diseases, it is the individual experience that helps science to advance, as patient organizations partner with experts (Rabeharisoa, 2008).

The immersion in biomedical culture and the use of its language is not restricted to scientific discussions nor used while in this space. Patient organizations adopt certain practices of biomedical culture even when communicating to patients, families and society. It is very common to observe physicians (and health professionals in general) to speak about a person with Down's syndrome, for instance, as "a Down", and sentences like "John, the Down", or "John is Down". The same type of behavior is witnessed on publications from patient organizations and their public on social networks: *Every family should have a Williams*, posted on Williams' syndrome patient organization on November 2014 or *her father is a DAAT*, observed on alpha-1 antitrypsin deficiency patient organizations on July 2015. In this last example, the acronym for the disease was sufficient to classify the person.

Some patient organizations frequently use this figure of speech while others are very aware of its consequences. To characterize a person as a disease is a narrowing portrait of a person and reiterates rare diseases/disability as a medical problem. Besides, this gives the impression that people with those diseases are worth less than the majority of society, as the only thing they may have is a disabled body.

Patient organizations also reproduce language mistakes rooted in biomedical discourse, which are specific to Portuguese. Two frequent errors are: (a) use the word pathology as a synonym for the word disease; and (b) refer to someone who has a disease as "the carrier of a disease", since a "carrier" is someone who has a deleterious allele for a genetic disease with autosomal recessive pattern.

The authority acquired while penetrating the biomedical culture warrants patient organizations to share information about health in a wider sense, such as vaccination calendar, the importance of regular exercise, screening tests for cancer, diabetes, hypertension, among others. The promotion of a healthy lifestyle by some associations is almost excessive. Apart from diseases that require dietary treatments, such as phenylketonuria, homocystinuria, Prader-Willi syndrome, the recommendations are trivial and reflect current cultural practices of self-care.

Even though this may be seen as distancing from medical power, it is an approximation to the biomedical paradigm (Crawford, 1980; Skrabanek, 1994). The idea that one must be responsible for its own health through the practice of exercises, by using vitamins and eating properly or by choosing holistic therapies is known as healthism (Crawford, 1980) and has emerged in the last century as a way to manage populations, by making individuals responsible for their choices and that has transformed health in a commodity.

These practices are supported by preventive measures of public health and are an expression of the responsible biological citizen.

GROUP IDENTITIES AND INDIVIDUAL'S SUBJECTIVITY

A group identity is elaborated and continuously molded by patient organizations as it is necessary to produce a space that will shelter patients and their families when they feel helpless. Biomedical institutions traditionally place people with rare diseases in an invisible space, on the grounds that rare diseases are infrequent, and do not produce a profitable market.

Health professionals are not familiarized with rare diseases and do not know how to investigate and to treat those patients. Huyard (2011b) indicates that patients seek in those organizations what they do not find in health professionals or other institutions, and this is one of the main reasons why people adhere to these organizations. In turn, patient organizations designate themselves as families, a concept that reinforces the feeling of belonging, therefore using emotional predicates in order to strengthen the public participation in the social movement.

The association of patients with Ehlers-Danlos syndrome represented this idea in a post published on October 2015 (Rodrigues, 2014). The author writes:

[…] beyond all the pain and symptoms that we have, we still need to suffer because of another problem… This is followed by the word 'pain', which the author uses as a puzzle for his next sentences lack of scientific knowledge by health professionals, institutional omission, and nonexistent social representation[1] *The author then finishes the post And this is how we feel… and this is how we are seen and treated. Or would it be untreated… whatever. [name of person] explained perfectly… a rare among the rare…*

The aforementioned post also introduces the category "to be rare." It is worth to note that not every patient organizations that take part in the social movement choose this representation. However, the ones that do so, classify the person with a rare disease as virtuous based on their accomplishments, suggesting they are some kind of super-heroes or that they may even have some essence of holiness. This way of framing people is filled with positivism, being also used to describe people with disabilities. The experience of living with a rare disease affects not only the individual but also every person, who has a relation to him/her, such as relatives and friends.

Many people with rare diseases wish to share life experiences with someone else who truly understands their reality (Huyard, 2009c), therefore groups or associations may be a way to fulfill this desire. The development of relations and identities sustained by biological characteristics was imagined by Paul Rabinow (1996) in the 1990s, as he analyzed the social consequences of the Human Genome Project:

In the future the new genetics will cease to be a biological metaphor for modern society and will become instead a circulation network of identity terms and restriction loci, around which and through which a truly new type of autoproduction will emerge, which I call 'biosociality' (Rabinow, 1996, p99)

The formulation of an identity based on biological aspects, such as the rarity of a disease define biosocial groups. The categorization of individuals by biological characteristics has been a common practice of many States throughout the 18th, 19th and 20th centuries and many State practices have defined citizenship in those nations, which is understood as biological citizenship. However, individuals have also taken part in the construction of these citizenships. More recently, actors of social movements in health have produced this kind of citizenship in order to assist with political and social demands. Even though biological citizenship may represent a group, we cannot underestimate its role as a guiding force of relations and choices at the individual level, as it is the individual who embodies this citizen (Rose & Novas, 2003).

An article about Angelman Syndrome with the following headline "Rare syndrome keeps a boy always 'happy'", posted on March 2013, serves as example on how biological citizenship may influence on individual level. Angelman Syndrome is a condition characterized by severe developmental delay, intellectual disability, severe speech impairment, gait ataxia, seizures and inappropriate behavior characterized by frequent and unprovoked laughter (Dagli, Mueller & Williams, 2017).

Unmotivated laughter is likely to be a manifestation of psychiatric diseases, such as mania and schizophrenia but also represents uncontrolled emotions. Nevertheless, the author of this post chose to associate the frequent laughter to the idea of unlimited happiness. On the one hand, this reaffirms that people with disabilities may experience blissful lives, on the other hand, this determines how life may be experienced and displaces those children from their humanity, as mood swings are a major part of the human being. Besides, it may even make it harder for families to deal with tantrums, a common behavior in some syndromes, as eternally happy people will never experience frustration or any other negative emotion, which is very far from the real life.

To adopt the name "rare disease" instead of Angelman syndrome (or any other disease) is a resource to emphasize the social movement around rare diseases, and to gather infrequent diseases under a name that represent them all, creating a larger group. In other words, when examined independently each disease represents a very small number of people. However, as there are more than 6000 rare diseases, this makes up to a large number of people affected by a rare disease in the country.

Considering that the frequency is 65/100.000, it is expected over 15 million people with a rare disease living in Brazil. In this sense, activists have been using the slogan rare diseases are rare, but patients with rare diseases are many to promote the cause. The politics of numbers as Rabeharisoa et al. (2014) point out is a strategy used by activists around the globe to push for policies that are focused on universal needs of people with rare diseases. Nevertheless, each disease has particularities that also need to be addressed, which those authors refer to as politics of singularization.

Very few associations do not use the term "rare diseases" to promote their causes, and usually they are related to hemophilia and cystic fibrosis. It is worth noting that the social movements in health that address those two diseases have been established in Brazil more than 15 years ago, *i.e.* many years before the rare diseases movement, and have been acknowledged by the State in public policies geared at cystic fibrosis and hemophilia. However, other disease groups already attained by public policies in the country chose to take part in the rare diseases movement, which implies that for some, to grant access to the health system and civil rights is not enough.

Organizations use patient's testimonials not only as a way to promote awareness campaigns or to construct a space where experiences may be shared, but also as a way to promote the discourses they identify with. Positive ideas are transmitted by narratives about rare diseases and disabilities in social networks. This is a manifestation of a positive society that tell their stories in a very transparent manner as argued by the philosopher Byung-Chul Han (2017), where there is no space for negativity, what makes it harder for people to deal with suffering. Besides, some characteristics of the social network reinforces the shallowness of communication. Facebook provides three main types of interaction: to comment on a post, to share a publication or "to like" a post. The majority of the public chooses to interact with organizations mainly by "likes" adding value to what is published and making the network interactions instantaneously. Information overflow, as stated by Han, impairs profound social transformations, as they fill emptiness and do not promote necessary reflections, which are the basis for a change (Han, 2017).

Coopman (2003) points out that cultural representations of disability are usually permeated by narratives considered pleasant by non-disabled. The narrative of overcoming is a frequent one, which brings disability close to the biomedical model, in the sense that there is something to be amended, usually by the individual's capability to triumph over his/her own problems. In rare diseases, not only disability shall be beaten, but also a poor medical prognosis or a certain expectancy of life established by previous scientific reports. These messages are usually transmitted by headlines stating that we need to improve ourselves or overcome the impossible, (audio-)visual content showing someone's resilience and life testimonials.

In the era that Olympic and Paralympic Games took place in Brazil, patient organizations hardly mentioned to the games on their pages. These few remarks included the participation of disabled people on Opening Ceremonies and the Olympic Torch Tour, the allocation of public funds in the organization of games in spite of investments in the public health system and the presence of Michael Phelps in the Olympic Games, a high performance athlete who supposedly has a rare disease. Some patient organizations describe Phelps as an athlete who has Marfan syndrome or Ehlers-Danlos syndrome due to his large wingspan. In turn, the public uses this image to relate himself or herself to a champion, maybe even some kind of God, through whom they expect to accomplish their own goals.

Patient organizations and their public also use the social network Facebook to elaborate discourses about diseases, which helps to provide meaning to illness. In this context, military metaphors are frequently observed. It is worth mentioning that they are so present in biomedical discourse. As Hodgkin (1985, p.1820) puts it: Medicine is war.

Metaphors are a kind of figurative language that organizes the conceptual system of human language, which situates an idea (an object) in certain words (a container) that relate in a certain space. They do not exist only in the cognitive domain, but they also affect our emotions and even simple acts in our daily lives (Lakoff & Johnsen, 2003).

Modern Medicine employs military language to describe diseases, illness, physiopathological processes, among others, since the discovery of microorganisms are regarded as the cause of some diseases, being located outside the body. Warlike metaphors recall the idea that men may control nature, in other words, that disease may be amenable to domination. In this sense, the physician would fight against disease and death to win over its patient. The passive patient no longer possesses his/her own body, which becomes a battlefield (Sontag, 2003). While placing bodies as places occupied by enemies (diseases and death) that must be eliminated, this metaphor produces two myths to deal with diseases - overcoming and cure, and only one possibility which is to win.

Patient organizations use words such as struggle, war, combat, warriors, weapon among others to describe illness, to mobilize resources for research of new drugs and the creation of public policies focused on treatment as in the following excerpts:

Spinal muscular atrophy, Spinraza (Nusinersen) and (patient organization name) in O Globo (a local newspaper) today. Our fight continues! Headline of a publication by the patient organization about a new drug for spinal muscular atrophy (SMA), published on December 2016. This post, then, presents the link to the journal website where one can find the newspaper article about the new drug.

The newspaper headline stated:

Ammunition against a fatal disease! and a fragment of the text: The genetic disease that most kills children around the world has, now, a rival able to protect its victims from the majority of its devastating sequels.

This article has had a major impact among spinal muscular atrophy patient organizations, and most of them published this piece. Nusinersen was released and approved for human use by the Federal Drug Administration in 2016. At that time, it was not registered in Brazil and patients and families with SMA started to work for the license and commercialization of this drug in the country.

SMA is a degenerative disease characterized mainly by muscle weakness. In the most severe form of the disease, type 0, children never achieve milestones, and usually die in the first year of life. In type 1, children can sit with support and do not survive to adulthood. In type 2, most children achieve adult life and depend on someone to help them with most activities of daily living. In types 3, life expectancy is not reduced but people may need help with some activities of daily living, even though they can walk independently. In type 4, the mildest form of the disease, symptoms manifest only in adults and patients, who are able to walk independently, and may need help with a few activities of daily life (Prior & Finanger, 2016).

Brazilian SMA patient organizations have carried out a campaign in favor of the drug since before its release in the American market. The message was that the disease triumphs. Many posts show children with SMA who passed away and the campaign slogan "Until when will we lose our children to SMA?" They also released statistical data about the disease in which they show numbers of the severe forms of the disease. The option to portray SMA as a severe and lethal disease has a political function. By appealing to a strong emotional message, associations gather more followers around the cause they defend, and promote the movement in favor of licensing the medication in the country as a first step to elaborate a policy that will allow for anyone with the disease to be treated through the public health system.

Patient organizations, and their Facebook pages, may be understood as communities of practice, as defined by Lawthorn and Chataika (2012) "a community of practice is a collection of people bound together by location, purpose, activity, values, desires, or perhaps labels" (Lawthorn & Chataika, 2012, p.235). These authors debate how groups of people with disabilities mediate disability as a political movement, but also as an identity movement, and that a community may include or exclude people based on its rhetoric. Therefore, the impact of these actions in people with SMA types 2, 3, 4 is unknown, as they do not seem represented by the organization. Besides, if they feel represented, what are the personal consequences of this kind of discourse?

The public engages in comments and argues that patient organizations are the leading way for them to guarantee their rights. On the one hand, this reinforces the idea that these organizations are major actors of social change and that their rhetoric is necessary. On the other hand, the choice of war metaphors reaffirms the passivity of the individual that has to deal with a disease, and this is an expression of the biomedical model. The relationship between the public and biomedical institutions is a hierarchical one, with patients submitting themselves to external control. This may be considered a conflicting attitude from patient organizations, especially when they act as lay experts. In other words, patient organizations question the power of biomedical institutions; however, they also promote this relation of power. These messages shape the illness experience and, considering that genetic rare diseases are chronic and for the majority of them, symptoms begin during infancy, the experience is shared by an entire family, and may present with negative outcomes (Helman, 2009; Sontag, 2003).

To understand rare diseases (or disability) as a medical issue may be an advantage as it provides an explanation to why a person is affected, extenuating the idea that a disease or a disability is a burden or a celestial punishment (Coopman, 2003). Most organizations explain, in a very superficial way, the genetic aspects of the disease and its heritability, what seems that they are just spreading superficial data. One of the most specific examples is the text published by Prader-Willi syndrome patient organization on the World Obesity Day:

Treat obesity with respect! Behind it, there is a genetic condition. People diagnosed with Prader-Willi syndrome have symptoms such as cognitive impairment, severe obesity and excessive eating, among others.

However, the purpose of this phrase might as well be to lessen the stigma of obesity and not of disability or of a rare disease. Contradicting what Coopman (2003) proposes, the explanation of rare diseases/disability as genetic diseases is perceived as a problem by some people, especially those affected by a neurodegenerative disease of autosomal dominant inheritance. Some of those disorders present symptoms only in adult life, usually by the time people already had children and the illness experience is marked by a family bearing witness to their loved ones slowly becoming disable and dependent.

The biggest problem we think, when we realize that this is a late-onset disease, is that we already had children, in other words, potentially new ataxic, since it is a disease passed on genetically. I already had grandchildren when I realized that. How I manage to redress this? It is to throw myself, to use me, my body, my soul, make me available to scientists to find a way to improve our quality of life or cure it [woman's testimony about Machado-Joseph disease that is part of a documentary called 'Quatro Heranças', published by spinocerebellar ataxia patient organization on June 2013].

My mother passed away at the age of 59 years old, she had already been having problems (…) she felt down, saying she tripped over something (…). At that time, the doctor diagnosed her with motor neuron disease, and told me it was a rare disease, that it manifested in children but also adults, that it was genetic (…) I didn't know it was hereditary until I found out I had a nephew grandchild with the same problem… very sad… [woman's testimony about Machado-Joseph disease commenting on the post about the documentary called 'Quatro Heranças', published on June 2013].

I live with this disease (Ataxia) and all the suffering it causes since I was a child, through my father. Hardly did I know that I had also inherited this disorder [woman's testimony posted on the page of the spinocerebellar ataxia patient organization on May 2016].

However, the link between rare disease/disability and genetic etiology is not enough reason to explain the disease in a family for some people. In those cases, the idea of a gift appears, reminding of a transcendent origin, particularly when it is the father or the mother who describes their children with a rare disease/disability.

(…) From this side, we keep moving forward in our mission, bursting in faith and with lots of resilience… concentrating our energies in good, positive ideas, always remembering to be grateful to our Father, for allowing us to learn a little, to evolve a little more, turning us into new people, and still having the privilege of being chosen to receive these angels. (…) a life's mission that will certainly bring us close to our Father. [Rett syndrome patient organization, October 2016]

It is possible to note religious thematic in many posts, mainly on those when some kind of protection is needed and when Christian virtues are mentioned. Angel is a word frequently used to describe a child, and they are the image of heavenly protection. Cardoso (2000) argues that the angel metaphor, traditionally linked to children with Down syndrome does not reduce the stigma associated to this condition. Gilbert (2012) indicates that this metaphor reinforces ideas of perfection and innocence, which have direct consequences on the lives of people with Down syndrome, who try to fit in this matrix. Children with rare diseases are also compared to angels, and while bringing valuable lessons to their parents, they impersonate the esteem and prosperity of a family. The analogy of being a transcendental being also makes us wonder if rhetoric about participation in society is a real one or if it is just an echo of a well-established discourse.

CONCLUSION

In summary, categories may simplify integration among different actors – patients, health professionals and representatives of the State and facilitate the social movement aimed at rare diseases. However, this is not without consequences neither for the group in the political sphere, nor for the individual. Each group should use simultaneously strategies in the 'politics of numbers' and the 'politics of singularization' in order to accomplish its goals.

Patient organizations are crafting the category of 'rare' in Brazil, and the social network is, without a doubt, one of the approaches that has been used to convey ideas and discourses. The concept of rare seems to be portrayed as a lack of knowledge about diseases and symptoms, challenging diagnosis, lack or unavailability of proper treatment and the need to persevere in the struggle to secure rights.

Even though the theme of rare diseases has recently emerged in the country, the discourses seem to mimic old beliefs about genetic diseases and disability. Discourses relate to ideas and concepts, which shape groups and individuals. It is not possible to interact with a group and not be influenced at some level by the ideas that circulate inside the group, with individual consequences.

It is possible to note that patient organizations, while using tactics of credibility, resemble biomedical institutions and reinforce the biomedical model of illness/disability. Activists seem to simultaneously criticize and relate to biomedical institutions, and while this may be a way it remains to know if this will be sufficient to advance major social transformations that are utterly necessary in Brazil.

REFERENCES

Aghamohammadi, A., Bahrami, A., Mamishi, S., Mohammadi, B., Abolhassani, H., Parveneh, N., & Razei, N. (2010). Impact of delayed diagnosis in children with primary antibody deficiencies. *Journal of Microbiology, Immunology, and Infection*, *44*(3), 229–234. doi:10.1016/j.jmii.2011.01.026 PMID:21524619

Arksey, H. (1994). Expert and lay participation in the construction of medical knowledge. *Sociology of Health & Illness*, *16*(4), 44–468. doi:10.1111/1467-9566.ep11347516

Armayones, M., Requena, S., Gómez-Zuñiga, B., Pousada, M., & Bañón, A. M. (2015). El uso de Facebook en asociaciones españolas de enfermedades raras: ¿cómo e para qué lo utilizan? *Gaceta Sanitaria*, *29*(5), 335–340. doi:10.1016/j.gaceta.2015.05.007 PMID:26145457

Barataud, B. (2001). *Cinq mille maladies rares, le choc de la génétique: constat, perspectives et possibilités d'évolution.* Retrieved from http://www.ladocumentationfrancaise.fr/rapports-publics/014000706/index.shtml

Bruni, S., Lavery, C., & Broomfield, A. (2016). The diagnostic journey of patients with mucopolysaccharidosis I: A real-world survey of patient and physician experiences. *Molecular Genetics and Metabolism Reports*, *8*, 67–73. doi:10.1016/j.ymgmr.2016.07.006 PMID:27536552

Budych, K., Helms, T. M., & Schultz, C. (2012). How do patients with rare diseases experience the medical encounter? Exploring role behaviour and its impact on patient-physician interaction. *Health Policy (Amsterdam)*, *105*(2-3), 154–164. doi:10.1016/j.healthpol.2012.02.018 PMID:22464590

Cardoso, M. H. C. A. (2000). *A herança arcaica de um modelo: História, Medicina e a síndrome de Down* (Doctoral dissertation). Retrieved from Biblioteca da Saúde da Mulher e da Criança, FIOCRUZ. (000043084)

Coopman, S. J. (2003). Communicating Disability: Metaphors of Oppression, *Metaphors of Empowerment. Annals of the International Communication Association*, *27*(1), 337–394. doi:10.1080/23808985.2003.11679030

Crawford, R. (1980). Healthism and the medicalization of everyday life. *International Journal of Health Services*, *10*(3), 365–388. doi:10.2190/3H2H-3XJN-3KAY-G9NY PMID:7419309

Dagli, A. I., Mueller, J., & Williams, C. A. Angelman Syndrome. (2017). In: M. P. Adam, H. H. Ardinger, R. A. Pagon, & S. E. Wallace (Eds.), *GeneReviews*. Retrieved from https://www.ncbi.nlm.nih.gov/books/NBK1144/

Dew, K., & Jutel, A. G. (2014). I am not a doctor, but…: The lay-professional relationship in diagnosis. In A. G. Jutel, & K. Dew (Eds.), *Social issues in diagnosis. Baltimore*, MD: Johns Hopkins University Press.

Dooms, M. M. (2016). Orphan devices: yesterday is history; tomorrow is mystery: towards a European orphan device directive? *Orphanet Journal of Rare Diseases*, *11*(1), 22. doi:10.118613023-016-0393-3 PMID:26939863

Engel, P. A., Bagal, S., Broback, M., & Boice, N. (2013). Physician and patient perceptions regarding training in rare diseases: The need for stronger educational initiatives for physicians. *The Journal of Rare Disorders*, *1*(2), 1–15. Retrieved from http://www.journalofraredisorders.com/Interface/errors/404.html?aspxerrorpath=/pub/IssuePDFs/Engel.pdf

Epstein, S. (1995). The construction of lay expertise: AIDS activism and the forging of credibility in the reform of clinical trials. *Science, Technology, & Human Values*, *20*(4), 408–437. doi:10.1177/016224399502000402 PMID:11653331

Epstein, S. (1996). *Impure science. AIDS, activism, and the politics of knowledge.* Berkley, CA: University of California Press.

EURORDIS - *European Organization for Rare Diseases.* (2018). *The voice of RARE DISEASE PATIENTS in Europe* [PDF file]. Retrieved from https://www.eurordis.org/publication/eurordis-leaflet

Fonseca, R. V. G. (2014). *A construção de uma Política Pública para doenças raras no Brasil* (Undergraduate degree dissertation). Retrieved from Biblioteca Digital da Produção Intelectual Discente. Retrieved from http://bdm.unb.br/handle/10483/8182

Forman, J., Taruscio, D., Llera, V. A., Barrera, L. A., Coté, T. R., Edfjäll, C., ... Tambuyzer, E. (2012). The need for worldwide policy and action plans for rare diseases. *Acta Paediatrica (Oslo, Norway)*, *101*(8), 805–807. doi:10.1111/j.1651-2227.2012.02705.x PMID:22519914

Frossard, V. C., & Dias, M. C. M. (2016). O impacto da internet na interação entre pacientes: Novos cenários em saúde. *Interface (Botucatu)*, *20*(57), 349–361. doi:10.1590/1807-57622014.1334

Gilbert, A. C. B. (2012). *Vértice do Impensável. Um estudo de narrativas em síndrome de Down.* Rio de Janeiro, Brazil: Editora Fiocruz. doi:10.7476/9788575415726

Giugliani, R., Vairo, F. P., Riegel, M., de Souza, C. F., Schwartz, I. V., & Pena, S. D. (2016). Rare disease landscape in Brazil: Report of a successful experience in inborn errors of metabolism. *Orphanet Journal of Rare Diseases*, *11*(1), 76. doi:10.118613023-016-0458-3 PMID:27282290

Gohn, M. G. (2011). Movimentos sociais na contemporaneidade. *Revista Brasileira de Educação*, *16*(47), 333–361. doi:10.1590/S1413-24782011000200005

Goodwin, J., Jasper, J. M., & Polletta, F. (2001). Introduction: why emotions matter. In J. Goodwin, J. M. Jasper, & F. Polletta (Eds.), *Passionate Politics. Emotions and social movements* (pp. 1–24). Chicago, IL: The University of Chicago Press. doi:10.7208/chicago/9780226304007.003.0001

Greene, J. A., & Podolsky, S. H. (2012). Reform, regulation, and pharmaceuticals – the Kefauver-Harris Amendments at 50. *The New England Journal of Medicine*, *367*(16), 1481–1482. doi:10.1056/NEJMp1210007 PMID:23075174

Hacking, I. (1999). *The social construction of what?* Cambridge, MA: Harvard University Press.

Han, B. (2017). *Sociedade da transparência* (E. P. Giachini, Trans.). Petrópolis, Brazil: Editora Vozes. (Original work published 2012)

Helman, C. G. (2009). *Cultura, Saúde e Doença* (5th ed.). (A. B. Bolner, Trans.). Porto Alegre, Brazil: Artmed. (Original work published 2007)

Héon-Klin, V. (2017). European Reference networks for rare diseases: What is the conceptual framework? *Orphanet Journal of Rare Diseases*, *12*(1), 137. doi:10.118613023-017-0676-3 PMID:28784158

Hodgkin, P. (1985). Medicine is war: And other medical metaphors. *British Medical Journal*, *291*(6511), 1820–1821. doi:10.1136/bmj.291.6511.1820 PMID:3936590

Huyard, C. (2009a). How did uncommon disorders become 'rare diseases'? History of a boundary object. *Sociology of Health & Illness*, *31*(4), 463–477. doi:10.1111/j.1467-9566.2008.01143.x PMID:19397760

Huyard, C. (2009b). Who rules rare disease associations? A framework to understand their action. *Sociology of Health & Illness*, *31*(7), 979–993. doi:10.1111/j.1467-9566.2009.01177.x PMID:19619152

Huyard, C. (2009c). What, if anything, is specific about having a rare disorder? Patients' judgments in being ill and being rare. *Health Expectations*, *12*(4), 361–370. doi:10.1111/j.1369-7625.2009.00552.x PMID:19840131

Huyard, C. (2011a). Quand la puissance publique fait surgir et équipe une mobilisation protestaire. *Revue Francaise de Science Politique*, *61*(2), 183–200. doi:10.3917/rfsp.612.0183

Huyard, C. (2011b). Porquoi s'associer? Quatre motifs d'entrée dans um collectif dans les associations de maladies rares. *Revue Francaise de Sociologie*, *52*(4), 719–745. doi:10.3917/rfs.524.0719

Ingelfinger, J. R., & Drazen, J. M. (2011). Patient organizations and research on rare diseases. *The New England Journal of Medicine*, *364*(17), 1670–1671. doi:10.1056/NEJMe1102290 PMID:21410388

Kozinets, R. V. (2005). *Netnography: redefined* (2nd ed.). London, UK: Sage.

Lakoff, G., & Johnsen, M. (2003). *Metaphors we live by* (2nd ed.). London, UK: The University Chicago Press. doi:10.7208/chicago/9780226470993.001.0001

Lawthom, R., & Chataika, T. (2012). Leave and Wenger, Communities of Practice and Disability. In D. Goodley, B. Hughes, & L. Davis (Eds.), *Disability and social theory. New developments and Directions* (pp. 233–251). New York, NY: Palgrave MacMillan. doi:10.1057/9781137023001_14

Lüchmann, L. H. H. (2014). Abordagens teóricas sobre o associativismo e seus efeitos democráticos. *Revista Brasileira de Ciências Sociais*, *29*(85), 159–178. doi:10.1590/S0102-69092014000200011

Melo, D. G., de Paula, P. K., de Araujo Rodrigues, S., de Avó, L. R. D. S., Germano, C. M. R., & Demarzo, M. M. P. (2015). Genetics in primary health care and the National Policy on Comprehensive Care for People with Rare Diseases in Brazil: Opportunities and challenges for professional education. *Journal of Community Genetics*, *6*(3), 231–240. doi:10.100712687-015-0224-6 PMID:25893505

Ministério da Saúde. (2014). *Portaria n° 199, de 30 de janeiro de 2014. Institui a Política Nacional de Atenção Integral às Pessoas com Doenças Raras, aprova Diretrizes para Atenção Integral às Pessoas com Doenças Raras no âmbito do Sistema Único de Saúde (SUS) e institui incentivos financeiros de custeio.* Brasília: Diário Oficial da União.

Oliveira, C. R. O., Guimarães, M. C. S., & Machado, R. (2012). Doenças raras como categoria de classificação emergente: o caso brasileiro. *DataGramaZero*, *13*(1), 1-10. Retrieved from http://www.brapci.inf.br/index.php/article/view/0000011723/611097bff4311db520c7ab0c01a792e4/

Osakabe, H. (2002). *Argumentação e discurso político* (2nd ed.). São Paulo, Brazil: Martins Fontes.

Passos-Bueno, M. R., Bertola, D., Horovitz, D. D. G., Ferraz, V. E. F., & Brito, L. A. (2014). Genetics and genomics in Brazil: A promising future. *Molecular Genetics & Genomic Medicine*, *2*(4), 280–291. doi:10.1002/mgg3.95 PMID:25077170

Polich, G. R. (2012). Rare disease patient groups as clinical researchers. *Drug Discovery Today*, *17*(3-4), 167–172. doi:10.1016/j.drudis.2011.09.020 PMID:22016088

Polletta, F., & Jasper, J. M. (2001). Collective identities and social movements. *Annual Review of Sociology*, *27*(1), 283–305. doi:10.1146/annurev.soc.27.1.283

Prior, L. (2003). Belief, knowledge and expertise: The emergence of the lay expert in medical sociology. *Sociology of Health & Illness*, *25*(3), 41–57. doi:10.1111/1467-9566.00339 PMID:14498929

Prior, T. W., & Finanger, E. (2016). Spinal Muscular Atrophy. In M. P. Adam, H. H. Ardinger, R. A. Pagon, & S. E. Wallace (Eds.), *GeneReviews*. Retrieved from https://www.ncbi.nlm.nih.gov/books/NBK1352/

Rabeharisoa, V. (2008). Experience, knowledge and empowerment: the increasing role of patient organizations in staging, weighting and circulating experience and knowledge In M. Akrich, J. Nunes, F. Paterson, & V. Rabeharisoa (Eds.), *The dynamics of patient organizations in Europe*. Retrieved from http://books.openedition.org/pressesmines/1588

Rabeharisoa, V., Callon, M., Filipe, A. M., Nunes, J. A., Paterson, F., & Vergnaud, F. (2014). From 'politics of numbers' to 'politics of singularisation': Patients' activism and engagement in research on rare diseases in France and Portugal. *Biosocieties*, *9*(2), 194–217. doi:10.1057/biosoc.2014.4

Rabinow, P. (1996). Artificiality and enlightenment: From sociobiology to biosociality. In *Essays on the Anthropology of Reason* (pp. 91–111). Princeton, NJ: Princeton University Press.

Rabinow, P. (1996). Artificiality and enlightenment: From sociobiology to biosociality. In J. X. Inda (Ed.), *Essays on the Anthropology of Reason* (pp. 91–111). Princeton, NJ: Princeton University Press.

Rath, A., Wakap, S. S. N., Demarest, S., & Lanneau, V. (2016). *Orphanet Report Series. Prevalence and incidence of rare diseases: bibliographic data.* Diseases listed by decreasing prevalence, incidence or number of published cases. Retrieved from https://www.orpha.net/consor/cgi-bin/Education_Home.php?lng=EN

Rodrigues, L. O. C. (2014, Dec. 1) *LOR Blog [web logcomment]*. Retrieved from http://lorcartunista.blogspot.com.br/

Rose, N. (2007). *The Politics of Life Itself.* Princeton, NJ: Princeton University Press. doi:10.1515/9781400827503

Rose, N., & Novas, C. (2003). Biological Citizenship. In A. Ong, & S. J. Collier (Eds.), *Global Assemblages: Technology, Politics, and Ethics as Anthropological Problems* (pp. 439–463). Oxford, UK: Blackwell Publishing.

Santos, G. C., Cagliari, C. I., & Teixeira, M. A. (2010). Rare diseases. Challenges for the public health sector in Brazil. Abstract retrieved from *VI International Conference on Rare Disease and Orphan Drugs*, P06.

Scheffer, M., Biancarelli, A., & Cassenote, A. (2018). *Demografia médica no Brasil 2018. São Paulo, Brazil.* SP: Conselho Regional de Medicina do Estado de São Paulo & Conselho Federal de Medicina.

Sergent, S. C. C., Cagliari, C. I., & Teixeira, M. A. (2010). GEDR – Rare diseases study group – Brazil. Abstract retrieved from *VI International Conference on Rare Disease and Orphan Drugs*, P09.

Skrabanek, P. (1994). *The death of human medicine and the rise of coercive healthism*. Suffolk, UK: St. Edmundsbury Press.

Sontag, S. (2007). *Doença como metáfora. AIDS e suas metáforas* (2nd ed.). (R. Figueiredo, & P. H. Britto, Trans.). São Paulo, Brazil: Companhia das Letras. (Original work published 1989)

Sontag, S. (2007). *Doença como metáfora. AIDS e suas metáforas* (2nd ed.). (R. Figueiredo, & P. H. Britto, Trans.). São Paulo, Brazil: Companhia das Letras. (Original work published 1989)

Streinraths, M., Vallance, H. D., & Davidson, G. F. (2008). Delays in diagnosing cystic fibrosis. Can we find ways to diagnose it earlier? *Canadian Family Physician Medecin de Famille Canadien*, *54*, 877–883. Retrieved from http://www.cfp.ca/content/54/6/877.long PMID:18556497

Tejada, P. (2010). *Rare Diseases Day. Report on the 2010 Campaign. 2010.* Krakow, Poland: European Organization for Rare Diseases; Retrieved from https://www.rarediseaseday.org/article/rare-disease-day-2010

Van de Bovenkamp, H. M., & Trappenburg, M. J. (2011). Government influence on patient organizations. *Health Care Analysis*, *19*(4), 329–351. doi:10.100710728-010-0155-7 PMID:20803075

Vieira, T., Schwartz, I., Muñoz, V., Pinto, L., Steiner, C., Ribeiro, M., ... Giugliani, R. (2008). Mucopolysaccharidoses in Brazil: What happens from birth to biochemical diagnosis? *American Journal of Medical Genetics*, *146A*(13), 1741–1747. doi:10.1002/ajmg.a.32320 PMID:18546277

Williams, P. H. (2011). Policy framework for rare disease health disparities. *Policy, Politics, & Nursing Practice*, *12*(2), 114–118. doi:10.1177/1527154411404243 PMID:21486874

Wilson, C. (2013). Orphan drugs and orphan drug legislation. In E. Hernberg-Ståhl, & M. Reljanović (Eds.), *Orphan Drugs Understanding the Rare Disease Market and Its Dynamics, Woodhead Publishing Series in Biomedicine*. Cambridge, UK: Woodhead Publishing. doi:10.1533/9781908818393.9

ADITIONAL READING

Akrich, M., Nunes, J., Paterson, F., & Rabeharisoa, V. (Eds.). (2008). *The dynamics of patient organizations in Europe*. Retrived from https://books.openedition.org/pressesmines/1577

Akrich, M., & Rabeharisoa, V. (2012). L'expertise profane dans les associations de patients, um outil de démocratie sanitaire. *Santé Publique*, *24*(1), 69–74. doi:10.3917pub.121.0069 PMID:22730612

Biehl, J., & Petryna, A. (2011). Bodies of rights and therapeutic markets. *Social Research*, *78*(2), 359–394. https://philpapers.org/rec/BIEBOR

Brown, P., & Zavestoski, S. (2004). Social movements in health: An introduction. *Sociology of Health & Illness*, *26*(6), 679–694. doi:10.1111/j.0141-9889.2004.00413.x PMID:15383036

Gibbon, S., & Novas, C. (Eds.). (2008). *Biosocialities, genetics and the social sciences*. New York: Routledge.

Lima, M. A. F. D., Gilbert, A. C. B., & Horovitz, D. D. G. (2018). Redes de tratamento e as associações de pacientes com doenças raras. *Ciencia & Saude Coletiva*, *23*(10), 3247–3256. doi:10.1590/1413-812320182310.14762018 PMID:30365844

Nunes, J. A., Matias, M., & Filipe, A. M. (2007). As organizações de pacientes como atores emergentes no espaço da saúde: O caso de Portugal. *Revista Eletrônica de Comunicação Informação & Inovação em Saúde*, *1*(1), 107–110. doi:10.29397/reciis.v1i1.894

Quackenbush, N. (2008). *Bodies in culture, culture in bodies: disability narratives and a rhetoric of resistance* (Doctoral dissertation). Retrieved from The University of Arizona. (659749949)

KEY TERMS AND DEFINITIONS

Disability: A physical, mental or emotional handicap.

Identity: A person's concept of self.

Lay Experts: Non-professionals who hold professional knowledge about a subject.

Netnography: Qualitative research method that adapts ethnography to Internet.

Patient Organizations: Group of people working together to pursue common goals.

Public Policy: Actions selected by governments to guide and determine present and future decisions.

Rare Diseases: A group of diseases, which are characterized by its low prevalence in a population.

Social Media: Platforms that provide the ability and tools to create and publish information though the Internet.

Social Movements in Health: Groups of people who organize themselves around a cause, specifically health themes, in order to gain political access.

ENDNOTES

1 In Portuguese, the word pain ("dor") has three letters that introduce each sentence: D = lack of scientific knowledge from health professionals ["Desconhecimento científico por parte dos profissionais de saúde"] O = Institutional Omission ["Omissão institucional"] R = Non-existent Social Representation["Representação social inexistente"]

Chapter 8
Challenges of Parents With Children With Rare Diseases in Portugal:
A Relational Perspective

Beatriz Moreira Silva Santos
University of Trás-Os-Montes and Alto Douro, Portugal

Cátia Filipa da Silva Ferreira
University of Trás-Os-Montes and Alto Douro, Portugal

Catarina Pinheiro Mota
University of Trás-Os-Montes and Alto Douro, Portugal & Center for Psychology, University of Porto. R, Alfredo Allen, Portugal

ABSTRACT

This chapter makes known the reality of Portuguese families with children diagnosed with a rare disease. The parenting, romantic attachment, coping and emotional regulation strategies, resilience, and personality characteristics of parental figures are the main focus of research carried out in Portugal. In this research participated 160 parental figures (99 mothers and 61 fathers) between 22 and 81 years old. It was found that the existence of a child with a rare disease in the family can give rise to a set of disparate feelings, where the parental figures have to reorganize themselves internally and externally to respond to the needs of the child. It is important to develop intervention programs that address the needs of the parental figures underlying the act of caring.

DOI: 10.4018/978-1-7998-2088-8.ch008

INTRODUCTION

Rare diseases reach significant numbers when observed globally (Luz, Silva, & DeMontigny, 2015). In the European Union, a rare disease assumes a proportion of 5 out of 10,000 people (Rare Disease UK, 2016; Silva & Sousa, 2015). But considering that there are over 7,000 different rare disease types, many of which are untitled and difficult to diagnose, these constitute 6 to 10% of diseases worldwide (Luz, et al., 2015; Pelentsov, Fielder, Laws, & Esterman, 2016b). In Portugal, there are about 800,000 patients with rare diseases and hundreds still to be diagnosed (Raríssimas, 2018).

The definition of rare diseases varies globally and is characterized by the low regularity with which they occur in the population, however, there is a wide range of different and increasingly numerous rare diseases (Dellve, Samuelsson, Tallborn, Fasth, & Hallberg, 2006; Schieppati, Henter, Daina, & Aperia, 2008). Rare diseases include, mostly, serious, degenerative or genetic diseases (Pelentsov et al., 2016b). They are often life threatening and can be debilitating as patients' quality of life is compromised due to the lack of autonomy and the high level of pain and suffering experienced by the rare disease patient and his family (Pelentsov et al., 2016b). Diagnoses and treatments for these diseases are uncertain and / or used too late due to the lack of information and scientific knowledge. The shortage of qualified health professionals and specialized support services also makes it difficult to make progress in the health of individuals with a rare disease (Luz, et al., 2015).

The issue of rare diseases, initially with an interest in medicine, has gained emphasis in addressing the social, economic, psychological and educational implications for patients and their caregivers (Pelentsov et al., 2016b; Waldboth, Patch, Mahrer-Imhof, & Metcalfe, 2016). However, there is still a lack of research in this area, namely studies addressing the relational and affective dynamics of parents, usually the primordial caregivers, in the circumstance of having a child with rare disease. This is why there is a need for reflection and dissemination of this theme (Pelentsov, Fielder, & Esterman, 2016a). This chapter aims to make known the emotional and relational experiences of parents of children with rare diseases, through a pilot research developed in Portugal. First, this chapter focuses on the experiences and difficulties of parental figures who have children with rare diseases. Next, the chapter focuses on the study with Portuguese families, where the main research results are presented. Finally, some intervention proposals with parental figures are suggested, in order to promoting their quality of life.

EXPERIENCES OF PARENTS WITH CHILDREN WITH RARE DISEASES

Taking care of a child involves a set of reorganizations in the roles of the members of the family, being necessary to offer an answer to the physical, affective and psychic needs of the child (Cruz, 2013). The birth of a child is a significant milestone in the dynamics of a family, where the parents build fantasies and expectations regarding the child (Soares, Araújo, & Bellato, 2016). The unexpected emergence of a rare disease in the child may trigger in the parental figures a grief process of the idealized child, developing feelings of anguish, hopelessness, impotence and doubt regarding the future of the family's dynamic and the idea of dealing with a child with special needs (Góes, 2006; Lucca & Petean, 2016; Milbrath, Motta, Gabatz, & Freitag, 2017). Many of the emotional difficulties experienced by parents of children with rare diseases are related to the difficulties of getting the correct diagnosis and finding information about the disease (Dellve et al., 2006). The fear of an uncertain or time-consuming diagnosis, the limited access to health information and resources, and the complexity of the access to support groups, are the main difficulties of the parental figures (Pelentsov et al., 2016a).

Parents of children with rare diseases tend to show more stress due to lack of competence and parental incapacity, emotion demands that are crucial for this context, and social isolation, lacking time for other activities necessary for the family, such as moments of rest, relaxation and leisure (Dellve et al., 2006). Coupled with the lack of time, marital dynamics may be compromised when a rare disease develops within the family. In a study conducted by Pelentsov et al. (2016a) with 23 parents with the purpose of understanding their experiences in caring for a child with a rare disease, it was found in some parents that the experience of caring for a special child had a positive impact on their relationship, strengthening the bound as a couple. However, difficulties in accepting the disease and dealing with the child's daily care needs can create a negative impact on most couples' love experiences.

The duration of the illness, uncertain and recurrent hospitalizations, and the high financial responsibilities can cause emotional instability and impair family integrity. Therefore, they are also considered as stress factors (Johnston et al., 2003; Monteiro, Matos, & Coelho, 2002; Theofanidis, 2007). Financial difficulties may be associated with the restrictions of the job functions of one of the couple's members to meet the special needs of the child (Farmer, Marien, Clark, Sherman, & Selva, 2004).

In order to deal with the reality of having a child with special needs, parents tend to seek information about the disease and other parental figures who experience similar situations (Luz, Carvalho, & Silva, 2011). The knowledge and contact with other similar cases can bring comfort and relief to the parents through the sharing of experiences, difficulties, and perspectives about the disease (Luz et al., 2011).

Pelentsov et al. (2016a) argue that sharing similar experiences between parental figures provides a shared social identity and a sense of belonging, reducing stress and improving the quality of care for a child with special needs.

Parents are increasingly turning to the internet to search for information about the rare disease of their children. In a study by Tozzi et al. (2013) with 516 parents, it was found that about 62% of parents considered that information found online about their child's disease was useful for making the diagnosis. Many parents of children with rare diseases consider the internet as an essential means of searching for information, since having knowledge about the disease offers the possibility to work with negative feelings and, consequently, accept reality (Gundersen, 2011).

Thus, parental figures become more adaptive in managing all their difficulties, as information about the disease and treatment, contact with other similar cases, and daily contact with the child increases (Luz et al., 2011).

PARENTS OF CHILDREN WITH RARE DISEASES: AN EXPLORATORY STUDY IN PORTUGAL

Given the gaps found in the Portuguese literature regarding the approach of relational experience of parents of children with rare diseases, the authors Ferreira and Mota (2018, 2019) and Santos and Mota (2018, 2019) developed an exploratory study in Portugal, with 160 parental figures (61 fathers and 99 mothers) aged 22 to 81, distributed throughout mainland Portugal.

The study included parents of children with 71 distinct rare diseases, predominantly Spina Bifida, Angelman Syndrome, Prader-Willi Syndrome, Peters Anomaly and Osteogenesis Imperfecta. The study included 23 parental figures who have a child with an undiagnosed or unknown condition. In this study, 124 parents reported that they would like more support in their child's illness process and 36 reported not needing support. Among those who would like more help, 32 highlight supports at State / financial level, 22 at the medical level and 15 at the scientific research level.

This research aimed to understand the experience of parents of children with rare diseases, in several aspects, particularly in terms of parenting, romantic attachment, coping and emotional regulation strategies, resilience and personality characteristics of parental figures.

This study assumes an innovative character due to the scarcity of national and international scientific studies in this field.

The results of this study are described in this chapter, in an integrative manner in the themes that the authors considered relevant to underline.

Results of the Exploratory Study in Portugal

Parenting in Rare Diseases

Parenting has been characterized by a complex process that contributes to the maturation of parental figures with regards to the development of skills to care for their child (Barroso & Machado, 2010; Cardoso & Silva, 2010). According to Cruz (2005, 2013), parenting includes various tasks designed to ensure the children's survival and to promote and support their physical, emotional and social development, using resources within and outside the family context. The main goal of parenting is the empowerment of parents to have the appropriate knowledge about their children's health and well-being, so they can become more independent to be integrated into society (Barroso & Machado, 2010; Cardoso & Silva, 2010; Hoghughi, 2004; Moreira & Ângelo, 2008).

The transition to parenting may not only bring unique and satisfying moments but may also confront the parents with new and unexpected demands. In this way, there is a risk of increasing stress levels and, consequently, deterioration of their health and well-being (Waldboth et al., 2016). In this way, the experience of parenting can involve positive or negative feelings and emotions. Giving birth to a child with a rare disease can become a painful and challenging event instead of being a source of joy and satisfaction (González-Lamuño & García, 2008). Parents of children with rare diseases face several challenges in their daily routine that may affect their parental role (Pelentsov et al., 2016a), requiring changes in the family dynamics and a redefinition of the parental identity (Maltby, Kristjanson, & Coleman, 2003; Meleis, Sawyer, Im, Messias, & Schumacher, 2000; Melnyk, Feinstein, Moldenhouer & Small, 2001). Given the rarity of their child's illness, the absence or inadequate provision of care may interfere with their child's physical and emotional development, leading to some considerable health and social problems (Demakakos, Pillas, Marmot, & Steptoe, 2016; Mooney-Doyle et al., 2015).

There is an essential factor that was shown to be related to the way that parental figures exercise their role, which is the absence or the presence of a diagnose that defines their child's rare disease. In a recent study, it was found that parents of children without a diagnosis of a rare disease reveal an approach based on unstable parenting practices, due to the lack of information on how to act on the reality of having a different child (Ferreira & Mota, 2019; Santos & Mota, 2018).

Families with little knowledge about their child's health status feel insecure in providing care and show difficulties in meeting their needs (Araújo, Collet, Moura, & Nóbrega, 2009; Nieweglowski, & More, 2008; Piccinini, Castro, & Alvarenga, 2003). Uncertainty regarding the diagnosis, the rarity of the disease, as well as the lack of information about it, may be related to the occurrence of high levels of parental stress, which may contribute to inadequate parenting, as parents express feelings of helplessness, anguish, uselessness and guilt for failing to meet their child's general needs (Góes, 2006; Lucca & Petean, 2016; Luz et al., 2015; Milbrath et al., 2017; Zurynski, Frith, Leonard, & Elliot, 2008). Thus, the exercise of inadequate parenting can lead to difficulties in the emotional regulation of parents, which in turn may lead to the use of more maladaptive coping strategies (Ferreira & Mota, 2019). The unpredictability associated with the disease process of a child with rare disease and the lack of guidance on caring may cause parents to experience significant physical and psychological overload, which may lead to emotional imbalance in caregivers. Being emotionally unbalanced, parents seem to have difficulty identifying effective strategies and, therefore, resort to maladaptive strategies as a way of denying or minimizing their suffering or simply because they consider that they are unable to deal with the problem (Ferreira & Mota, 2019).

On the other hand, parents having access to some information about the diagnosis, treatment and / or prognosis of their child's disease becomes essential for providing appropriate care to the special needs of the child, enabling them to develop fully and better adaptation to the disease process (Aymé, 2000; Yeh, Lee, Chen, & Li, 2000). Thus, it is clear that parents who are more informed about their child's diagnosis have greater control over the situation and more potential for care compared to parents of children without diagnosed disease.

The research carried out in Portugal, also revealed differences between fathers and mothers of children with rare diseases in parenting (Santos & Mota, 2018).

In recent decades, the increasing number of mothers in the labor market has led to greater involvement of parents in childcare, changing the distribution of parental responsibilities (Doucet, 2001). However, some authors feel that the disparities between fathers and mothers persist with regard to the commitment to care for their children (Keller & Honig, 2004; Pelchat, Lefebvre, & Perreault, 2003). Particularly, given the existence of a child with a rare disease in the family, most of the time, and depending on the degree of severity of the disease, one of the couple's members, mostly the mother figure, has to leave their professional activity for effectively respond to all the demands and challenges underlying the diagnosis of a rare disease (Farmer et al., 2004). The literature has described that a greater involvement of the mother in the care provided to the rare disease afflicted child seems to potentiate the development of higher stress levels in the mothers, due to the demanding and constant care underlying the existence of a child with a rare disease (Albuquerque, Pereira, Fonseca, & Carnavarro, 2015). However, the continuous satisfaction of the needs of the child, on the part of the mother, seems to promote the attachments between both, enhancing greater affective availability, emotional support, sensitivity and acceptance of the child. In turn, the lower involvement of the father figure in the care of a rare child seems to make them less sensitive in their ability to correctly

Figure 1. Parenting: Differences in diagnosis and gender

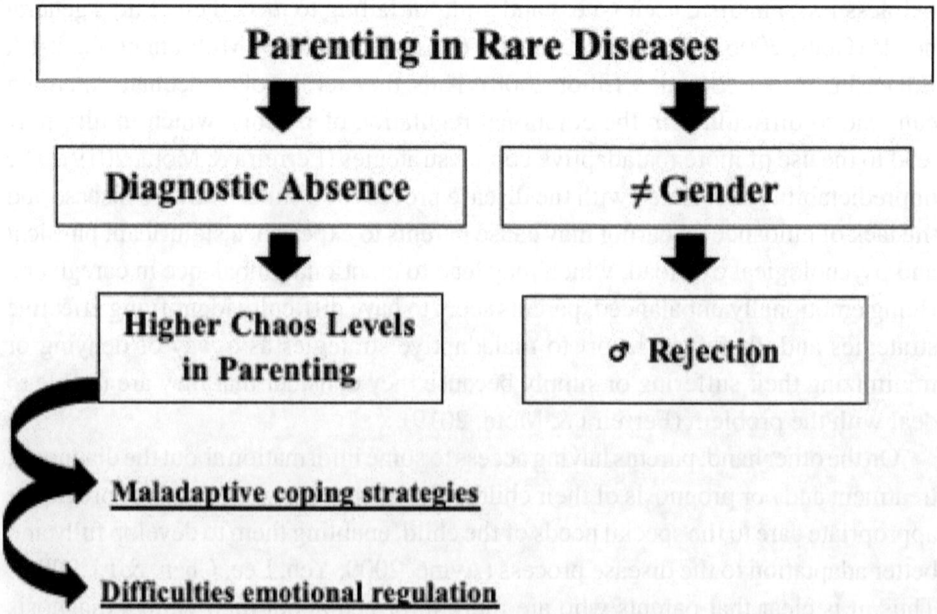

perceive and interpret the child's signs and respond appropriately (Pelchat et al., 2003). This may arise, in the exercise of parenting, feelings of rejection, hostility and non-acceptance of the child (Figure 1).

The gender differences in parenting and how parental figures adapt to the emergence of a rare disease in the family may be related to the quality of the relationship that parents of children with rare diseases have with their own attachment figures. The literature suggests that the safety of parenting relationships is often associated with more available, responsive, and sensitive parenting (Ainsworth & Bell, 1969; Ainsworth, Blehar, Waters, & Wall, 1978; Bell & Ainsworth, 1972). On the other hand, the existence of an insecure attachment, marked by excessive control and overprotection by parental figures, seems to hinder the development of an individual's autonomy and personal identity, triggering a more fragile and unstable internal structure (Bowlby, 1969). In the present investigation, it was found that parents of children with rare diseases who have seen their process of exploration of the world and self-withdrawn and inhibited by their parental figures seem to exercise parenting based on rejection, punitive disciplinary practices and hostility, not being so available to meet the needs of their children with rare disease (Ferreira & Mota, 2018). Parental figures who care for a child with a rare disease, and that have experienced constraints in their individuality and autonomy development in their childhood, may find it more difficult to cope with the challenge of parenting and, especially, with the unexpected emergence of an illness in their child. This event may cause feelings of powerlessness and insecurity in developing appropriate parenting skills to care for a different child (Ferreira & Mota, 2018).

Challenges in the Romantic Relationships

The existence of a child with a severe illness in the family represents one of the most distressing and disabling life events, especially for parental figures. This may change the dynamics of the couple relationship through, for example, intensifying conflicts (Gaither, Bingen, & Hopkins, 2000). However, the literature points to different conclusions regarding the impact that the existence of a child with a rare disease can have in the couples romantic relationship. Most studies have shown that some parents experience negative effects in the marital relationship because of their child's disease, especially, in terms of love satisfaction between the couple (Pelentsov et al., 2016a). However, other parents seem to express positive effects, where the child disease provides greater unity and cohesion between the couple (Katz, 2002; Pelentsov et al., 2016a). This variability of the impact of a serious illness of a child in the marital relationship may be related to the quality of the bond that is established between the loving couple, which in turn may contribute to the development of resilience in parental figures. Romantic relationships can be attachment relationships, where individuals tend to seek closeness with their love partner at times of greatest need, in order to alleviate negative feelings of distress and to promote comfort and a sense of security (Mikulincer & Shaver, 2014). Thus, in the presence of stress and threat situations, such as the existence of a rare disease within the family, positive experiences with a romantic attachment figure make it possible to develop feelings of confidence and security to cope with adversity (Bartholomew & Horowitz, 1991). A secure romantic attachment relationship, based on trust, mutual support, emotional availability and open communication in feelings and thoughts, not only contributes to greater marital satisfaction, but also helps parents to deal with their child's illness in a more adaptable way (Wijnberg-Williams, Van de Wiel, Kamps, & Hoekstra-Webers, 2015).

On the other hand, an insecurity romantic attachment between the couple, seems to be associated with lower levels of resilience in parental figures. Martins, Moreira and Canavarro (2016) argue that the establishment of an insecure romantic attachment based on avoidance of the romantic couple is related to higher levels of parental stress and lower family cohesion, enhancing the development of lower levels of resilience in parents.

The present study about the experience of parents of children with rare diseases emphasizes the importance of having a secure romantic attachment between the couple, in order to face the adversities of caring for a different child.

Research shows that even in situations of high levels of rejection in parenting, the existence of a high level of trust in the romantic relationship may promote better adaptation of the parental figures to the inherent difficulties when it comes to caring for a child with a rare illness and, consequently, enhance the development of parental resilience (Santos & Mota, 2018). Luther (2007) points out that the existence of a romantic relationship where support prevails, especially emotional support between the couple, is an important factor for the development of resilience. In addition, other authors report that having a good relationship with the romantic partner is associated with lower levels of parental stress (Mulsow, Caldera, Pursley, Reifman, & Huston, 2002; Williford, Calkins, & Keane, 2007). The results obtained in the Portuguese population case suggest that the presence of trust and security in romantic relationships between couples of children with rare diseases occupies a prominent place in the development of resilience of the parental figures (Santos & Mota, 2018). Even though, there are moments of hostility and rejection towards the rare disease child, the presence of an accessible and responsive loving couple seems to play a secure grounding role in times of environmental exploration, and to be a source of security and protection in more disturbing times (Figure 2).

The existence of a supportive and secure partner, probably, enhances the sharing of tasks that are inherent to the special childcare, allowing to regulate stress levels and, consequently, a better adaptation to the child's disease process (Kersh, Hedvat, Hauser-Cram, & Warfield, 2006). The presence of a secure romantic attachment figure may help emerge in the parenting figures a more confident and more secure view relatively to themselves and their future, enhancing the development of a more cohesive internal structure to cope with vicissitudes. On the other hand, the existence of a secure base may reduce, in parenting figures, the feeling of isolation, as well as promote the sharing of feelings and tasks referring to the child with rare disease, enhancing the joint construction and resignification of feelings related to the child, which may lead to personal and family growth (Santos & Mota, 2018).

The research carried out in Portugal, also reveals that fathers denote higher levels of dependence on romantic relationship compared to mothers. For males, the scarce time shared with the partner without the presence of the child is the greatest difficulty imposed on the romantic relationship between the couple. In this specific context with children with rare diseases, male figures may feel more insecure and, therefore, denote a greater emotional and physical need for closeness with their partner, and maybe underlying in the romantic relationship greater separation anxiety issues and fear of loss (Santos & Mota, 2018).

Figure 2. The importance of Romantic Attachment (RA) in the association between parenting and resilience

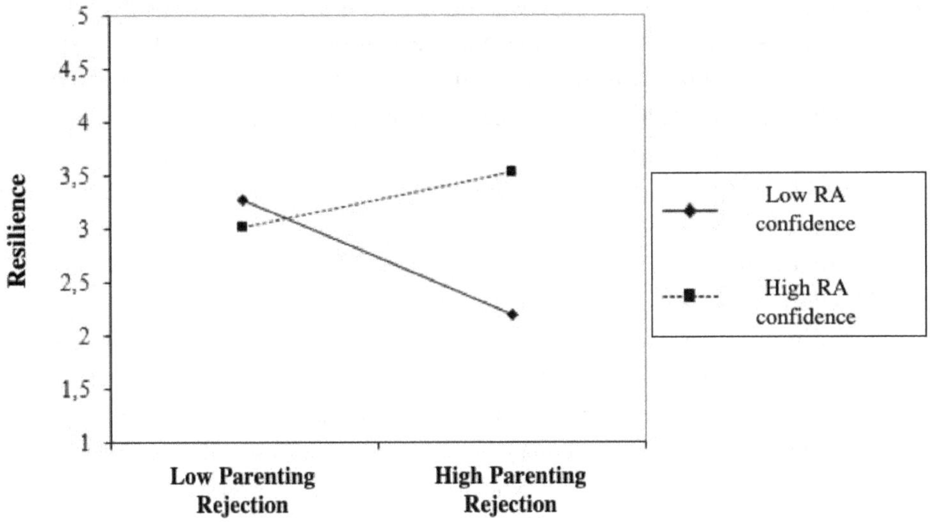

Resilience Promoting Factors in Rare Diseases

Family adjustment, in particular parental figures, to a child with a rare disease seems to be a dynamic process that occurs due to the balance between changes in the health condition of the child with the rare disease, the stage of development where the child is at, and the different needs of the family (Smith, Cheater, & Bekker, 2013). By focusing on the accomplishments of their children with a rare condition, most parents can adapt and face life with the vicissitudes inherent to the daily life of a child with this condition. The sense of control over caring for a different child may come from caring routines that strengthen the parent-child bond, allowing parents to become more flexible about care and treatment regimens (Smith et al., 2013). Caring for a child with a rare disease can trigger constructive and positive reactions. These arise with no sense of response to some motivations, such as the desire to feel needed and protect another human being, as well as to acquire a sense of personal worth, executed by success, when facing the challenges and tasks of raising a child with a rare disease (Zagalo Cardoso, 2001).

In a study by Strehle and Middlemiss (2007) with parents of 32 children with 4q deletion syndrome (rare chromosomal disease, mostly not hereditary, and characterized by symptoms as skeletal abnormalities, heart defects, intellectual disability, developmental delay, and short stature), to understand how parents view the situation of having a child with rare genetic disease, it was found that in most cases, caring for and educating a child with a rare condition has provided other insights into their potential as caregivers. The results also pointed out that parents became more positive and began autonomously looking for new information about their children's disease as they grew older. Zagalo-Cardoso (2001) suggests that some parents can transform the experience of caring for a child with some rare disease into a unique personal fulfillment and satisfying experience.

Although family adaptation to a child with rare disease is a complex and multidimensional phenomenon (Dellve et al., 2006), as it exerts changes in all dimensions of caregivers' lives, especially parental figures, it should be noted that the different living circumstances of parents may be related to how they adjust to a child with rare disease.

According to Taanila, Kokkonen and Jarvelin (1996), in the specific case of rare diseases, the existence of certain internal and external resources, such as the acceptance of the disease by parental figures, cohesive intrafamily relationships and knowledge about the disease may provide a positive adaptation to the situation of having a different child. On the other hand, poor family cohesion, weak marital commitment, difficulty in administering care, as well as the emotional difficulties that the situation entails, can jeopardize the adaptation to a child with a rare disease. Thus, it is clear that while some factors harm, others favor the adjustment of parental figures to a different child, with families that may be more vulnerable than others.

Diseases considered rare can be an ongoing learning experience, not only for those affected but also for their families (Luz et al., 2015). This learning may be related to the development of new health skills by parents, as well as caring skills to exercise more appropriate parenting (Schieppati et al., 2008). Pelentsov and colleagues (2016b) reported that many parents of children with a rare disease feel that they have no alternative but to assume the role of "expert" in all aspects of their children's health. The authors considered that despite parents' difficulties, most parents may be able to assess their children's health needs, deal with emergencies when they arise, adapt care, discuss the disease with health professionals and make decisions.

In the present study, it was found that there are no differences between mothers and fathers in terms of resilience (Santos & Mota, 2019). However, research points out that the differences between parental figures lie in how they adapt and deal with the existence of a rare illness in the family; where mothers seem to resort more to social support (e.g. friends and extended family), indicating greater need for contact with other parental figures who are in the same situation (Brazil & Krueger, 2002; Gray, 2003), fathers seem to resort mostly to strategies based on solving concrete problems (Dulac, 2001). It is, usually, the mother who mainly takes care of the daily duties, subjecting herself to a significant physical and psychological burden (Silva, Brito, Sousa, & France, 2010). Mothers seem to adopt strategies that allow them to reduce the demands of daily tasks concerning the act of caring and, consequently,

Figure 3. Variation of coping strategies with age and gender

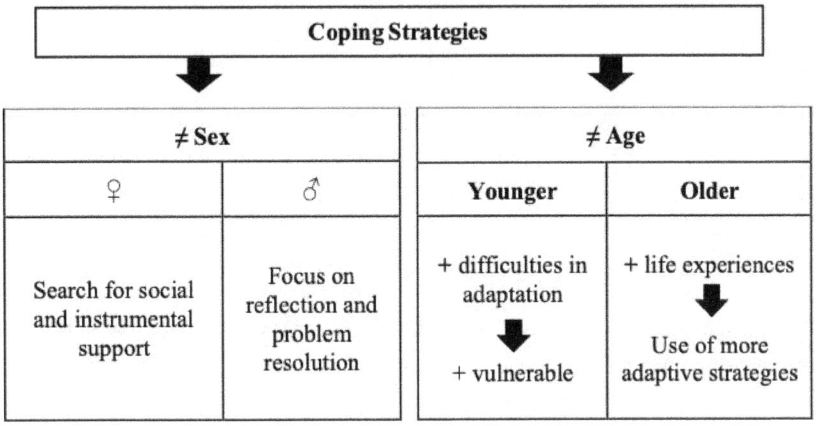

improve their well-being and quality of life, promoting greater integration and adaptation to the new family dynamics, more optimism about the progress of the child illness, greater emotional stability, and an interest in understanding their child's clinical situation in more detail (Ferreira & Mota, 2019) (Figure 3).

Another relevant result of the present investigation is associated with the age of the parental figures. Younger parents seem to have higher levels of stress in the face of illness due to their lack of preparedness to care for their special needs children, and their poor life experience, making them more vulnerable. On the contrary, older parents seem to adopt adaptive coping strategies focused on accepting the disease process, since they have more life experience and, at the same time, an emotional experience more open and willing to face possible adverse situations (Ferreira & Mota, 2018) (Figure 3).

In order to understand the resilience process of families with children with rare diseases, it has also become essential to understand which protective / individual factors parental figures have, particularly their personality characteristics (Laranjeira, 2007; Masten, 2001). The present research suggests that more assertive and socially active, loving, competent and determined parents, as well as creative and open to new experiences, are more likely to develop higher levels of resilience. Parents who denote these emotionally adjusted personality traits are more likely to accept their child's illness, be more willing to look for other sources of rare disease information and demonstrate greater ability to manage internal and external resources, enhancing a better adaptation to the whole process (Santos & Mota, 2019). On the other hand, parents of children with rare diseases who have individual characteristics based on emotional lability and melancholy, as well as anxious and depressive personality traits,

Table 1. Resilience variation with personality characteristics and gender

Personality Characteristics	Resilience Process
- Agreeableness **- Openness to Experience** **- Extraversion** - Conscientiousness	Resilience
- Neuroticism	Resilience
≠ Sex	
♀ Openness to Experience	No significant differences

seem to be less resilient (Santos & Mota, 2019). Being the exercise of parenting itself a challenging experience in the life of parental figures, the birth of a different child and, consequently, the care of the child with rare disease seems to be a triggering factor of high levels of anxiety, feelings of anguish and disorientation (Griffith et al., 2011). Thus, it is clear that parental figures with a more fragile personality structure may be more vulnerable to anxiogenic events, notably to the process of adaptation of the rare disease of the child.

This study also revealed important data regarding differences in personality characteristics between fathers and mothers. It was found that mothers have more personality traits based on imagination, intellectual curiosity and creativity compared to fathers (Santos & Mota, 2019). Mothers who have a child with a rare disease tend to seek more information about the disease by investigating and contacting similar cases in order to promote understanding of the disease and the provision of parental care (Brazil & Krueger, 2002; Gray, 2003). This search for new information about the disease and the desire for contact with other parental figures may meet a personality more open to new experiences based on social interaction and curiosity. On the other hand, these personality traits may stem from the fact that the mother figure spends more time on caring for the child with the rare disease and, therefore, often has to offer different and diverse responses, improvising the care (Santos & Mota, 2019). This is due to the unpredictability and often lack of knowledge of the tasks underlying parenting when a different child exists (Table 1).

CONCLUSION AND FUTURE RESEARCH DIRECTIONS

Throughout the theoretical review in this chapter, it was possible to realize the important role that the family plays in the overall development of a child.

The transition to parenting, along with the birth of a child with a rare condition, can be considered too stressful and full of shifts, changes and challenges. In this situation, parents will need to develop adequate parenting skills and strategies to cope, appropriately, with the demands associated with these events.

The pilot research hereby described and carried out in Portugal with parents of children with rare diseases came to draw attention to the difficulties that the parental figures find in the process of caring for a child with rare disease. In addition, this research highlights that the way that the care is exercised to the child, the individual characteristics of the parents, and the quality of the romantic attachment between the parents can contribute to overcoming the challenges of caring for a different child. This investigation also highlights the coping strategies used by caregivers and the difficulties of emotional regulation associated with the existence of a child with a rare disease. It is noteworthy, above all, the perception of the family, more specifically of the parents, about their potential as caregivers of a child with a rare disease, in a multidimensional perspective, leading to a broader and more practical knowledge about the reality of these families. This knowledge can contribute to provide a response to the needs and concerns pointed by the parental figures, in the sense of a more effective intervention with this population.

It is, therefore, essential to emphasize the need to create support guides or specific intervention programs for parental figures, involving multiple interventional dimensions, at the emotional, relational and family level, based on the provision of information about the disease, as well as the best way to provide parental care. The implementation of this type of intervention programs would be an added value in providing support to parents of children with rare diseases, encouraging them for a current and future experience with higher quality. In addition, it would be pertinent to create protocols with associations for individuals with rare diseases, in order to provide caregivers with individual or group psychological support consultations for further decentralization and / or adaptation to the disease process. The implementation of these protocols could be an opportunity to promote the awareness of health professionals for the need for more effective monitoring of parental figures, not only at the emotional level, but also in the level of practical competences.

In future investigations, it would be relevant to consider other relational variables, such as the specificities inherent to the rare genetic disease and the characteristics of the child with the disease, for a better understanding of the experiences of parental figures. It would also be relevant to carry studies that addressed another target population namely, to understand the experience of individuals with siblings with a rare disease.

In addition, a comparative study could be interesting, specifically comparing the experience of parents with children with a rare congenital disease with the experience of parents with children with a rare acquired disease. In the context of rare diseases, the creation of a mobile phone application or app could also be relevant to improve and promote communication between parents of children with rare diseases. This application would aim to facilitate and establish direct contact between families and health professionals, work as a social network between parents with children with rare diseases to share experiences and at the same time, promote their appreciation and personal investment, as well as the decentralization of the child's disease.

As explored in the literature review, unfamiliarity of information about the rare disease of children may be a factor of great vulnerability for parents, where the use of technology and online research may play a key role in coping and accepting disease.

Investing in rare disease research and the underlying difficulties for caregivers, as well as implementing intervention programs tailored to the needs of parental figures, could be a relevant step towards providing multi-valued support to parents of children with rare diseases, where the rarity factor constitutes a differentiating aspect and turns the act of caring extremely difficult.

REFERENCES

Ainsworth, M., Blehar, M., Waters, E., & Wall, S. (1978). *Patterns of attachment: A psychological study of the strange situation*. Hillsdale, NJ: Erlbaum.

Ainsworth, M. D. S. (1991). Attachments and other affectional bonds across the life cycle. In C. M. Parkes, J. Stevenson-Hinde, & P. Marris (Eds.), *Attachment across the life cycle* (pp. 33–51). New York: Routledge.

Ainsworth, M. D. S., & Bell, S. M. (1969). Some contemporary patterns of mother-infant interaction in the feeding situation. In A. Ambrose (Ed.), *Stimulation in early infancy* (pp. 133–170). San Diego, CA: Academic Press.

Ainsworth, M. D. S., & Bell, S. M. (1969). Some contemporary patterns of mother-infant interaction in the feeding situation. In A. Ambrose (Ed.), *Stimulation in early infancy* (pp. 133–170). San Diego, CA: Academic Press.

Albuquerque, S., Pereira, M., Fonseca, A., & Carnavarro, M. (2015). Resiliência, stresse parental e sobrecarga de pais de crianças com diagnóstico de anomalia congénita. [Resilience, parental stress and overload of parents of children diagnosed with congnital anomaly]. *Psychologica, 58*(2), 7-23. doi: -2_1. doi:10.14195/1647-8606_58

Almeida, B., & Melgaço, P. (2016). Quando a criança nasce doente: A subjetividade do infante e as relações familiares. *Psicologia em Revista, 22*(2), 356–373. doi:10.5752/P.1678-9523.2016V22N2P356

Araújo, Y. B., Collet, N., Moura, F. M., & Nóbrega, R. D. (2009). Conhecimento da família acerca da condição crônica na infância. [Family knowledge about chronic condition in childhood]. *Texto & Contexto Enfermagem, 18*(3), 498–505. doi:10.1590/S0104-07072009000300013

Aymé, S. (2000). *Les injustices de la naissance*. Paris, France: Hachette Littératures.

Barroso, R., & Machado, C. (2010). Definições, dimensões e determinantes da parentalidade. [Definitions, dimensions, and determinants of parenting]. *Psychologica, 1*(52), 211–229. doi:10.14195/1647-8606_52-1_10

Bartholomew, K., & Horowitz, L. M. (1991). Attachment styles among young adults: A test of a four-category model. *Journal of Personality and Social Psychology, 61*(2), 226–244. doi:10.1037/0022-3514.61.2.226 PMID:1920064

Bell, S. M., & Ainsworth, M. D. S. (1972). Infant crying and maternal responsiveness. *Child Development, 43*(4), 1171–1190. doi:10.2307/1127506 PMID:4643768

Bowlby, J. (1969). Attachment and loss: Vol. 1. *Attachment*. New York: Basic Books.

Bowlby, J. (1971). Attachment and loss: Attachment (vol. 1). Harmandsworth: Penguin Books.

Bowlby, J. (1973). *Attachment and loss: Separation, anxiety, and anger* (Vol. 2). New York: Basic Books.

Bowlby, J. (1981). Attachment and Loss: Loss, Sadness, and Depression (Vol. 3). Middesex: Penguin Books.

Bowlby, J. (1988). *A secure base: Parent-child attachment and healthy human development*. London, UK: Basic Books.

Brazil, K., & Krueger, P. (2002). Patterns of family adaptation to childhood asthma. *Journal of Pediatric Nursing, 17*(3), 167–173. doi:10.1053/jpdn.2002.124110 PMID:12094358

Bruce, J. E., Quirke, S., & Shaw, S. R. (2010). Families of children with genetic disorders. In *P. McCabe, & S. Shaw (Eds.), Genetic and acquired disorders: Current topics and interventions for educators* (pp. 59–67). Thousand Oaks, CA: Corwin.

Cardoso, A., & Silva, A. P. (2010). Representing nursing knowledge on maternal and neonatal health: A study on the cultural suitability of ICNP. *International Nursing Review*, *57*(4), 426–434. doi:10.1111/j.1466-7657.2010.00829.x PMID:21050193

Cruz, O. (2005). *Parentalidade* [Parenting]. Coimbra, Portugal: Quarteto.

Cruz, O. (2013). *Parentalidade* [Parenting]. Porto, Portugal: Livpsic.

Dellve, L., Samuelsson, L., Tallborn, A., Fasth, A., & Hallberg, L. (2006). Stress and well-being among parents of children with rare diseases: A prospective intervention study. *Journal of Advanced Nursing*, *53*(4), 392–402. doi:10.1111/j.1365-2648.2006.03736.x PMID:16448482

Demakakos, P., Pillas, D., Marmot, M., & Steptoe, A. (2016). Parenting style in childhood and mortality risk at older ages: A longitudinal cohort study. *The British Journal of Psychiatry*, *211*(6), 1–7. doi:10.1192/bjp.bp.115.163543 PMID:26941265

Doucet, A. (2001). You see the need perhaps more clearly than I have. *Journal of Family Issues*, *22*(3), 328–357. doi:10.1177/019251301022003004

Dulac, G. (2001). Les stéréotypes sociaux sur les rôles et l'implication des pères dans les services à la famille. *Défi Jeunesse*, *7*(2), 26–32.

Farmer, J., Marien, W., Clark, M., Sherman, A., & Selva, T. (2004). Primary care supports for children with chronic health conditions: Identifying and predicting unmet family needs. *Journal of Pediatric Psychology*, *29*(5), 355–367. doi:10.1093/jpepsy/jsh039 PMID:15187174

Ferreira, C., & Mota, C. P. (2018). *Vinculação aos pais, parentalidade e estratégias de coping na vivência de pais de filhos com doenças raras*. [Parental attachment, parenting and coping strategies in the experience of parents of children with rare diseases]. Poster presented at *4.º Congresso da Ordem dos Psicólogos Portugueses*, September 12-15, 2018, Braga, Portugal.

Ferreira, C., & Mota, C. P. (2019). *Parentalidade e coping na vivência de pais com filhos com doenças raras: papel mediador da regulação emocional.* [Parenting and coping in the experience of parents with children with rare diseases: Mediating role of emotional regulation]. Oral Communication at table #8 "Intervenção em situações de doença crónica e hospitalização" at the X Congresso Internacional de Psicologia da Criança e do Adolescente - "Psicoterapia e outras abordagens terapêuticas", April 10-11, 2019 at Universidade Lusíada de Lisboa, Portugal.

Gaither, R., Bingen, K., & Hopkins, J. (2000). When the bough breaks: The relationship between chronic illness in children and couple functioning. In K. Schmaling, & T. Sher (Eds.), *The Psychology of Couples and Illness: Theory, Research, & Practice* (pp. 337–365). Washington, DC: American Psychological Association. doi:10.1037/10360-012

Góes, F. A. D. B. (2006). Um encontro inesperado: Os pais e seu filho com deficiência mental. [An unexpected encounter: Parents and their mentally disabled child]. *Psicologia: Ciência e Profissão, 26*(3), 450–461. doi:10.1590/S1414-98932006000300009

González-Lamuño, D., & García, M. F. (2008). Enfermedades raras en pediatría. [Gobierno de Navarra: Departamento de Salud.]. *Anales del Sistema Sanitario de Navarra, 31*, 21–29. doi:10.4321/S1137-66272008000400003 PMID:18953370

Gray, D. E. (2003). Gender and coping: The parents of children with high functioning autism. *Social Science & Medicine, 56*(3), 631–642. doi:10.1016/S0277-9536(02)00059-X PMID:12570979

Griffith, G. M., Hastings, R. P., Nash, S., Petalas, M., Oliver, C., Howlin, P., ... Tunnicliffe, P. (2011). You have to sit and explain it all, and explain yourself: Mother's experiences of support services for their offspring with a rare genetic intellectual disability syndrome. *Journal of Genetic Counseling, 20*(2), 165–177. doi:10.100710897-010-9339-4 PMID:21203808

Gundersen, T. (2011). 'One wants to know what a chromosome is': The internet as a coping resource when adjusting to life parenting a child with a rare genetic disorder. *Sociology of Health & Illness, 33*(1), 81–95. doi:10.1111/j.1467-9566.2010.01277.x PMID:20937053

Hazan, C., & Shaver, P. (1987). Romantic love conceptualized as an attachment process. *Journal of Personality and Social Psychology, 52*(3), 511–524. doi:10.1037/0022-3514.52.3.511 PMID:3572722

Hazan, C., & Shaver, P. (1990). Love and work: An attachment-based theoretical perspective. *Journal of Personality and Social Psychology*, *52*, 511–524. doi:10.1037/0022-3514.52.3.511 PMID:3572722

Hoghughi, M. (2004). Parenting: an introduction. In M. Hoghughi, & N. Long (Eds.), *Theory and research for practice* (pp. 1–18). Handbook of parenting London, UK: Sage.

Johnston, C., Hessl, D., Blasey, C., Eliez, S., Erba, H., Dyer-Friedman, J., ... Reiss, A. (2003). Factors associated with parenting stress in mothers of children with Fragile X syndrome. *Developmental and Behavioral Pediatrics*, *24*(4), 267–275. doi:10.1097/00004703-200308000-00008 PMID:12915799

Katz, S. (2002). Gender differences in adapting to a child's chronic illness: A causal model. *Journal of Pediatric Nursing*, *17*(4), 257–269. doi:10.1053/jpdn.2002.126709 PMID:12219325

Keller, D., & Honig, A. S. (2004). Maternal and paternal stress in families with schoolaged children with disabilities. *The American Journal of Orthopsychiatry*, *74*(3), 337–348. doi:10.1037/0002-9432.74.3.337 PMID:15291710

Kersh, J., Hedvat, T. T., Hauser-Cram, P., & Warfield, M. E. (2006). The contribution of marital quality to the wellbeing of parents of children with developmental disabilities. *Journal of Intellectual Disability Research, 50*, 883-893. doi: /. doi:10.1111/j.1365-2788.2006.00906.x

Laranjeira, C. (2007). Do vulnerável ser ao resiliente envelhecer: Revisão de literatura. [From vulnerable being to resilient aging: literature review]. *Psicologia: Teoria e Pesquisa (Brasília)*, *23*(3), 327–332. doi:10.1590/S0102-37722007000300012

Lucca, S. A. D., & Petean, E. B. L. (2016). Fatherhood: Experiences of fathers of boys diagnosed with Duchenne Muscular Dystrophy. *Ciencia & Saude Coletiva*, *21*(10), 3081–3089. doi:10.1590/1413-812320152110.20302016 PMID:27783781

Luther, S. (2007). Resilience in development: a synthesis of research across 5 decades. Developmental Psychopathology Vol. 3: Risk, Disorder, and Adaptation (2nd ed.) (Eds. D. Cicchetti, & D. J. Cohen), pp. 739–95. Hoboken, NJ: John Wiley & Sons.

Luz, G., Carvalho, M., & Silva, M. (2011). O significado de uma organização de apoio aos portadores e familiares de fibrose cística na perspectiva das famílias. [The meaning of a support organization for cystic fibrosis patients and families from the perspective of families]. *Texto & Contexto Enfermagem*, *20*(1), 127–134. doi:10.1590/S0104-07072011000100015

Luz, G., Silva, M. R. S., & DeMontigny, F. (2015). Doenças raras: Itinerário diagnóstico e terapêutico das famílias de pessoas afetadas. [Rare diseases: diagnostic and therapeutic itinerary of families of affected people]. *Acta Paulista de Enfermagem*, *28*(5), 395–400. doi:10.1590/1982-0194201500067

Maltby, H. J., Kristjanson, L., & Coleman, M. E. (2003). The parenting competency framework: Learning to be a parent of a child with asthma. *International Journal of Nursing Practice*, *9*(6), 368–373. doi:10.1046/j.1440-172X.2003.00445.x PMID:14984073

Martins, T. C., Moreira, H., & Canavarro, M. C. (2016). Adult attachment and dyadic adjustment: The mediating role of shame. *The Journal of Psychology*, *150*(5), 560–575. doi:10.1080/00223980.2015.1114461 PMID:26759960

Masten, A. S., & Powell, J. L. (2003). A resilience framework for research, policy, and practice: Contributions from project competence. In S. S. Luthar (Ed.), Resilience and vulnerability: Adaptation in the context of childhood adversities (pp. 1-25). New York.

Meleis, A. I., Sawyer, L. M., Im, E. O., Messias, D. K. H., & Schumacher, K. (2000). Experiencing transitions: An emerging middle-range theory. *Advances in Nursing Science*, *23*(1), 12–28. doi:10.1097/00012272-200009000-00006 PMID:10970036

Melnyk, B. M., Feinstein, N. F., Moldenhouer, Z., & Small, L. (2001). Coping in parents of children who are chronically ill: Strategies for assessment and intervention. *Pediatric Nursing*, *27*(6), 547–557. PMID:12024526

Mikulincer, M., & Shaver, P. R. (2014). Attachment bonds in romantic relationships. In M. Mikulincer, & P. R. Shaver (Eds.), *Mechanisms of social connection: from brain to group* (pp. 273–290). Washington, DC: American Psychological Association. doi:10.1037/14250-000

Milbrath, V. M., Motta, M. D. G. C., Gabatz, R. I. B., & Freitag, V. L. (2017). O nascimento de um filho com paralisia cerebral: Um tempo presente inesperado. [The birth of a child with cerebral palsy: An unexpected present tense]. *Revista Interdisciplinar em Cultura e Sociedade*, *3*, 47–60.

Monteiro, M., Matos, A. P., & Coelho, R. (2002). A adaptação psicológica de mães cujos filhos apresentam paralisia cerebral: Revisão da literatura. [Psychological adaptation of mothers whose children have cerebral palsy: literature review]. *Revista Portuguesa de Psicossomática*, *4*(2), 149–178.

Mooney-Doyle, K., Deatrick, J. A., & Horowitz, J. A. (2015). Tasks and communication as an avenue to enhance parenting of children birth-5years: An integrative review. *Journal of Pediatric Nursing*, *30*(1), 184–207. doi:10.1016/j.pedn.2014.03.002 PMID:24680918

Moreira, P. L., & Angelo, M. (2008). Tornar-se mãe de criança com câncer: Construindo a parentalidade. [Becoming a mother of a child with cancer: Building parenting]. *Revista Latino-Americana de Enfermagem*, *16*(3), 355–361. doi:10.1590/S0104-11692008000300004 PMID:18695806

Mulsow, M., Caldera, Y. M., Pursley, M., Reifman, A., & Huston, A. C. (2002). Multilevel factors influencing maternal stress during the first three years. *Journal of Marriage and the Family*, *64*(4), 944–956. doi:10.1111/j.1741-3737.2002.00944.x

Nieweglowski, V. H., & More, C. L. O. O. (2008). Comunicação equipe-família em unidade de terapia intensiva pediátrica: Impacto no processo de hospitalização. [Team-family communication in a pediatric intensive care unit: impact on the hospitalization process]. *Estudos de Psicologia*, *25*(1), 111–122. doi:10.1590/S0103-166X2008000100011

Pelchat, D., Lefebvre, H., & Perreault, M. (2003). Differences and similarities between mothers and fathers experiences of parenting a child with a disability. *Journal of Child Health Care*, *7*(4), 231–247. doi:10.1177/13674935030074001 PMID:14636429

Pelentsov, L. J., Fielder, A. L., & Esterman, A. J. (2016a). The supportive care needs of parents with a child with a rare disease: A qualitative descriptive study. *Journal of Pediatric Nursing*, *31*(3), 207–218. doi:10.1016/j.pedn.2015.10.022 PMID:26651231

Pelentsov, L. J., Fielder, A. L., Laws, T. A., & Esterman, A. J. (2016b). The supportive care needs of parents with a child with a rare disease: Results of an online survey. *BMC Family Practice*, *17*(1), 207–218. doi:10.118612875-016-0488-x PMID:27439905

Pelentsov, L. J., Fielder, A. L., Laws, T. A., & Esterman, A. J. (2016b). The supportive care needs of parents with a child with a rare disease: Results of an online survey. *BMC Family Practice*, *17*(1), 207–218. doi:10.118612875-016-0488-x PMID:27439905

Piccinini, C. A., Castro, E. K., Alvarenga, P., Vargas, S., & Oliveira, V. Z. (2003). A doença crônica orgânica na infância e as práticas educativas maternas. [Chronic organic disease in childhood and maternal educational practices]. *Estudos de Psicologia*, *8*(1), 75–83. doi:10.1590/S1413-294X2003000100009

Rare Disease UK. (2016). Acedido a 12 de maio de 2017 em https://www.raredisease.org.uk/what-is-a-rare-disease/

Ioana – *Associação nacional de deficiências mentais e raras*. (2018). Acedido a 16 de junho de 2018 em http://www.rarissimas.pt/index.php

Santos, B., & Mota, C. P. (2018). *Parentalidade e resiliência em pais de filhos com doenças raras: O efeito moderador da vinculação amorosa.* [Parenting and resilience in parents of children with rare diseases: The moderating effect of romantic attachment]. Comunicação oral apresentada no 4º Congresso da Ordem dos Psicólogos, de 12 a 15 de setembro, Braga.

Santos, B., & Mota, C. P. (2019). *Personalidade e resiliência em pais de filhos com doenças raras: Efeito mediador da vinculação amorosa.* [Personality and resilience in parents of children with rare diseases: Mediating effect of romantic attachment]. Comunicação oral no âmbito da mesa 8 "Intervenção em situações de doença crónica e hospitalização" no X Congresso Internacional de Psicologia da Criança e do Adolescente - "Psicoterapia e outras abordagens terapêuticas", que se realizou nos dias 10 e 11 de abril de 2019 na Universidade Lusíada de Lisboa.

Schieppati, A., Henter, J., Daina, E., & Aperia, A. (2008). Why rare diseases are an important medical and social issue. *Essay Focus*, *371*(9629), 2039–2041. doi:10.1016/S0140-6736(08)60872-7 PMID:18555915

Silva, C. X., Brito, E. D., Sousa, F. S., & França, I. S. X. (2010). Criança com paralisia cerebral: Qual o impacto na vida do cuidador? [Child with cerebral palsy: what is the impact on the caregiver's life?]. *Revista da Rede de Enfermagem do Nordeste*, *11*, 204–214.

Silva, E., & Sousa, T. (2015). Avaliação econômica no âmbito das doenças raras: Isto é possível? *Cadernos de Saude Publica*, *31*(3), 1–11. doi:10.1590/0102-311X00213813 PMID:25859711

Smith, J., Cheater, F., & Bekker, H. (2013). Parents' experiences of living with a child with a long-term condition: A rapid structured review of the literature. *Health Expectations*, *18*(4), 452–474. doi:10.1111/hex.12040 PMID:23311692

Soares, J., Araújo, L., & Bellato, R. (2016). Cuidar na situação de adoecimento raro: Vivência da família e sua busca por amparo dos serviços de saúde. [Caring for a rare illness: Family experience and their search for support from health services]. *Revista Saúde e Sociedade*, *25*(4), 1017–1030. doi:10.1590/S0104-12902016162301

Strehle, E., & Middlemiss, P. (2007). Children with 4q-syndrome: The parents' perspective. *Journal of Genetic Counseling*, *18*(2), 189–199. PMID:17710871

Taanila, A., Kokkonen, J., & Jarvelin, M. (1996). The long-term effects of children's early-onset disability on marital relationships. *Developmental Medicine and Child Neurology*, *38*(7), 567–577. doi:10.1111/j.1469-8749.1996.tb12121.x PMID:8674907

Theofanidis, D. (2007). Chronic illness in childhood: Psychosocial adaptation and nursing support for the child and family. *Health Science Journal*, *2*, 1–8.

Tozzi, A., Mingarelli, R., Agricola, E., Gonfiantini, M., Pandolfi, E., Carloni, E., ... Dallapiccola, B. (2013). The internet user profile of Italian families of patients with rare diseases: A web survey. *Orphanet Journal of Rare Diseases*, *8*(76), 1–8. doi:10.1186/1750-1172-8-76 PMID:23680013

Waldboth, V., Patch, C., Mahrer-Imhof, R., & Metcalfe, A. (2016). Living a normal life in an extraordinary way: A systematic review investigating experiences of families of young people's transition into adulthood when affected by a genetic and chronic childhood condition. *International Journal of Nursing Studies*, *62*, 44–59. doi:10.1016/j.ijnurstu.2016.07.007 PMID:27450665

Wijnberg-Williams, J., Van de Wiel, M., Kamps, W., & Hoekstra-Weebers, M. (2015). Effects of communication styles on marital satisfaction and distress of parents of pediatric cancer patients: A prospective longitudinal study. *Psycho-Oncology*, *24*(1), 106–112. doi:10.1002/pon.3617 PMID:25045011

Williford, A. P., Calkins, S. D., & Keane, S. P. (2007). Predicting change in parenting stress across early childhood: Child and maternal factors. *Journal of Abnormal Child Psychology*, *35*(2), 251–263. doi:10.100710802-006-9082-3 PMID:17186365

Yeh, C. H., Lee, T. T., Chen, M. L., & Li, W. (2000). Adaptational process of parents of pediatric oncology patients. *Pediatric Hematology and Oncology*, *17*(2), 119–131. doi:10.1080/088800100276479 PMID:10734654

Zagalo-Cardoso, J. A. (2001). Doenças genéticas: Impacto psicológico e representações sociais. [Genetic diseases: Psychological impact and social representations] In *M. C. Canavarro (Org.), Psicologia da Gravidez e da Maternidade* (pp. 211–235). Coimbra, Portugal: Quarteto Editora.

Zurynski, Y., Frith, K., Leonard, H., & Elliott, E. (2008). Rare childhood diseases: How should we respond? *Archives of Disease in Childhood*, *93*(12), 1071–1074. doi:10.1136/adc.2007.134940 PMID:18684747

KEY TERMS AND DEFINITIONS

Attachment: Concept developed by John Bowlby that explains the innate disposition of the human being to establish affective bonds and close relationships with the primordial figures.

Coping: Set of strategies that individuals use in order to adapt and manage certain life circumstances, perceived as adverse.

Emotional Regulation: Processes, intrinsic and extrinsic, through which individuals exert an effect on experiencing and expressing emotions in order to achieve emotional stability in an adverse situation.

Parenting: Set of tasks inherent in parenting to promote the development of their children as fully as possible, using resources within and outside the family.

Personality: Set of patterns of behaviors, thoughts, feelings and attitudes that are inherent in an individual and that tend to vary with each individual, making the subject a unique organism.

Rare diseases: Serious, degenerative or genetic diseases that are generally life threatening and can be debilitating as their quality of life is compromised due to lack of autonomy and the high level of pain and suffering experienced by the individual rare disease patient and his family.

Resilience: Set of adaptive processes that promote encouragement, resistance and empowerment in the face of traumatic and / or stressful situations.

Chapter 9
Neuropsychiatry in Late Onset Tay-Sachs Disease:
Key Features and Possible Etiology of Psychosis

Natan Gadoth
Department of Neurology, Maynei Hayeshua Medical Center, Bnei Barak and the Sackler Faculty of Medicine, Tel Aviv University, Israel

ABSTRACT

The neuropsychiatric adult onset Tay-Sachs disease is relatively unknown. Although clinical features and mode of presentation are variable, there are common symptoms and signs of, for example, spinocerebellar atrophy, motor neuron disease, psychiatric disorder, and neuroimaging features of cerebellar atrophy. This chapter reviews the neuropsychiatric features of Late Onset Tay-Sachs disease, discussing possible interconnections between psychosis and the cerebellum in this disease. Understanding this interlink offers some important insights into the rarity of the disease that together with the diverse clinical onset and manifestations are responsible for a marked delay in diagnosis and even misdiagnosis. Genetic testing for the activity of Hexosaminidase A, prompted by the presence of cerebellar atrophy will establish the diagnosis. In all, the combination of cerebellar degeneration together with atypical psychiatric features is in line with the ongoing assumption that the cerebellum and its thalamo-cortical outflow are responsible for psychosis, and in particular, schizophrenia.

DOI: 10.4018/978-1-7998-2088-8.ch009

INTRODUCTION

Rare genetic diseases present a diagnostic challenge since the clinical manifestations are complex (Maddalena, Bale, Das, Grody, & Richards, 2005; Zelnik et al., 2000) and variable due to slow progression of the disease as the patients get older, heterogeneity of the genetic defects responsible for a particular syndrome and or variable deficiency of a specific enzyme (Hechtman, & Kaplan, 1993).

A diagnosis of rare yet "undiagnosed" diseases is very often reached retrospectively, after "accidently" reading a case report describing identical clinical features to those of a particular "undiagnosed or misdiagnosed" patient (Kielgman, Bordini, Basel, & Nocton, 2017; Ramoni et al., 2017).

Late Onset Tay-Sachs (LOTS) disease fits perfectly into this framework. It is very rare, with a progressive complex and variable clinical course which appears as the patients are getting older and the presence of heterogeneous mutations which are responsible for different degrees of enzyme deficiency (Neudofer et al., 2005; Rucker et al., 2004). While the neurological characteristics of LOTS may resemble motor neuron disease (Amyotrophic Lateral Sclerosis [ALS] - like, Spinal muscular atrophy [SMA] - like) (MacQueen, Rosebush, & Mazurek, 1998), they can also include psychiatric, cognitive and movement disorders. Thus, familiarity with the complex clinical pictures of LOTS is essential for the early diagnosis, avoiding unnecessary, time consuming and frequently costly tests.

The combination of early onset psychosis and cerebellar atrophy is present in the majority of the patients (Streifler, Golomb, & Gadoth, 1989). Brain imaging in late-onset GM2 gangliosidosis is intriguing since the cerebellum and its thalamo-cortical pathways are implicated in the etiology of psychosis, and in particular, in schizophrenia.

In this chapter, the neuropsychiatric features of LOTS are reviewed and the possible link between psychosis and the cerebellum as manifested in this disease are discussed. The review carried out provides an example in which different knowledge basis are necessary to dialogue within the scientific community to advance on different aspects of a rare disease.

TOWARDS THE RARE NEURONOPATHY GM2 GLANGLIOSIDOSIS

GM2 gangliosidosis is a rare neurometabolic lysosomal storage disease. The lysosomes are cytoplasmic membrane bound organelles that contain a variety of enzymes (hydrolases) necessary for breaking down complex macromolecules. A deficiency of a single lysosomal enzyme will cause storage of a macromolecule which, is the substrate for this enzyme within the lysosome. GM2 together with three other gangliosides are major components of the brain, accounting for more than 90% of its total ganglioside fraction. G refers to 'ganglioside', the M to monosialic (i.e., it has one sialic acid), and 2 is due to the fact that it was the second monosialic ganglioside discovered.

Although the functions of gangliosides are not fully understood, they are involved in ion transport, binding of neurotransmitters and cell adhesion. Hexosaminidase, a lysosomal enzyme necessary for degradation (breakdown) of GM2, is presented in the form of the isoenzymes Hexosaminidase A (Hex-A) and Hexosaminidase B (Hex-B). While both isoenzymes can hydrolyze a wide spectrum of macromolecules, only HEX-A is able to hydrolyze GM2 (Ferreira &, Gah, 2017). Deficient activity of HEX-A results in storage of GM2 within neurons, a condition known as neuronopathy, in contrast to neuropathy which is a disorder of peripheral nerves. It was found that the content of GM2 within the gray matter of the brain where the neurons are located is 100-300 times greater than the normal levels. The affected neurons take a ballooned appearance due the accumulation of the storage lipid material (GM2) (Figure 1). GM2 storage is caused by total deficiency of Hex-A, partial deficiency of Hex-A, a combined deficiency of Hex A and B, known as Sandhoff disease and a deficiency of the non-catalytic GM2 activator which manifest similarly to infantile TSD.

All the above-mentioned enzymes are responsible for degradation of GM2 (Lemieux et al., 2006; Navon, & Proia, 1989; Sandhoff, Harzer, Wässle, & Jatzkewitz, 1971; Zaroff et al., 2004).

Three clinical forms of this storage are known, each with a different age of onset and clinical course:

- **Infantile Tay - Sachs disease (TSD):** The classical infantile form known by the eponym Tay - Sachs disease (TSD), is characterized by very low or absent activity of Hex-A (Fernandes Filho & Shapiro, 2004; Kaback et al., 1993; O'Brien et al., 1971; Schnet, et al., 1970), as shown in Figure 2. Less known are the juvenile (subacute) and adult (chronic) subtypes of GM2, in which residual Hex-A activity is present and the age of onset is either during late childhood or adulthood;
- **Juvenile Tay-Sachs Disease (TSD):** The Juvenile form presents in late childhood with progressive spasticity and rigidity, seizures and severe cognitive decline leading to vegetative state between the ages of 5 and 15 years old (Maegawa et al., 2006; Neurodorfer, & Kolodny, 2004);
- **The adult onset form (LOTS)**: The adult onset form (LOTS) presents, during the second decade of life, with motor clumsiness and peculiar form of "stutter like" dysarthria which is a motor speech disorder that results from

Figure 1. The Mechanism of GM2 storage in LOTS. Source: Author's ownership

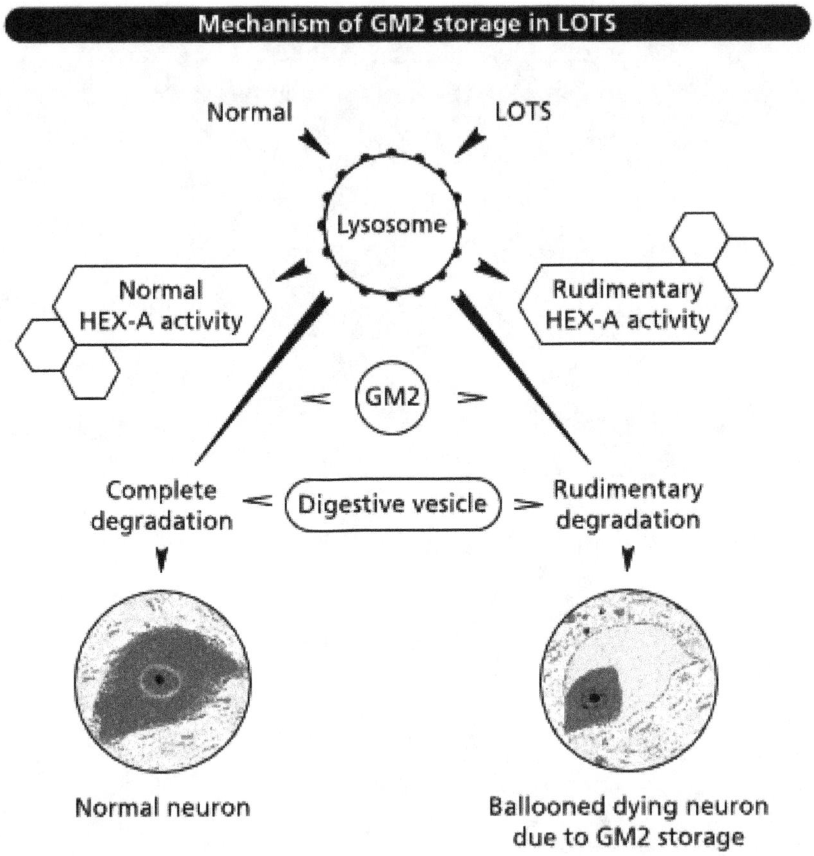

damage to the brain area responsible for function of the muscles involved in speech production and manifests by poor articulation of phonemes. Psychiatric impairment is quite common and may be the presenting sign. Slow neurological deterioration comprising cerebellar, pyramidal, extrapyramidal and lower-motor neuron symptoms and signs is the rule. The correct diagnosis is often delayed until the 3rd - 4th decades of life (Neurodorfer, & Kolodny, 2004; Regier, 2016; Rucker et al., 2004).

Figure 2. Thin layer chromatography showing the presence of both Hex-A and Hex-B in the normal subject (N) and lack of Hex-A with preserved Hex-B in a patient with TSD. Courtesy of Prof. R. Navon

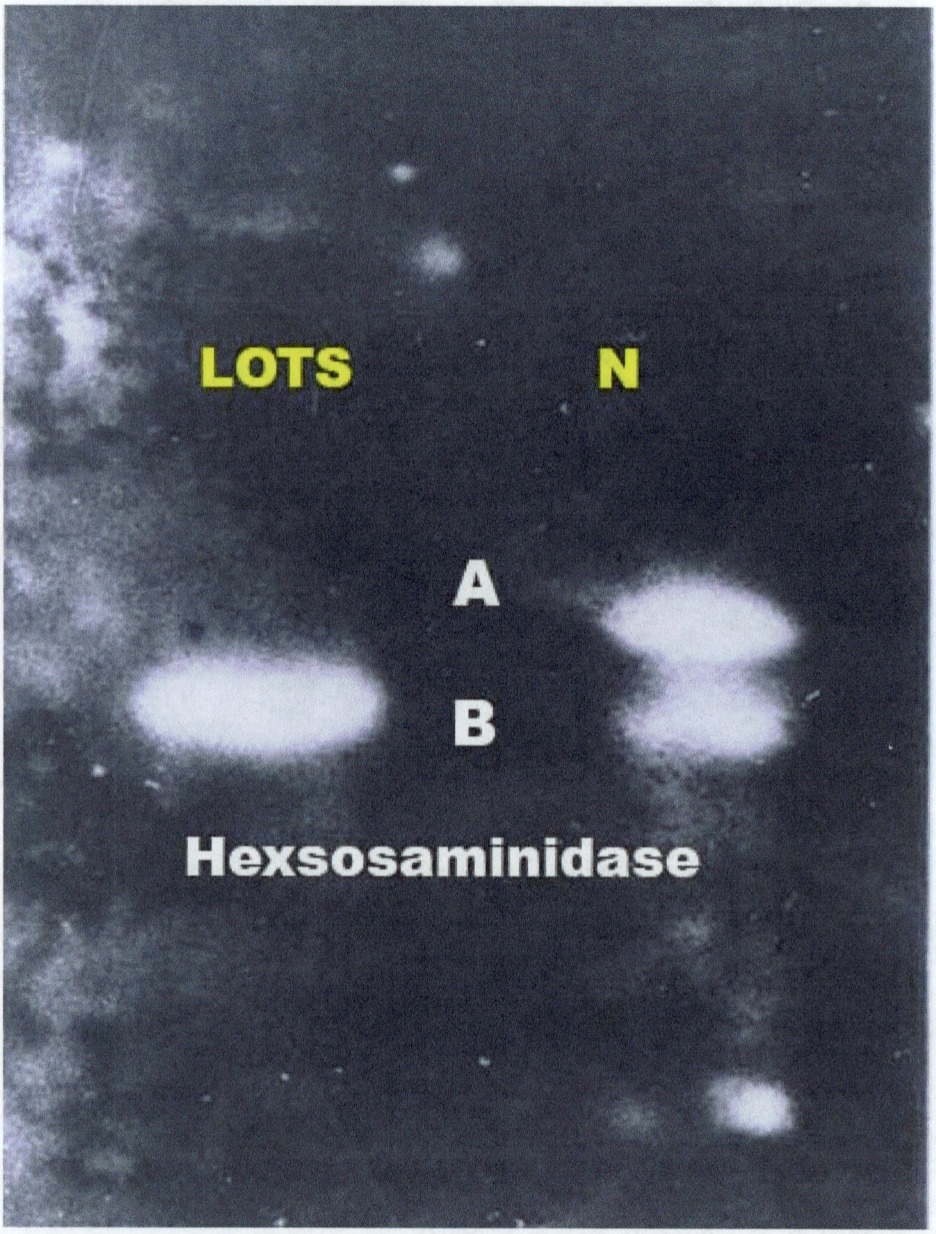

The exact prevalence of this form of GM2 (LOTS) is not known since many cases who have been classified as adult onset GM2 had their first symptoms during early childhood with shortened life expectancy. While Neudorfer and colleagues (2005), have noted the estimated incidence of LOTS in Ashkenazi Jews of 1 in 135,000, Maier and colleagues (2017), gave an estimate of 1 in 300,000 in people of non-Jewish extraction.

All forms of GM2 gangliosidosis are inherited in an autosomal recessive pattern which refers to the state that each parents of a patient with LOTS carry in his cells a normal copy and a mutated copy of Hex-A, and their affected child will carry in each cell a pair of mutated Hex A, one from the father and the other from the mother. Both Jewish and non-Jewish patients share the variable clinical features of LOTS. However, Jewish Ashkenazi patients with LOTS are compound heterozygotes (in each cell the pair of mutated genes are not identical) for the Gly269- Ser point mutation together with one of the allelic infantile Tay-Sachs mutations, whereas the mutations found in Non-Jewish patients are highly heterogeneous (Akli et al.1993).

Since LOTS is extremely rare, the following case report of a recently evaluated patient may serve the inexperienced reader by enhancing his ability to reach an early clinical diagnosis. This patient was first examined in the author's clinic during January 2018.

Demonstrative Case Report

As mentioned above, the following case report illustrates a scenario in which a patient was diagnosed with Late Onset Tay-Sachs Disease (LOTS):

A 50-year-old single man was born in Latvia. The non-consanguineous healthy parents are of Ashkenazi Jewish extraction. A 57-year-old brother suffers from "psychiatric symptoms" and coordination problems but refuses any form of medical care. The patient's life history since his mother's pregnancy, delivery and early psychomotor development was unremarkable. Speech onset was delayed in the form stuttering. He completed 9 years of public school, where he was described as clumsy with poor achievements in gymnastics. At the age of 14 years old, the parents divorced. Soon after, he experienced his first attack of "paranoid psychosis" during a febrile illness for which he was hospitalized in a psychiatric institution for 1 year.

During the next 7 years, he continued drug treatment for episodes of "depression". The family immigrated to Israel when he was 21 years old and soon after he was diagnosed with late onset Tay-Sachs Disease, confirmed by Hexosaminidase- A deficiency in the serum and white blood cells (3.4% and 5.8% respectively). Two-point mutations at different exons in the HEXA gene were detected. Exons are regions

Figure 3. Brain MRI: (A) Sagittal and (B) Axial views. Note cerebellar cortical atrophy (arrows)
Source: Author's ownership. Patient's MRI with the patient and guardian (mother) permission

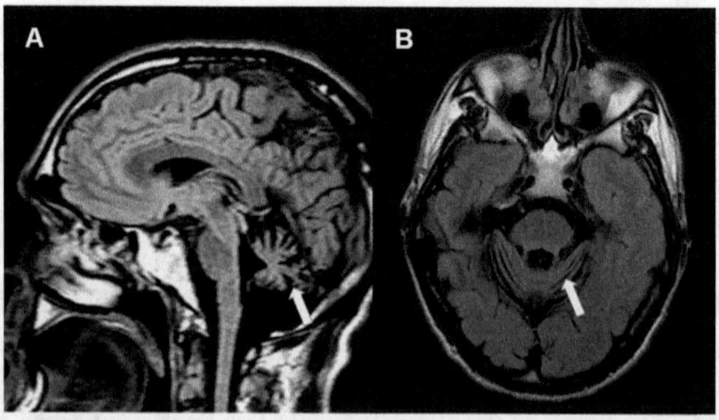

of the gene which will be expressed (Gilbert 1978). Motor functions deteriorated at the age of 36 years with difficulties in getting up from bed and standing up from sitting position, frequent falls, swallowing problems and cognitive decline. At the age of 42 years, he was hospitalized in a rehabilitation center. Dysarthria, hand tremor, facial muscle twitching, symmetrical muscle wasting with proximal weakness due to lower neuron motor disease mimicking spinal muscular atrophy, increased muscle tone, truncal ataxia (inability to maintain a stable body posture and stance caused mostly by damage to the cerebellum), diminished deep tendon reflexes, partial sphincter control, and dysphagia mainly for liquids were noted. Cognitive functions were summarized as difficulties in short and long-term memory and abstract thinking. On his latest evaluation in our clinic during January 2018, worsening of truncal ataxia and dysarthria were noted. Brain CT and Magnetic Resonance Imaging (MRI) disclosed prominent cerebellar, cortical and vermis atrophy (Figure 3). Electroencephalogram (EEG) was normal.

Over the years, he was followed closely by several psychiatrists and had to be hospitalized several times for either a prolonged psychotic episode or bouts of depression.

Methotrimeprazine (RonexineR), Fluvoxamine (FavoxilR), Risperidone (RisperdalR), Sodium Valproate (DepaleptR), Lithium Carbonate, Clonazepam (ClonexR), Citalopram Hydrochloride (RecitalR), Brotizolam (BondorminR), in variable combinations and dosage were administered for extended periods. Risperdone and valproic acid were the most often combination used. The onset of orobucal dyskinesia in the form of unusual and unintended involuntary and uncontrolled nature which was considered as tardive improved by dose reduction of Risperdone. There was no long-term beneficial effect of those drugs on the nature, severity or frequency of psychiatric flare-ups.

LITERATURE REVIEW AND DISCUSSION

The onset of psychotic episodes (Osher et al., 2011) alternating with periods of depressed mood (Shaphiro, Logigian, Kolodny, & Pastores, 2008), starting during the second decade of life and the poor response to a variety of antipsychotic drugs (Shapiro, Hatters-Friedman, Fernandes-Filho, Anthony, & Natowicz, 2006), is rather the rule in LOTS.

The combination of progressive cerebellar, pyramidal, extrapyramidal, lower motor neuron and psychiatric symptoms and signs described above, together with radiological cerebellar atrophy which is present in almost all patients published so far, regardless of the neurological presentation, is unique for this form of GM2 (Argov, & Navon, 1984; Lemieux et al., 2006; Navon, & Proia, 1989; Yokoyama et al., 2014). Even if not all the above-mentioned clinical features are present at onset, most of them will manifest along with aging and disease progression.

Psychiatric impairment was already mentioned in few early case reports (*e.g.* - Johnson, 1986; Rapin, Suzuki, Suzuki, & Valsamis 1976 [case 3]; Yaffe et al. 1979; Streifler, Golomb, & Gadoth, 1989; Oates, Bosch, & Hart,1986). It is worth noting that Navon and her colleagues (Navon, Argov & Frisch, 1986) were pioneers to recognize that psychiatric impairment should be considered as an integral part of the complex clinical picture of the disease. Indeed, they found that 30% of their patients suffered from drug resistant psychosis at the time of their evaluation. They have also noted that the presence of psychiatric impairment predicted a worse clinical course.

In a literature review of the psychiatric manifestation of LOTS published in 1998, MacQueen, Rosebush, and Mazurek (1998) were able to identify 63 published cases of LOTS and added a single personal patient. Mental status was mentioned in 39 of those patients, out of those, 21 (54%) suffered from psychosis, mainly in the form of "hebephrenic schizophrenia" (disorganized schizophrenia). Mood disorder was present in 18 patients (27%), mainly in the form of early onset monopolar depression, evolving to overt hebephrenia. The detailed clinical - psychiatric features, course and treatment were available for only 8 patients, of those 3 were diagnosed and treated in the authors' group of research and medical center (Streifler et al., 1989). The characteristic clinical course in those patients were quite similar to the course of the patient described hereby. Recurrent prolonged bouts of acute psychosis characterized by marked disorganized thinking, agitation, hallucinations and delusions, paranoid and manic behavior intermingled with episodes of atypical depressive bouts, and less frequently catatonic state or manic behavior, are some of the characteristic observed (Rosebush et al., 1995).

In the same vein, a similar proportion of patients with psychosis was later reported by Zaroff and colleagues (2004), Shapiro, Pastores, Giantess, Luzy, and Kolodny, (2009), Osher et al. (2015), and somewhat lower in non-Jewish patients (Jahnová et al. 2019).

The cerebellum was traditionally considered as the center for motor learning and control (Albus, 1971). In the last years, ample evidence for the possible role of the cerebellum in cognition emerged from evolutional and developmental neurobiology as well as anatomical and neuroimaging studies (Moberget et al. 2019). Moreover, it was recognized that symptoms and signs of schizophrenia can be explained by cerebellar abnormalities (Andreasen 1999; Andreasen et al. 1999).

More recent research has pointed out that abnormalities in the Cortico-Cerebellar -Thalamic -Cortical Circuit (CCTCC) may be responsible for schizophrenia (Andreasen & Pierson, 2008). Indeed, hyperconnectivity of this circuit was recently shown to predict the later development of psychosis in individuals at clinical high risk for psychosis display and patients with schizophrenia (Cao et al. 2018). To supplement those data is the fact that cerebellar structural abnormalities are present in schizophrenia in the form of decreased size of Purkinje cells (Tran, Smutzer, Doty, & Arnold, 1998), and decrease blood flow and atrophy of the vermis (Heath, Franklin, & Shraberg, 1979). In addition, recent neuroimaging studies emphasized the role of the cerebello-thalamic pathway in psychosis (Bernard, Orr, & Mittal, 2017).

Considering all the above together with the fact that in the infantile form of GM2 (Brismar, et al. 1990) and more recently in LOTS (Lee at al. 2008), cerebello-thalamic outflow is progressively impaired, and, subsequently, one would expect that the patients will be not only at high risk to develop psychosis but also suffer from severe organic psychosis. The fact that psychosis is part of the clinical picture of other hereditary metabolic disorders affecting the cerebellum such as Machado-Joseph Disease (SCA III), (Braga-Neto, et al.,2016), cerebro-tendinous-xanthomatosis, metachromatic leukodystrophy and Neiman-Pick disease Type C (Demily, & Sedel, 2014), is in line with the above mentioned assumptions. Moreover, even acquired structural cerebellar damage such as stroke can cause psychosis (Liao, Wei, & Chen, 2018).

Nevertheless, not all published patients with LOTS suffered from psychosis. Most of them who were considered as "atypical" were young non-Jewish patients who carried for several years a diagnosis of ALS-like or SMA-like disorder (Table 1).

When psychosis is not part of the clinical picture the diagnosis is often delayed. The case report by Deik (2014) is a good example of the complexity of LOTS without psychosis. This Jewish female presented as her early twenties with motor difficulties which progressed to marked gait problems at the age of 28 years when neurological

Table 1. Non-Jewish LOTS patients with motor neuron like disease without psychosis

Author	Ethnic Origin / Gender	Age of onset / Diagnosis (y)	Diagnosis
Maier, (2017)	Romanian /M	17 / 32	Anterior horn cell disease
Jahnova, (2019) (patient 1) (patient 2)	Czech / F Czech / F	15 / 18 17 / 20	Proximal lower extremity weakness
Prihodova, (2013) (patient 1) (patients 2)	Slovak / F Slovak / F	10 / 17 10 / 29	Spinal Muscular Atrophy III like
Barritt, (2017)	Hungarian / M	14 / 35	ALS like
Navon (1997)	Ukraine / F	10 / 20	Spinal Muscular Atrophy III like
Zamrozik (2013)	Polish / M	30 / 39	Spinal Muscular Atrophy like

evaluation including muscle biopsy, normal brain MRI and electrodiagnostic study which was summarized as "chronic neuropathy". At age of 30 years her progressive gait disability prompted a second evaluation including electrodiagnosis summarized as "variant of SMA." Progressive cerebellar impairment started during late 40s, which led to a third evaluation at the age of 52 years including documentation of cerebellar atrophy on brain MRI, electrodiagnosis of "chronic, generalized motor axonopathy" and comprehensive spinocerebellar ataxia (SCA) and recessive ataxia panels which was negative for known mutation. She was finally diagnosed with LOTS at the age of 53 years.

Most of the patients who were considered as "atypical" were non-Jewish, without psychosis who suffered from progressive motor neuron disease mimicking spinal muscular atrophy or ALS (see Table 1). It is quite possible that those few cases may either develop psychosis as the disease progress or may carry mutations which are not associated with psychosis. This assumption deserves further research.

CONCLUSION

This chapter reviews the neuropsychiatric features of Late Onset Tay Sachs (LOTS) disease, discussing possible interconnections between psychosis and the cerebellum and its thalamo-cortical outflow. Given that LOTS is a very rare disease, with a progressive complex and variable clinical course and the presence of heterogeneous mutations that affect neural-motor functions, this study gives a further insight into early onset psychosis.

The study identified begins by providing an overview of the rare neuronopathy GM2 gangliosidosis traditionally known as Tay-Sachs Disease. Although more attention has focused on Infantile Tay-Sachs Disease (TSD), less known were the Juvenile (subacute) and adult (chronic) subtypes of GM2, in which residual Hex-A activity is present and the age of onset is either during late childhood or adulthood.

As illustrated in a demonstrative case report (authors' patient), no long-term beneficial effect has been shown with the administration of a set of drugs on the nature, severity or frequency of psychiatric flare-ups, suggesting a poor response to a variety of antipsychotic drugs.

Based on the literature review, psychiatric manifestation in LOTS often occur. In other words, mental disorders and psychosis are very likely to manifest, mainly in the form of "hebephrenic schizophrenia" (disorganized schizophrenia), mood disorders, monopolar depression and evolve to overt hebephrenia. Patients tended to exhibit disorganized thinking, agitation, hallucinations and delusions, paranoid and manic behavior intermingled with episodes of atypical depressive bouts, and less frequently catatonic state or manic behavior.

In addition, one may suppose that once cerebello-thalamic outflow has been shown progressively impaired in TSD, these patients will be not only at high risk to develop psychosis but also will suffer from severe organic psychosis.

The review carried out provides an example in which different knowledge basis are necessary to dialogue within the scientific community to advance on different aspects of a rare diseases.

ACKNOWLEDGMENT

Funding: This research received no specific grants from any funding agency in the public, commercial, or not-for-profit sectors.

The author wishes to thank Mrs G. Gadoth for assistance with the artwork presented in this chapter.

Disclosure Statement: The author reports no conflict of interest.

REFERENCES

Akli, S., Chomel, J. C., Lacorte, J. M., Bachner, L., Kahn, A., & Poenaru, L. (1993). Ten novel mutations in the HEXA gene in non-Jewish Tay-Sachs patients. *Human Molecular Genetics*, *2*(1), 61–67. doi:10.1093/hmg/2.1.61 PMID:8490625

Albus., J.S. (1971). A theory of cerebellar function. *Mathematical Bioscience 10*(1-2), 25-61. (71)90051-4 doi:10.1016/0025-5564

Andreasen, N. C. (1999). A unitary model of schizophrenia: Bleuler's "fragmented phrene" as schizencephaly. *Archives of General Psychiatry*, *56*(9), 781–787. doi:10.1001/archpsyc.56.9.781 PMID:12884883

Andreasen, N. C., Nopoulos, P., O'Leary, D. S., Miller, D. D., Wassink, T., & Flaum, M. (1999). Defining the phenotype of schizophrenia: Cognitive dysmetria and its neural mechanisms. *Biological Psychiatry*, *46*(7), 908–920. doi:10.1016/S0006-3223(99)00152-3 PMID:10509174

Andreasen, N. C., & Pierson, R. (2008). The role of the cerebellum in schizophrenia. *Biological Psychiatry*, *64*(2), 81–88. doi:10.1016/j.biopsych.2008.01.003 PMID:18395701

Argov, Z., & Navon, R. (1984). Clinical and genetic variations in the syndrome of adult GM2 gangliodosis resulting from hexosaminidase a deficiency. *Annals of Neurology*, *16*(1), 14–20. doi:10.1002/ana.410160105 PMID:6235771

Barritt, A. W., Anderson, S. J., Leigh, P. N., & Ridha, B. H. (2017). Late-onset Tay-Sachs disease. *Practical Neurology*, *17*(5), 396–399. doi:10.1136/practneurol-2017-001665 PMID:28739864

Bernard, J. A., Orr, J. M., & Mittal, V. A. (2017). Cerebello-thalamo-cortical networks predict positive symptom progression in individuals at ultra-high risk for psychosis. *NeuroImage. Clinical*, *14*, 622–628. doi:10.1016/j.nicl.2017.03.001 PMID:28348953

Braga-Neto, P., Pedroso, J. L., Gadelha, A., Laureano, M. R., de Souza Noto, C., Garrido, G. J., & Barsottini, O. G. (2016). Psychosis in Machado-Joseph Disease: Clinical Correlates, Pathophysiological Discussion, and Functional Brain Imaging. Expanding the Cerebellar Cognitive Affective Syndrome. *Cerebellum 15*(40), 483-490. doi:10.100712311-015-0716-2

Brismar, J., Brismar, G., Coates, R., Gascon, G., & Ozand, P. (1990). Increased density of the thalamus on CT scans in patients with GM2 gangliosidoses. *AJNR. American Journal of Neuroradiology*, *11*(1), 125–130. PMID:2105593

Cao, H., Chén, O. Y., Chung, Y., Forsyth, J. K., McEwen, S. C., Gee, D. G., & Mirzakhanian, H. (2018). Cerebello-thalamo-cortical hyperconnectivity as a state-independent functional neural signature for psychosis prediction and characterization. *Nature Communications*, *9*(1), 3836. doi:10.103841467-018-06350-7 PMID:30242220

Deik, A., & Saunders-Pullman, R. (2014). Atypical presentation of late-onset Tay-Sachs disease. *Muscle & Nerve*, *49*(5), 768–771. doi:10.1002/mus.24146 PMID:24327357

Demily, C., & Sedel, F. (2014). Psychiatric manifestations of treatable hereditary metabolic disorders in adults. *Annals of General Psychiatry*, *13*(1), 27. doi:10.118612991-014-0027-x PMID:25478001

Dykens, E. M. (2013). Aging in rare intellectual disability syndromes. *Developmental Disabilities Research Reviews*, *18*(1), 75–83. doi:10.1002/ddrr.1130 PMID:23949831

Fernandes Filho, J. A., & Shapiro, B. E. (2004). Tay - Sachs disease. *Archives of Neurology*, *61*(9), 1466. doi:10.1001/archneur.61.9.1466 PMID:15364698

Ferreira, C. R., & Gah, W. A. (2017). Lysosomal storage diseases. Translational science of rare diseases. 2(1-2): 1-71. doi:. doi:10.3233/TRD-160005

Gilbert, W. (1978). Why genes in pieces? *Nature*, *271*(5645), 501. doi:10.1038/271501a0 PMID:622185

Heath, R., Franklin, D., & Strasberg, D. (1979). Gross pathology of the cerebellum in patients diagnosed and treated as functional psychiatric disorders. *The Journal of Nervous and Mental Disease*, *167*(1), 585–592. doi:10.1097/00005053-197910000-00001 PMID:573778

Hechtman, P., & Kaplan, F. (1993). Tay–Sachs Disease Screening and Diagnosis: Evolving Technologies. *DNA and Cell Biology*, *12*(8), 651–665. doi:10.1089/dna.1993.12.651 PMID:8397824

Jahnová, H., Poupětová, H., Jirečková, J., Vlášková, H., Košťálová, E., Mazanec, R., & Magner, M. (2019). Amyotrophy, cerebellar impairment and psychiatric disease are the main symptoms in a cohort of 14 Czech patients with the late-onset form of Tay-Sachs disease. *Journal of Neurology*, *266*(8), 1953–1959. doi:10.100700415-019-09364-3 PMID:31076878

Johnson, W. G. (1981). The clinical spectrum of hexosaminidase deficiency diseases. *Neurology*, *31*(11), 1453–1456. doi:10.1212/WNL.31.11.1453 PMID:7198192

Kaback, M., Lim-Steele, J., Dabholkar, D., Brown, D., Levy, N., & Zeiger, K. (1993). Tay-Sachs disease—carrier screening, prenatal diagnosis, and the molecular era: An international perspective, 1970 to 1993. *Journal of the American Medical Association, 270*(19), 2307–2315. doi:10.1001/jama.1993.03510190063028 PMID:8230592

Kliegman, R. M., Bordini, B. J., Basel, D., & Nocton, J. J. (2017). How Doctors Think. *Pediatric Clinics of North America, 64*(1), 1–15. doi:10.1016/j.pcl.2016.08.002 PMID:27894438

Lee, S. M., Lee, M. J., Lee, J. S., Kim, H. D., Lee, J. S., Kim, J., ... Lee, Y. M. (2008). Newly observed thalamic involvement and mutations of the HEXA gene in a Korean patient with juvenile GM2 gangliosidosis. *Metabolic Brain Disease, 23*(3), 235–242. doi:10.100711011-008-9090-9 PMID:18648917

Lemieux, M. J., Mark, B. L., Cherney, M. M., Withers, S. G., Mahuran, D. J., & James, M. N. G. (2006). Crystallographic Structure of Human β-Hexosaminidase A: Interpretation of Tay-Sachs Mutations and Loss of GM2 Ganglioside Hydrolysis. *Journal of Molecular Biology, 359*(4), 913–929. doi:10.1016/j.jmb.2006.04.004 PMID:16698036

Liao, P. C., Wei, C. J., & Chen, P. H. (2018). Onset of psychosis following strokes to the cerebellum and thalamus. *Psychosomatics, 59*(4), 413–414. doi:10.1016/j.psym.2017.09.001 PMID:29054750

MacQueen, G. M., Rosebush, P. I., & Mazurek, M. F. (1998). Neuropsychiatric Aspects of the Adult Variant of Tay - Sachs disease. *The Journal of Neuropsychiatry and Clinical Neurosciences, 10*(1), 10–19. doi:10.1176/jnp.10.1.10 PMID:9547461

Maddalena, A., Bale, S., Das, S., Grody, W., & Richards, S. (2005). Technical Standards and Guidelines: Molecular Genetic Testing for Ultra-Rare Disorders. *Genetics in Medicine, 7*(8), 571–583. doi:10.1097/01.GIM.0000182738.95726.ca PMID:16247296

Maegawa, G. H., Stockley, T., Tropak, M., Banwell, B., Blaser, S., Kok, F., & Clarke, J. T. (2006). The natural history of juvenile or subacute GM2 gangliosidosis: 21 new cases and literature review of 134 previously reported. *Pediatrics, 118*(5), e1550–e1562. doi:10.1542/peds.2006-0588 PMID:17015493

Maier, S., Bajko, Z., Moţăţăianu, A., Stoian, A., Şchiopu, B., & Bălaşa, R. (2017). Late Onset Tay - Sachs disease in a Non-Jewish Patient: Case Report. *Acta Medica Marisiensis, 63*(4), 199–203. doi:10.1515/amma-2017-0034

Moberget, T., Alnæs, D., Kaufmann, T., Doan, N. T., Córdova-Palomera, A., Norbom, L. B., ... Westlye, L. T. (2019). Cerebellar Gray Matter Volume Is Associated with Cognitive Function and Psychopathology in Adolescence. *Biological Psychiatry*, *86*(1), 65–75. doi:10.1016/j.biopsych.2019.01.019 PMID:30850129

Navon, R., Argov, Z., Frisch, A., Opitz, J. M., & Reynolds, J. F. (1986). Hexosaminidase A deficiency in adults. *American Journal of Medical Genetics*, *24*(1), 179–196. doi:10.1002/ajmg.1320240123 PMID:2939718

Navon, R., Khosravi, R., Melki, J., Drucker, L., Fontaine, B., Turpin, J. C., & Baumann, N. (1997). Juvenile-onset spinal muscular atrophy caused by compound heterozygosity for mutations in the HEXA gene. *Annals of Neurology*, *41*(5), 631–638. doi:10.1002/ana.410410512 PMID:9153525

Navon, R., & Proia, R. (1989). The mutations in Ashkenazi Jews with adult GM2 gangliosidosis, the adult form of Tay-Sachs disease. *Science*, *243*(4897), 1471–1474. doi:10.1126cience.2522679 PMID:2522679

Neudorfer, O., & Kolodny, E. H. (2004). Late-onset Tay-Sachs disease. *The Israel Medical Association Journal*, *6*(2), 107–111. PMID:14986470

Neudorfer, O., Pastores, G. M., Zeng, B. J., Gianutsos, J., Zaroff, C. M., & Kolodny, E. H. (2005). Late-onset Tay-Sachs disease: Phenotypic characterization and genotypic correlations in 21 affected patients. *Genetics in Medicine*, *7*(2), 119–123. doi:10.1097/01.GIM.0000154300.84107.75 PMID:15714079

O'Brien, J. S., Okada, S., Fillerup, D. L., Veath, M. L., Adornato, B., Brenner, P. H., & Leroy, J. G. (1971). Tay-Sachs disease: Prenatal diagnosis. *Science*, *172*(3978), 61–64. doi:10.1126cience.172.3978.61 PMID:5546285

Oates, C. E., Bosch, P., & Hart, M. N. (1986). Movement disorders associated with chronic GM2 gangliosidosis. *European Neurology*, *25*(2), 154–159. doi:10.1159/000116100 PMID:3081350

Osher, E., Fattal-Valevski, A., Sagie, L., Urshanski, N., Amir-Levi, Y., Katzburg, S., & Elstein, D. (2011). Pyrimethamine increases β-hexosaminidase A activity in patients with Late Onset Tay Sachs. *Molecular Genetics and Metabolism*, *102*(3), 356–363. doi:10.1016/j.ymgme.2010.11.163 PMID:21185210

Osher, E., Fattal-Valevski, A., Sagie, L., Urshanski, N., Sagiv, N., Peleg, L., & Stern, N. (2015). Effect of cyclic, low dose pyrimethamine treatment in patients with Late Onset Tay Sachs: An open label, extended pilot study. *Orphanet Journal of Rare Diseases*, *10*(1), 45. doi:10.118613023-015-0260-7 PMID:25896637

Prihodova, I., Kalincik, T., Poupetova, H., & Nevsimalova, S. (2013). Late-onset Tay–Sachs disease can mimic spinal muscular atrophy type III—two case reports. *Ceská a Slovenská Neurologie a Neurochirurgie*, *76/109*(2), 221–224. Retrieved from https://www.ncbi.nlm.nih.gov/pubmed/27491214

Ramoni, R. B., Mulvihill, J. J., Adams, D. R., Allard, P., Ashley, E. A., Bernstein, J. A., & McCray, A. T. (2017). The Undiagnosed Diseases Network: Accelerating Discovery about Health and Disease. *American Journal of Human Genetics*, *100*(2), 185–192. doi:10.1016/j.ajhg.2017.01.006 PMID:28157539

Rapin, I., Suzuki, K., Suzuki, K., & Valsamis, M. P. (1976). Adult (chronic) GM2 gangliosidosis: Atypical spinocerebellar degeneration in a Jewish sibship. *Archives of Neurology*, *33*(2), 120–130. doi:10.1001/archneur.1976.00500020048008 PMID:175770

Regier, D. S., Proia, R. L., D'Azzo, A., & Tifft, C. J. (2016). The GM1 and GM2 Gangliosidoses: Natural History and Progress toward Therapy. *Periaortic Endocrinology Reviews*, *13*(S1), 663–673. PMID:27491214

Rosebush, P. I., MacQueen, G. M., Clarke, J. T. R., Callahan, J. W., Strasberg, P. M., & Mazurek, M. F. (1995). Late-onset Tay-Sachs disease presenting as catatonic schizophrenia: Diagnostic and treatment issues. *The Journal of Clinical Psychiatry*, *56*(8), 347–353. PMID:7635850

Rucker, J. C., Shapiro, B. E., Han, Y. H., Kumar, A. N., Garbutt, S., Keller, E. L., & Leigh, R. J. (2004). Neuro-ophthalmology of late-onset Tay-Sachs disease (LOTS). *Neurology*, *63*(10), 1918–1926. doi:10.1212/01.WNL.0000144275.76658.F4 PMID:15557512

Sandhoff, K., Harzer, K., Wässle, W., & Jatzkewitz, H. (1971). Enzyme Alterations and Lipid Storage in Three Variants of Tay-Sachs Disease. *Journal of Neurochemistry*, *18*(12), 2469–2489. doi:10.1111/j.1471-4159.1971.tb00204.x PMID:5135907

Schneck, L., Friedland, J., Valenti, C., Adachi, M., Amsterdam, D., & Volk, B. W. (1970). Prenatal diagnosis of Tay-Sachs disease. *Lancet*, *295*(7647), 582–584. doi:10.1016/S0140-6736(70)91624-7 PMID:4190540

Shapiro, B. E., Hatters-Friedman, S., Fernandes-Filho, J. A., Anthony, K., & Natowicz, M. R. (2006). Late-onset Tay–Sachs disease: Adverse effects of medications and implications for treatment. *Neurology*, *67*(5), 875–877. doi:10.1212/01.wnl.0000233847.72349.b6 PMID:16966555

Shapiro, B. E., Logigian, E. L., Kolodny, E. H., & Pastores, G. M. (2008). Late-onset Tay–Sachs disease: The spectrum of peripheral neuropathy in 30 affected patients. *Muscle & Nerve*, *38*(2), 1012–1015. doi:10.1002/mus.21061 PMID:18642377

Shapiro, B. E., Pastores, G. M., Gianutsos, J., Luzy, C., & Kolodny, E. H. (2009). Miglustat in late-onset Tay-Sachs disease: A 12-month, randomized, controlled clinical study with 24 months of extended treatment. *Genetics in Medicine*, *11*(6), 425–433. doi:10.1097/GIM.0b013e3181a1b5c5 PMID:19346952

Streifler, J., Golomb, M., & Gadoth, N. (1989). Psychiatric Features of Adult GM2. *The British Journal of Psychiatry*, *155*(1), 410–413. doi:10.1192/bjp.155.3.410 PMID:2611559

Tran, K. D., Smutzer, G. S., Doty, R. L., & Arnold, S. E. (1998). Reduced Purkinje cell size in the cerebellar vermis of elderly patients with schizophrenia. *The American Journal of Psychiatry*, *155*(9), 1288–1290. doi:10.1176/ajp.155.9.1288 PMID:9734558

Yaffe, M. G., Kaback, M. M., Goldberg, M., Miles, J., Itabashi, H., McIntyre, H., & Mohandas, T. (1979). An amyotrophic lateral sclerosis-like syndrome with hexosaminidase - A deficiency: A new type of GM2 ganglisidosis [Abstract]. *Neurology*, *29*(1), 611.

Yokoyama, T., Nakamura, S., Horiuchi, E., Ishiyama, M., Kawashima, R., Nakamura, K., & Yagishita, S. (2014). Late onset GM2 gangliosidosis presenting with motor neuron disease: An autopsy case. *Neuropathology*, *34*(3), 304–308. doi:10.1111/neup.12088 PMID:24354582

Zaroff, C. M., Neudorfer, O., Morrison, C., Pastores, G. M., Rubin, H., & Kolodny, E. H. (2004). Neuropsychological assessment of patients with late onset GM2 gangliosidosis. *Neurology*, *62*(12), 2283–2286. doi:10.1212/01.WNL.0000130498.19019.02 PMID:15210895

Zelnik, N., Khazanov, V., Sheinkman, A., Karpati, A. M., & Peleg, L. (2000). Clinical Manifestations of Psychiatric Patients Who Are Carriers of Tay - Sachs disease. *Neuropsychobiology*, *41*(3), 127–131. doi:10.1159/000026644 PMID:10754426

KEY TERMS AND DEFINITIONS

Adult Onset Tay-Sachs Disease: A very rare, with a progressive complex and variable clinical course due to aging and the presence of heterogeneous mutations which are responsible for different degrees of enzyme deficiency.

Ganglioside: The name ganglioside was first used in 1942 to lipids newly isolated from ganglion cells of the brain. A ganglioside is a molecule composed of a glycosphingolipid (ceramide and oligosaccharide) with one or more sialic acids (e.g. n-acetylneuraminic acid, NANA) linked on the sugar chain. GM2 is a type of ganglioside. G refers to ganglioside, the M is for monosialic (it has one sialic acid), and 2 refers to the fact that it was the second monosialic ganglioside discovered. It is associated with GM2 gangliosidoses.

GM2 Gangliosidosis: A very rare neuronopathy, in which intraliposomal storage of GM2 ganglioside is caused by a total or relative deficiency of the lysosomal enzyme β- hexosaminidase A (Hex-A). This enzyme catalyzes the biodegradation of the gangliosides. The GM2 gangliosidoses consist of three related genetic disorders: Tay–Sachs disease, AB variant, and Sandhoff disease.

Hexosaminidase A (HEX-A): Alpha-polypeptide enzyme encoded in Human gene HEXA, chromosome 15. Hexosaminidase A deficiency caused by mutations in the HEXA gene, is an inherited disease that causes brain and other nerve cells to die.

Chapter 10
Portraying Rare and Misdiagnosed Diseases in Movies:
A Content Analysis, 1980–2018

Liliana Vale Costa
https://orcid.org/0000-0003-2451-3073
University of Aveiro, Portugal & DigiMedia, Portugal

Ana Isabel Veloso
https://orcid.org/0000-0002-5070-0756
University of Aveiro, Portugal & DigiMedia, Portugal

ABSTRACT

This chapter examines the portrayal of rare and misdiagnosed diseases in 9 movies from 1980 to 2018. The analysis embodies the representation of rare diseases and the suggested audiovisual strategies to comprehend the message conveyed. Most of the movies introduced the disease by highlighting its symptoms. The binomial culture of cure and care often emerges, as well as the patient's desire for the mundane pleasures in life and over dependence in a health system. The high hopes in research advances and lack of information are majorly covered in the caregivers' attempts to seek tests and drug trials and their mediator's role in patient-physician interactions. The audiovisual strategies adopted vary between the accelerated montage to communicate the contrast between the frenetic side of everyday life and the patient's process of coping with the disease, deep focus from patients to parents, and close-ups to show the individual's reactions and perspectives.

DOI: 10.4018/978-1-7998-2088-8.ch010

INTRODUCTION

In an increasingly visual-oriented society, scholars (*e.g.* Grushka, 2009; McDonagh, Goggin,& Squier, 2005; Miguel, 2016; Müller, 2008; Sweeny, 2004) have been more and more interested in the way that visuals can facilitate individuals' "meaning-making" (Fei, 2007; Harrison, 2003) through the use of such elements as semiotics, perceptual theory, psychosocial factors and aesthetics that are often used to transmit pieces of data, information and emotion in multiple media (Hortin,1994). Indeed, visual composition, syntax and elements are so omnipresent in the representation of an individual's actions, objects and symbols that they may consciously or unconsciously have a strong impact on empathic relationships, actions, self-perception, decision-making and behavior change (Gumpert & Cathcart, 1985; Hortin,1994; Messaris, 1998).

In the medical context, visual language is also used to transmit information about, for example, the portrayal of common symptoms and the representation of a certain disease (i.e. representation in medical literature, arts of Italian Renaissance, epidemic cartoons and TV series) (Gilman, 1998). But also in cartographies of epidemics (Koch, 2011), wayfinding, labelling and signage design in health care environments (Delvin, 2014; Hashim, Alkaabi, & Bharwani, 2014; Pati, Harvey Jr., Willis, & Pati, 2015) and in media campaigns (Randolph & Viswanath, 2004; Wakefield, Loken, & Homik, 2010). In these different media, health-related communication may also rely on allegories (e.g. Niemiec, 2010), parallels (Eysenbach, 2008; Koplan, 2003), non-verbal – *e.g.* gestures (Asan, Young, Chewning, & Montague, 2015; Bickmore et al., 2010), and metaphors (Krieger, Parrott, & Nussbaum, 2010). As Evers (1969, p.34, cf Hortin,1994, p.16) puts it:

Movies, photographs, commercials and even printed statements are representations of reality. They are metaphors, and therefore must be understood as metaphorical points of view. That is what mediacy is about (Evers, 1969, p.34 cf Hortin, 1994, p.16)

The use of movies in the medical context and its impact on stigma and attitudes towards certain illnesses or health education have been widely covered (e.g. Banos, 2007; Damjanović, Vuković, Jovanović, & Jašović-Gašić, 2009; Pirkis, Blood, Francis, & McCallum, 2006). However, its use to foster discussion, create awareness towards orphan drugs and demystify the challenges of rare disease research have been quite overlooked.

The aim of this chapter is to examine the portrayal of rare and misdiagnosed diseases in movies from 1980 to 2018. In specific, the messages that are transmitted relative to the disease, ethical dilemmas, interaction among different health stakeholders, and the audiovisual strategies used to convey such messages (camera movements, color, lighting, montage, among others).

This chapter is structured as follow: The next section discusses the use of movies to convey health-related information, providing a brief overview of cinematography in the story-making process. The International Rare Disease Festival is presented as an example of an initiative that is paving the way into the use of movies as a *medium* to meet this purpose. It proceeds with the process of movie selection, the content categories used and data collection. The results section examines the way rare diseases are portrayed in movies and the audiovisual strategies used. The chapter concludes by summarizing the main audiovisual strategies used in movies and its purpose to convey a certain meaning to the information provided and portrayal of rare diseases.

HEALTH-RELATED INFORMATION IN MOVIES

A considerable amount of literature has been published about the use of movies to medical education – *e.g.,* González-Blasco, Delgado-Marroquín, Moreto and Altisent (2019), Membrives, Isem, and Matheu (2016) and Ali (2014). Indeed, movies can play a prominent role in fostering information literacy in the context of health considering the fact that they communicate a story visually and may elicit emotions with a strong impact on decision-making and behavior change. However, it is worth noting that cinema *verité* continues to challenge health representation in such medium, being it often influenced by collective myths, fantasies and stigma.

Some of the common health-related themes covered in movies are:

- **Psychiatry education and therapist-patient relationships:** psychiatry disorders that are covered in movies are varied – e.g. delirium, dementia, schizophrenia, addiction, mood and personality disorders (Byrne, 2009; Cape, 2009; Dave & Tandon, 2011; Tobia, et al., 2016; Wilson, Heath, Heath, Gallagher, & Huthwaite, 2014). There is a general perspective of distrust in people diagnosed with a mental illness and a dualism between facts and fiction and the demonization of psychosis (Byrne, 2009; Datta, 2009; Gabbard, 2001; Hyler & Moore, 1996; Menon, & Ranjith, 2009; Tobia et al., 2016), in which doctor-patient relationships are explored (Virzi, et al., 2011);

- **Dermatology portrayal:** a study conducted by Vail Reese (1995) relative to the portrayal of skin and cutaneous diseases has revealed that skin abnormalities are used as a representation of evil and villains in filmmaking (e.g. skin diseases, facial acne, albinism, rosacea…). The misrepresentations of skin conditions and diseases in cinema often influence stigmatization, attitude and demand for plastic surgery;
- **Teaching Psychopathology:** one of the common topics covered in the movies has been the risks of depression, suicide, posttraumatic stress, personality disorders (Hyler & Moore, 1996), human consciousness and death representation (Knox, 2006; Jung, 2012);
- **Cine-film medical teaching:** cinefilms and documentaries have been often used in order to show cinematography surgeries (Krementsov, 2015) and medical operations (Essex-Lopresti, 1998; Van Dijck, 2002);
- ***Cinema verité* and health dilemmas:** beyond ethical concerns, the tension and confronts between health professionals, patients, caregivers and society in health-related decision making have been often explored (Little, Kahn, & Green, 1999). The ethical dimension and confidentiality are often a topic that emerges in movies that cover health-related information (González-Blasco, Delgado-Marroquín, Moreto, & Altisent, 2019);
- **Cinematic depictions of Physicians/Psychiatrists and Stereotypic representation of diseases:** physicians and, especially, psychiatrists are often represented characters, whom are feared, heroic or evil (Cashman, 2019; Gabbard & Gabbard, 1999; Kalra, 2012; Scott, 2014), and these myths and fantasies may have an impact on patients daily basis and interactions with their physician/psychiatrist (Gabbard, 2001; Kelly, 2006). There are also a number of stereotypic representation of diseases in the movies, for example, multiple sclerosis (Karenberg, 2008) and oncological diseases (De Fiore, et al., 2014);
- **Fostering observational learning and empathy:** movies may act as imagery symbols and metaphors, inciting emotions, empathy with the characters (understand the character's motivation and behavior) (Akram, O'Brien, O'Neill, & Latham, 2009) and observational learning (Schulenberg, 2003).

In the subsections that follow, the process of story-making through cinematography will be introduced and current work undertaken in the portrayal of rare diseases in movies will be presented.

Story-Making Through Cinematography

The process of telling stories and providing meaning to actions through moving images has evolved throughout time. In fact, cinema has adopted a visual language to communicate ideas, actions, emotions and tones, in which the process of telling through moving pictures is the subject of interest to the cinematography field.

The linear Aristotelian narrative structure (i.e. from the exposition/inciting moment, climax and resolution) has evolved to integrate both an illusion of continuity and a spatial, temporal and linear discontinuity (Sesonke, 1980), delving into a much more dialectical approach. Specifically, the Gestalt Law of Perceptual Closure is essential to understand this illusion of continuity in the presentation of different pieces of information that are perceived as a whole (Coren & Girgus, 1980).

As Eisenstein (1938/42, p.32 cf Barry, 1994, p.129) puts it:

[…] the spectator is compelled to proceed along that self-same road that the author travelled in creating the image … the spectator not only sees the represented elements of the finished work, but also experiences the dynamic process of the emergence and assembly of the image just as it was experienced by the author […] (Eisenstein, 1938/42, p.32 cf Barry, 1994, p.129)

For that, *montage* had been a key tool to story-making, reinforcing the visual tension between past and present, space and rhythm. The following are some of the montage techniques:

- **Parallel montage:** parallel montage occurs when two geographically distance actions are perceived as simultaneous;
- **Accelerated montage:** accelerated montage refers to the process of shortening the video length or duration and increase the speed, in order to transmit the idea of excitement and rhythm;
- **Montage of attraction:** montage of attraction is relative to the use of objects, expressions and ideas organized in a certain sequence in order to produce specific stimuli, elicit certain emotion and change the viewer's perception (Begin, 2006; Kuiper, 1961). In this type of montage, the Kuleshov Effect is often used, in which the viewers' perception towards a certain sequence of shots is changed, in comparison with a single shot (Prince & Hensley, 1992).

If, on the one hand, cinema can present viewers with illusory effects and play with some psychology theories (e.g. *Kuleshov Effect, Object petit a*), on the other hand, this medium also represents everyday life by establishing interrelationships among one's reality, society, and symbols in a plain *simulacra*, as posited by Baudrillard

(1994). Movies can also unravel some 'truths' by documenting life-as-it-is. This principle of unraveling the 'truth', through a *Kino-Eye*, is defended by Dziva Vertov (1984, p.66). In his book *Kino-eye: the writings of Dziga Vertov*, he writes:

The establishment of a visual (kino-eye) and auditory (radio-ear) class bond between the proletariats of all nations and lands on a platform of the communist decoding of world relations. The decoding of life as it is. [...] Instead of surrogates for life (theoretical presentations, film-drama, etc.) carefully selected, recorded, and organized facts (major or minor) from the lives of the workers themselves as well as from those of their class enemies. (Vertov, 1984, p.66)

Having present these diverse perspectives towards movie pictures and given that one of the main goals of this chapter is to identify the audiovisual strategies used to convey certain messages, a brief overview of some strategies beyond montage and its possible meaning are provided below:

- **Different shots for different situations and inherent meaning:** A movie scene can embody different shots: (a) Wide and distant shots may be used to show the environment or transmit isolation with the reinforcement of the color scheme (cool or warm); (b) Establishing shots open the scene and inform the viewer about the location (possibly creating some ambiguity between telepresence and self-awareness); and (c) Close-ups to show character's reactions;
- **Point-of view shots (POVs) to communicate the character's interactions with others and conflicts:** POVs aim to involve the viewers in the story by seeing and experiencing what the character is seeing and representing, in an empathic interaction. Some of the cinematic elements that are often used are: (a) over-the-shoulder (OTS) by filming over the shoulder of an actor; and (b) glancing into a rear-view mirror in order to unravel key elements that can impact on the whole story;
- **Interplay of Visual Principles:** A set of visual principles also apply to the cinematographic language – *e.g.* unity (the organization of elements in such a way that is perceived as only one single unit), balanced vs unbalanced composition in *mis-en-scène* (placing on the frame), rhythm and directionality (by creating patterns through the use of repetition and indicate the direction where the viewer should look at through camera movements, eyes pointing the direction and visual weight), Proportion (through deep focus, proximity and distortion of angle lenses), Contrast (allude to emotional and spatial relationships through the use of light and shadow), Emphasis (e.g. Hitchcock's

basic rule - the importance of an object in the story should match its size in the frame); and Hierarchy (e.g. depth of field and camera angles);

- **Communicating through Space Compression and Expansion, Camera Movements and Positive/Negative Spaces:** Space compression can communicate the tightness of a place and a claustrophobic environment, whereas its expansion distorts it. Camera movements direct the viewer's gaze direction to what is happening (e.g. panning, tilt, move in/out, zoom in/out, punch-in and moving shots) and positive-negative space often suggests if it is in or out of balance depending on a distant or closer viewpoint or an active/observational role from the viewer.

Other strategies related with sound, lightening, directing and editing may follow but for this chapter they are not covered, as the essential has been introduced in order to provide the general context of this study. The following section presents the Rare Disease Film Festival as an example of an initiative that intertwines movie-making and rare diseases.

The Rare Disease Film Festival

The Rare Disease Film Festival is an event that gathers filmmakers, patients, caregivers, researchers, patient advocates, health professionals, researchers and general community to discuss and share their experiences and stories about rare diseases.

Such initiative shows the movies, short movies, documentaries and short animations that fosters conversations and collaborations between stakeholders with different experiences and knowledge basis, paving the way into research and science support. All the information is compiled in the website https://www.rarediseasefilmfestival.com (Figure 1).

Among the diseases covered in these films are: Batten, Sanfilippo, Epidermolysis bullosa, GAN, Angelman's Syndrome, PACs1 Syndrome, Goldenhar Syndrome, Congenital Disorders of Glycosylation, GM1 Gangliosidosis, Vader syndrome, Charcot-Marie-Tooth Syndrome, Sickle Cell Anemia, Spina Bifida, Autism, Lafora Disease, SMA, PGAD, Pfeiffer Syndrome, Cystic fibrosis, Wilson Disease, Duchenne and Becker muscular dystrophy, MS Multiple Sclerosis, Bosch-Boonstra-Schaaf Optic Atrophy Syndrome (BBSOAS), Friedreich's ataxia, Hemophilia, Fraser Syndrome, Synesthesia, Myotubular Myopathy, Tay-Sachs, GM1, leukodystrophy, Huntington's Disease, Von Hippel-Lindau Syndrome (VHL), Cerebral palsy, USP7, Degenerative Neurological Disorder, NGLY1, Menkes Syndrome (Menkes Disease), Fragile X, Niemann Pick type c, Mitochondrial Disease and Hunter Syndrome MPS.

Figure 1. Rare Disease Film Festival, https://www.rarediseasefilmfestival.com (Access Date: August 23, 2019)

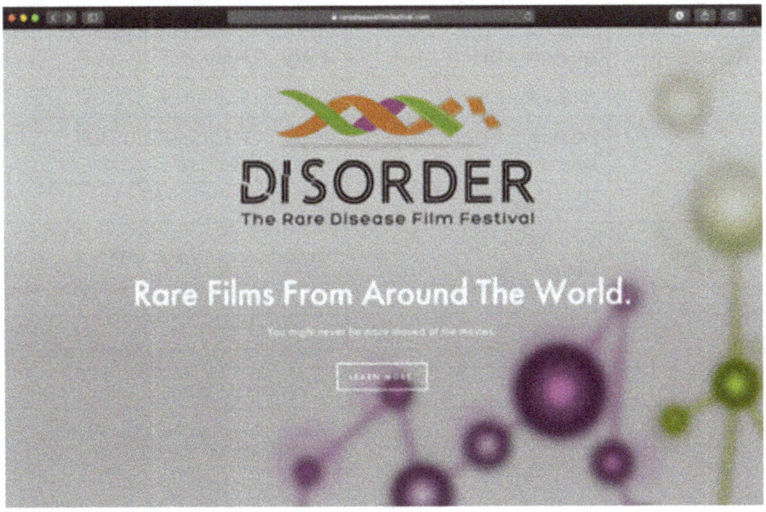

From this website, the movies 'Cuerdas (2014)', 'Imagine (2015)', and 'Ian (2018)' were selected considering that they were available on the website and did not follow the format of a health or advocacy group campaign, which was not the focus of this chapter, and a thorough analysis from the advertising and marketing lenses would be needed.

METHOD

This chapter examines the portrayal of rare and misdiagnosed diseases in movies from 1980 to 2018. A content analysis was performed in order to get insights into the messages that are transmitted, and the audiovisual strategies used to convey such messages. Therefore, the imdb and rare disease festival database were searched in order to find movie titles addressing "rare diseases", excluding foundation campaigns.

Out of 29 movies, twenty were excluded owing to lack of access or its focus, leaving 9. Table 1 gives an account of the selected movies. The inclusion criteria were: (a) Being published in imdb and rare disease festival database from 1980 to 2018; and (b) reference to the term "rare disease" in the title or movie description. The exclusion criteria were: (a) Lack of access; and (b) Focus on foundation campaigns.

Table 1. Movies depicting rare or misdiagnosed diseases selected for content analysis

Year	Movie	Genre	Rare or Misdiagnosed Disease Portrayed
1980	The Elephant Man[1]	Biography/Drama	Proteus Syndrome[2]
1992	Lorenzo Oil[3]	Biography/Drama	Adrenoleukodystrophy (ALD) [4]
2013	Life According to Sam[5]	Documentary, Biography/ Drama	Progeria or Hutchinson-Gilford Progeria Syndrome[6]
2014	Cuerdas[7]	Animation	N/A (Palsy)
2015	Imagine[8]	Short Movie Biography/ Drama	Niemann-Pick Type C (NPC) [9]
2015	In Crystal Skin[10]	Documentary	Epidermolysis bullosa (EB)[11]
2016	Brain on Fire[12]	Biography/Drama	Anti-NMDA receptor encephalitis[13]
2018	Ian[14]	Animation	N/A (Cerebral Palsy)
2018	Midnight Sun[15]	Drama/Romance	Xeroderma pigmentosum (XP) [16]

The video scripts were re-read and analyzed, aiming at identifying the interactions, values and attitudes of different role characters towards rare and misdiagnosed diseases. Data was qualitatively analyzed.

It is worth noting that although the animations are not specific in terms of the disease covered, they were the only movies in the category 'Animation' that were highlighted in the website of the Rare Disease Film Festival and covered the socio-cultural aspect of the pediatric patients' limitations and disease coping.

Content Categories

The content analysis embodied the following categories:

- **Portrayed Rare Disease:** This category refers to the way rare diseases and associated health stakeholders are represented in the movies, namely, the disease description and symptoms, ethical dilemmas, physician-caregiver-patient communication, patients' self-image and integration in society, the role of the caregiver, use of information search tools, and the advancements/ challenges found in research;
- **Audiovisual strategies used:** This category embodies camera movements, color and lighting, sound, montage techniques, composition, camera shots and angles.

Both verbal and nonverbal messages were taken into account and after viewing each movie and re-reading video script, each passage that supported each category was highlighted with a side note. In the end, all notes and statements from each movie were compared in order to find repetitive patterns.

A total of 458 minutes from the 9 movies were analyzed from June 15, 2019 to August 10, 2019.

Data Analysis

Following the pre-determined categories (i.e. Portrayed Rare Diseases and Audiovisual Strategies), the *corpus* of analysis (text and video clips) were coded and compared.

RESULTS

Based on the content analysis performed in this study, Table 2 shows an overview of the portrayed rare diseases and audiovisual strategies used in movies from 1980 to 2018.

As shown in Table 2, most of the movies introduced the disease by highlighting its symptoms. For example:

It is believed that the main character (Joseph Merrick) had Proteus Syndrome[2] that is characterized by skeletal and blood vessel malformations, tumors, tissue overgrowth and pulmonary disease – i.e. "[...] the alarming curvature of the spine [...] the looseness of the skin and the varying fibers/tumors that cover 90% of the body[...] The patient also suffers from chronic bronchitis [...]" – In The Elephant Man (1980)

The main character is diagnosed with Adrenoleukodystrophy (ALD) that is X-linked recessive genetic occurring only in males whose mother is a defective gene carrier. It is often characterized by adrenal insufficiency, abnormalities in blood pressure, attention deficit and progressive loss of vision, cognitive, motor and intellectual capacities. – In 'Lorenzo Oil' (1992)

The main character is diagnosed with Xeroderma pigmentosum (XP) that is characterized by the sensitivity to DNA to ultraviolet radiation, leading to its damage and affect the skin, eyelids, eyes' surface, tip of the tongue and may possibly lead to neurodegeneration and hearing loss – i.e. "[...]XP, which means a severe sensitivity to sunlight. If sunlight so much as glances off my skin. I'll get skin cancer, and my body can't repair the damage so my brain starts to fail – which could mean hearing loss, difficulty in hearing loss, difficulty in walking and swallowing, movement

Table 2. Overview of the Portrayed Rare Diseases and Audiovisual strategies used in movies

Movie	Portrayed Rare Disease	Audiovisual strategies used
The Elephant Man (1980) [1]	• It is believed that the main character (Joseph Merrick) had Proteus Syndrome[2] that is characterized by skeletal and blood vessel malformations, tumors, tissue overgrowth and pulmonary disease – i.e. "[…] the alarming curvature of the spine […] the looseness of the skin and the varying fibers-tumors that cover 90% of the body[…] The patient also suffers from chronic bronchitis […]" • Culture of cure vs Culture of care – i.e. "If loving kindness can be called care and practical concern, then I did show loving kindness […]", "We can care for you, but we can't cure you." • Physician-patient communication (diagnosis process): 1.Reference to a caregiver as a mediator ("your owner tells me – I mean, the man who looks after you"), 2. Use of non-verbal communication (e.g. nodding); 3. Assessment of a congenital and hereditary disease ("Have you always been the way you are now?, […] Are your parents still alive?") and pain ("Are you in any pain?") • Patient's desire for a normal life – i.e. "I wish… I could sleep…like normal people." • Integration in society and self-image – i.e. "He is a freak!", "[…] under no circumstances…whatsoever…are any mirrors to be brought […].", "He's so ugly.", "I am not an animal. I am a human being!" • Vulnerability from others who take advantage from the patient and condition – i.e. "But all you do us profit from another man's misery", "On the move again… my treasure", "People pay to see your monster."	• Merrick's body is presented as *"object petit a"* (Lacan, 1901) in the first part of the movie, by being absent from the visual field, inaccessible – *i.e.* film-cuts as a character (Treves) walk, forbidden symbols "No entry" and initial failed encounters with Merrick, who remains hidden (180° movement camera when the main character is exposed, in-front camera when he is hidden), curtains and spotlights • Close-ups of characters' reactions – *e.g.* begin to cry when there is a close-up, emotional character engagement (Kember, 2004). • Morale fable by emerging bioethical and socio-ethical – protection vs exploitation, moral worth, Merrick's death • Contrast between light/white (effect) and black/shadow/darkness (tension) • Sound repetition – *i.e. breath, heartbeat, clock ticking, footsteps, mechanical sounds* (Fernandes, 2015)
Movie	**Portrayed Rare Disease**	**Audiovisual strategies used**
Lorenzo Oil (1992) [3]	•The main character is diagnosed with Adrenoleukodystrophy (ALD) [4] that is X-linked recessive genetic occurring only in males whose mother is a defective gene carrier. It is often characterized by adrenal insufficiency, abnormalities in blood pressure, attention deficit and progressive loss of vision, cognitive, motor and intellectual capacities. In the movie, teachers notice that something is strange in Lorenzo's behavior, confusion with the Attention Deficit Hyperactivity Disorder (ADHD) and suggest a special aid class, which parents refuse. There is some uncertainty revealed during the diagnosis process, "It's quite rare. The leukodystrophies […] ALD is an inborn error of metabolism that causes a degeneration of the brain. It only affects males, usually between the ages of five and ten. Its progress is relentless. The end is inevitable.", "Well, to be honest, we're not quite certain just how it works." •Physician-caregiver communication: 1. Confront with the lack of information, time and health stakeholders' pace to treat the disease – "[…] the doctors are in the dark."; "[…] they will tell us in their own time.", "So what you're saying is that our children are in the service of medical science. How foolish of me. I always assumed...that medical science was in the service of the sufferers.", "There's no mathematical certainty. And because we deal with human beings who suffer, it can appear heartless." •The need of different knowledge bases to understand the disease – i.e. "[…] we need a command of genetics, biochemistry… microbiology, neurology […]"; "All these experts, working in isolation, each one on his own piece of the jigsaw" •Lack of investment in rare diseases, "Ours is what is known as an orphan disease. It's too small to be noticed, too small to be funded…" • The caregiver's role and emotional burnout – i.e. "She doesn't want nobody. She's too angry."; "Our parents suffer enough without being made the victims of false hopes."	• Morale fable by emerging ethical concerns regarding life-prolonging in child; • Dramatic opera music – anticipate the patient diagnosis and is life-threatening; •Montage by attraction – *e.g.* between dad's face and the studies relative to ALD; • 'Ghosting' between research books (such words as mute, coma, death) and Lorenzo's dad. Recency effect - Repetition of the word 'death'; •After searching for the disease in the library for the first time – there is a scene of the father in the stairs, using the bird's Eye View (aka Top Shot) as he was lost in an information labyrinth; • Vignette of a number of male ALD patients who used Lorenzo's Oil; • Side Dolly camera movement between the hospital corridor and the Lorenzo's mother on the phone, showing the contrast between one's passivity and proactivity; • Close-ups in the boy's mother in order to show their emotions – e.g. intense sense of sadness, guilty, tiredness, despair; • Choosing the Lorenzo's anniversary as a landmark to the change in his condition (indicate "time passing by").
Movie	**Portrayed Rare Disease**	**Audiovisual strategies used**

continued on following page

Table 2. Continued

Movie	Portrayed Rare Disease	Audiovisual strategies used
Life According to Sam (2013) [5]	• The main character Sam is diagnosed with Progeria or Hutchinson-Gilford Progeria Syndrome[6] that is characterized by premature ageing – "What is aging in Sam, is aging in all of us. But in his body, the process is accelerated. There is no cure for progeria.", "Progeria is known as a pre-ageing syndrome. It doesn't age all the senses because a 13 year- old has a 13-year old mind and doesn't have cataracts and does not have cancer or other problems. But from the cardiovascular point of view, these kids all develop cardiovascular disease." • Hope in research advancements and lack of funding, "The physician was sorry, but there was no research" • Lack of information about the disease, "When Sam was diagnosed with Progeria in 1998, there was nothing out there. There was no research going on, treatment, cure, or foundation to go to." • Patient's desire for a normal life, e.g. "I wish I could ride any roller coaster […]", "I kind of just want my mom to be done with progeria for her sake […]" • Dependence on a health system – medication and clinical trials, "The gold standard of a clinical trial is testing the drug on hundred, if not to say, thousands of people and half of the people get the drug and half doesn't […]"	• Close-ups and extreme close-ups to show an intimate interaction with the character; • Use a "shallow" depth of field - limit the audience can see beyond the focus (i.e., fingers, hands, eyes) and create a very "tactile" world, within the character's 'bubble'; • Follow the characters very close to reinforce this intimacy.
Short Movie Imagine (2015) [8]	• The main character is diagnosed with Niemann-Pick Type C (NPC) [9] that is characterized by the body's inability to transport cholesterol and fatty substances, resulting in the its accumulation in body and brain tissues. The disease symptoms and information are referred: "[…] type of neurodegenerative disease which means Millie will start to decline both mentally and physically eventually."; "I am finding so hard to learn. To concentrate […] I keep coughing when I am eating [...] I keep forgetting things […] I have physiotherapy now […] and I have to have speech therapy now."; "How are the seizures? She's having 5 maybe 6 a day."; "Damage done is irreversible." •Physician-caregiver communication: 1. Disbelief in the physician - "[…] It can't be true. He's wrong, isn't he?", 2. Ask for validation/ a 'second' opinion and (re-)test, 3. Confrontation ("And how are you coping with them?" "How do you think?), • The caregiver's role and emotional burnout – i.e. "Tablets help me sleep", "She cries a lot.", "I work part time now." • Use of Search Engine Optimization (SEO) tools to obtain further information about the disease and trials – i.e. "Leave it. You will only upset yourself again. Trials in America in America, something called cyclodextrin, we could go there."	• The narrator of the story is the patient – repeats the opening statement at different stages of the disease ("My name is Miller. I'm 10 years old") and creates awareness to the short life period of these patients by ending with the statement ("I'm 10 years old. I will always be 10 years old."); * Deep focus from the patient with the nurse to the parents and physician; *Confront between the parents and the physician: Over-the shoulder the physician to focus on the parents' reactions and close-up of the physician; Close-ups following the direction of the characters' looking at – from mother to father, from one to the other, to physician, to the patient who remains distant with the nursing care.
Movie	**Portrayed Rare Disease**	**Audiovisual strategies used**
Short Movie Imagine (2015) [8]	• Integration in society and self-image – i.e. "I am not sure what is wrong with me, but I know I am not like the others."	* Use of repetition and accelerated montage to show the frenetic rhythm of school and daily life activities; * Use of close-ups to show different perspectives, and parent's emotions and feelings from the parents; **Mise-en-scene* (e.g. photographs, ballerina box) * Light and temperature – bluish and grey

continued on following page

Table 2. Continued

Movie	Portrayed Rare Disease	Audiovisual strategies used
In Crystal Skin (2015) [10]	• The main character has Epidermolysis bullosa (EB) [11] that is characterized by mechanical trauma and blister formation. This also may embody scars, musculoskeletal deformities and affect respiratory, gastrointestinal and genitourinary tracts (NORD). Although the disease is not mentioned, in the film, it shows the daily-life of a girl with EB with the wounds being treated by her mother and feeling of tiredness – "In the mornings when I wake up sometimes I don't like to go to school…because the cold makes me very tired. My mom gets mad because she doesn't want me to stay in bed."; "I have my days when I'm delicate and other days when I'm doing much better." * The important role of the caregiver and emotional burnout – e.g. "When Maria Alejandra was born, I had to become another part of her. I'm always with her, helping her."; "My relationship with my Mom. She's my best friend. She's my gift. She's the one I love the most."; "When she has many wounds and doesn't want to go to school, I want to run away."	* Medium and long shots in order to show the whole environment, surroundings and all conditions; *Parallel montage (e.g. empty swings whereas the little girl is at home); *Low angle shot (upshot) to transmit the message of the importance of school to this family and the teacher as an authority. Natural setting as the place for shooting.
Brain on Fire (2016) [12]	• The main character is diagnosed with the autoimmune disorder with rare diagnosis Anti-NMDA receptor encephalitis that is characterized by the lack of NMDA receptors that control the brain's electrical impulses, having an impact on reality perception, patients' memory, sleep, speech, vision, hearing, movement and leading to seizures. In patient's words: "I feel really sick. You know, my head hurts, my stomach hurts, and my hand's numb […]", "Have you ever been trapped? Lost in your own body?", "I guess, you could say that I've had these flu-like symptoms. I've had a lot of numbness on my left arm and leg. I feel my head really fuzzy all the time." • Misdiagnosed disease – *e.g.* "How many people, do you think throughout history were diagnosed as schizophrenic, psychotic, bipolar, or maybe just being crazy, when they had something that could've been so easily diagnosed?", "Any history of Lyme disease?"	• Camera – from inside to outside vs outside to inside separated by a window – 'care watch'. Close-up following a gestalt approach; • Choosing Susannah's anniversary as a landmark to the change in his condition (indicate "time passing by") • The patient begins to tell her story (Patient story) but with the evolvement of the disease her voice is replaced by dialogues and dialogues between her parents and doctors.
Brain on Fire (2016) [12]	• Use of Search Engine Optimization (SEO) tools to obtain further information about the disease – *e.g.* "I googled it." •Physician-caregiver communication: 1. Disbelief in the physician "This ain't some kids club, where you get to play doctor! This is my daughter's life!"; 2. Excess of medicines: "I'm gonna give you a prescription for Olanzapine. It's an anti-psychotic prescribed to treat mood and thought disorders. Take these pills and check back in with me."; "she takes the anti-seizure meds I'd prescribed, and everything should be fine.", "I'm gonna prescribe a Haloperidol. It should sedate her and also we could do some further testing." • Integration in society and self-image – i.e. "It just feels weird.", "She looks hungover.", "I don't think she's acting normal, but I don't think she's on drugs.", "I'm looking in her eyes, she's looking at me. And I can tell that she's not there."	• Ghost effect – spinning in chair to indicate change and confusion. Predominance of white and blue – clinical ambience. Following shots many camera shootings from one side of the window to the other as the spectator had also the role to surveil the patient and her strange behavior, 'keeping an eye on her'. • In some scenes, the character appears in front of the camera and then there is a smooth zoom-out, suggesting that she must be left behind by the spectator, with her own thoughts.
Midnight Sun (2018)	• The main character is diagnosed with Xeroderma Pigmentosum (XP) that is characterized by the sensitivity to DNA to ultraviolet radiation, leading to its damage and affect the skin, eyelids, eyes' surface, tip of the tongue and may possibly lead to neurodegeneration and hearing loss – i.e. "[...]XP, which means a severe sensitivity to sunlight. If sunlight so much as glances off my skin. I'll get skin cancer, and my body can't repair the damage so my brain starts to fail – which could mean hearing loss, difficulty in hearing loss, difficulty in walking and swallowing, movement problems, loss of intellectual functions and capacity for speech, seizures and, oh yeah, death.", "XP generally lies dormant until a triggering event." • Physician-caregiver communication (check status information): 1. Assess changes in a patient's condition – "Have you noticed any changes in her motor function?", 2. The need of the patients to be present in physician-caregiver communication "[…] but she should be coming to these appointments with you." That evolves; 3. Reported symptoms – *i.e.* "If you notice any symptoms, Katie – unexpected shaking, muscle pain, loss of motor function – you have to promise to tell me immediately."; • Use of Search Engine Optimization (SEO) tools to obtain further information about the disease. The important role of the caregiver in assisting the patient is recognized – e.g. "I did everything I was supposed to […]." • Integration in society and self-image – i.e. "When you tell someone you're sick, then you start to become more likely a disease and less like a person." Hope in research advancements and lack of funding – i.e. "People aren't exactly flocking to fund for a disease that affects only one in a million […] drug trial ran out of money […]."	• Outdoor and indoor scenes are arranged in a comparative way – what is happening in the neighborhood and indoor. The window is the symbolic object that establishes the connection between inside and outside. Then, the perspective changes from indoor to outdoor at night. • Traditional emotional arc (A young girl has XP and can't be out in the sunlight; despite being advised by her caregiver, she fails with it one day and her life is at risk. She realizes that she wants to adhere to a memorable experience outside with friends (go sailing), even if that means accelerating the process of dying; • Accelerated montage in which increasing speed is given when Kate goes out and having fun; • Morale socio-ethical – Kate's death
Animation "Cuerdas"[7](2014) and "Ian" (2018)	• Although there is not a specific disease represented in these animation (palsy + cerebral palsy), both animations cover integration in society and self-image.	• Set scene: School Playground; • The interrelationships between the environment and groups/social interactions are represented through wide and medium shots; *The effect of the environment and groups on the individual are reinforced with camera close-ups.

problems, loss of intellectual functions and capacity for speech, seizures and, oh yeah, death.", "XP generally lies dormant until a triggering event."- In Midnight Sun (2018)

The binomial culture of cure and care is often emerged, as well as the patient's desire for the mundane pleasures in life and overly dependence in a health system. The following passages are illustrative of these observations:

Culture of cure vs Culture of care – i.e. "If loving kindness can be called care and practical concern, then I did show loving kindness [...]", "We can care for you, but we can't cure you." – In 'The Elephant Man' (1980)

Patient's desire for a normal life, e.g. "I wish I could ride any roller coaster [...]", "I kind of just want my mom to be done with progeria for her sake [...]" – In 'Life According to Sam' (2013)

Furthermore, the high hopes in research advances and lack of information are majorly covered in the caregivers' attempts to seek for tests and drug trials and their mediator's role in patients-physician's interactions.

Hope in research advancements and lack of funding – i.e. "People aren't exactly flocking to fund for a disease that affects only one in a million [...] drug trial ran out of money [...]" – In Midnight Sun (2018)

Dependence on a health system – medication and clinical trials, "The gold standard of a clinical trial is testing the drug on hundred, if not to say, thousands of people and half of the people get the drug and half doesn't [...]"-In Life According to Sam (2013)

Use of Search Engine Optimization (SEO) tools to obtain further information about the disease and trials – i.e. "Leave it. You will only upset yourself again. Trials in America in America, something called cyclodextrin, we could go there." – In the Short Movie 'Imagine' (2015)

The audiovisual strategies adopted also vary between the accelerated montage to communicate the contrast between the frenetic side of everyday life and the patient's process of coping with the disease, deep focus from patients to parents, and close-ups to show the individual's reactions and perspectives. The following are some of the examples:

Use of repetition and accelerated montage to show the frenetic rhythm of school and daily life activities. Deep focus from the patient with the nurse to the parents and physician. – In the Short Movie 'Imagine' (2015)

Accelerated montage in which increasing speed is given when Kate goes out and having fun. – In 'Midnight Sun' (2018)

Close-ups in the boy's mother in order to show their emotions – e.g. intense sense of sadness, guilty, tiredness, despair. In 'Lorenzo Oil' (1992)

In summary, the portrayal of rare diseases in movies generally follow the structure: (a) Present the disease by showing its common symptoms; (b) Cover the antagonism between a culture of cure and a culture of care; (c) Explore the high hopes in research advances and the lack of information by showing the caregivers' attempts to seek for tests and drug trials and mediator's role in patients-physician's interactions. Relative to the audiovisual strategies adopted, they vary between accelerated montage to communicate the contrast between the frenetic side of everyday life and the patient's process of coping with the disease, deep focus from patients to parents, and close-ups to show the individual's reactions and perspectives.

CONCLUSION

This chapter set out to examine the portrayal of rare and misdiagnosed diseases in 9 movies from 1980 to 2018, by analyzing the representation of rare diseases and the suggested audiovisual strategies to comprehend the message conveyed.

Most of the movies that were reviewed introduced the disease by highlighting its symptoms. The binomial culture of cure and care has often emerged, as well as the patient's desire for the mundane pleasures in life and overly dependence in a health system. In addition, the high hopes in research advances and lack of information were majorly covered in the caregivers' attempts to seek for tests and drug trials and their mediator's role in patients-physician's interactions.

Regarding the audiovisual strategies adopted in most movies, they vary between the accelerated montage to communicate the contrast between the frenetic side of everyday life and the patient's process of coping with the disease, deep focus from patients to parents, and close-ups to show the individual's reactions and perspectives.

In sum, the chapter suggests several courses of action for understanding the audiovisual strategies that are often used to communicate a story visually and foster individual's "meaning-making" within the health sector. Important limitations of this study, however, should be noted.

Firstly, the sampling of the movies was limited to those that were found in the imdb and rare disease festival databases and which the authors had access to. Surveying rare diseases of only 9 movies may have, therefore, biased the prevalence of the strategies and language used. Considering the age gap of the movies analyzed, future considerations would be also interesting in to dividing the topics portrayed in the movies by decade and rare conditions portrayed.

Secondly, the rare diseases which were analyzed seem to be focused into the ones of morphological or physical disabilities. Authors should consider cinematographic content that approaches also metabolic and mental disorders.

Future studies need to be extended to the search of other databases and compare the strategies used to communicate the message in different video formats – *e.g. documentaries, short movies, movies, animations, campaigns* and compare the strategies used with the end-user's attention, using eye-tracking. The authors of this Chapter are carrying out work in this area by analyzing audiovisual strategies and health-related communication within an online community context.

ACKNOWLEDGMENT

This work was supported by Fundação para a Ciência e Tecnologia and ESF under Community Support Framework III – the project SEDUCE 2.0 nr. POCI-01-0145-FEDER-031696.

REFERENCES

Akram, A., O'Brien, A., O'Neill, A., & Latham, R. (2009). Crossing the line–learning psychiatry at the movies. *International Review of Psychiatry (Abingdon, England)*, *21*(3), 267–268. doi:10.1080/09540260902746880 PMID:19459104

Ali, K. (2014). From lecture halls to cinema screens: Learning about the psyche through films. *Medical Humanities*, *40*(1), 69–69. doi:10.1136/medhum-2013-010479 PMID:24298043

Asan, O., Young, H. N., Chewning, B., & Montague, E. (2015). How physician electronic health record screen sharing affects patient and doctor non-verbal communication in primary care. *Patient Education and Counseling*, *98*(3), 310–316. doi:10.1016/j.pec.2014.11.024 PMID:25534022

Banos, J. E. (2007). How literature and popular movies can help in medical education: Applications for teaching the doctor-patient relationship. *Medical Education*, *41*(9), 918. doi:10.1111/j.1365-2923.2007.02829.x PMID:17727535

Barry, A. (1994). Perceptual Aesthetics and Visual Language. In D. Moore, & F. M. Dwyer (Eds.), *Visual Literacy: A Spectrum of Visual Learning, Englewood Cliffs*. New Jersey: Educational Technology Publications.

Baudrillard, J. (1994). *Simulacra and Simulation*. United States of America: The University of Michigan.

Begin, P. (2006). Buñuel, Eisenstein, and the 'Montage of Attractions': An Approach to Film in Theory and Practice. *Bulletin of Spanish Studies*, *83*(8), 1113–1132. doi:10.1080/14753820601073613

Bickmore, T. W., Pfeifer, L. M., Byron, D., Forsythe, S., Henault, L. E., Jack, B. W., ... Paasche-Orlow, M. K. (2010). Usability of conversational agents by patients with inadequate health literacy: Evidence from two clinical trials. *Journal of Health Communication*, *15*(sup2S2), 197–210. doi:10.1080/10810730.2010.499991 PMID:20845204

Biesecker, L. G. (2001). The multifaceted challenges of Proteus syndrome. *Journal of the American Medical Association*, *285*(17), 2240–2243. doi:10.1001/jama.285.17.2240 PMID:11325326

Byrne, P. (2009). Why psychiatrists should watch films (or What has cinema ever done for psychiatry?). *Advances in Psychiatric Treatment*, *15*(4), 286–296. doi:10.1192/apt.bp.107.005306

Cape, G. (2009). Movies as a vehicle to teach addiction medicine. *International Review of Psychiatry (Abingdon, England)*, *21*(3), 213–217. doi:10.1080/09540260902747094 PMID:19459096

Cashman, C. R. (2019). Golden Ages and Silver Screens: The Construction of the Physician Hero in 1930-1940 American Cinema. *The Journal of Medical Humanities*, 1–16. doi:10.100710912-019-09554-0 PMID:30838501

Cohen, J. M. (1988). Understanding Proteus syndrome, unmasking the elephant man, and stemming elephant fever. *Neurofibromatosis*, *1*(5-6), 260–280. PMID:3152479

Coren, S., & Girgus, J. S. (1980). Principles of perceptual organization and spatial distortion: The gestalt illusions. *Journal of Experimental Psychology. Human Perception and Performance*, *6*(3), 404–412. doi:10.1037/0096-1523.6.3.404 PMID:6447756

Damjanović, A., Vuković, O., Jovanović, A. A., & Jašović-Gašić, M. (2009). Psychiatry and movies. *Psychiatria Danubina*, *21*(2), 230–235. PMID:19556954

Datta, V. (2009). Madness and the movies: An undergraduate module for medical students. *International Review of Psychiatry (Abingdon, England)*, *21*(3), 261–266. doi:10.1080/09540260902748001 PMID:19459103

Dave, S., & Tandon, K. (2011). Cinemeducation in psychiatry. *Advances in Psychiatric Treatment*, *17*(4), 301–308. doi:10.1192/apt.bp.107.004945

De Fiore, L., Costantini, A., Di, M. M., Gori, S., Lorusso, D., Rosti, G., & Pinto, C. (2014). Cancer on the big screen. How and when movies deal with oncological diseases. *Recenti Progressi in Medicina*, *105*(5), 198–209. doi:10.1701/1493.16455 PMID:24873943

Devlin, A. (2014). Wayfinding in healthcare facilities: Contributions from environmental psychology. *Behavioral Science*, *4*(4), 423–436. doi:10.3390/bs4040423 PMID:25431446

Essex-Lopresti, M. (1998). The medical film 1897-1997: Part I. The first half-century. *The Journal of Audiovisual Media in Medicine*, *21*(1), 7–12. doi:10.3109/17453059609063115 PMID:9764516

Eysenbach, G. (2008). *Credibility of health information and digital media: New perspectives and implications for youth.* Digital media, youth, and credibility, 123-154.

Fei, V. L. (2007). The visual semantics stratum: making meaning in sequential images. In T. D. Royce, & W. L. Bowcher (Eds.), *New directions in the analysis of multimodal discourse* (pp. 195–213). Mahwah, NJ: Lawrence Erlbaum.

Fernandes, I. (2011*). The Elephant Man (1980) by David Lynch: from 'freak' and clinical case to allegory. Cine Qua Non - Bilingual Arts Magazine, #9*. Lisboa, Portugal: CEAUL. 2015. 54-75. Retrieved from http://hdl.handle.net/10451/29473 (Access date: August 13, 2019)

Gabbard, G. (2001). Psychotherapy in Hollywood cinema. *Australasian Psychiatry*, *9*(4), 365–369. doi:10.1046/j.1440-1665.2001.00365.x

Gabbard, G., & Gabbard, K. (1999). *Psychiatry and the Cinema* (2nd ed.). Washington, DC: American Psychiatric Press.

Gilman, S. L. (1988). *Disease and representation: Images of illness from madness to AIDS*. Ithaca, NY: Cornell University Press.

González-Blasco, P., Delgado-Marroquín, M. T., Moreto, G., & Altisent, R. (2019). Vocación y profesionalismo: Reflexiones de los estudiantes catalizadas por el cine de Spielberg. *Educación Médica*, *20*(4), 249–255. doi:10.1016/j.edumed.2018.10.001

Grushka, K. (2009). Meaning and identities: A visual performative pedagogy for socio-cultural learning. *Curriculum Journal*, *20*(3), 237–251. doi:10.1080/09585170903195860

Gumpert, G., & Cathcart, R. (1985). Media grammars, generations, and media gaps. *Critical Studies in Media Communication*, *2*(1), 23–35. doi:10.1080/15295038509360059

Harrison, C. (2003). Visual social semiotics: Understanding how still images make meaning. *Technical Communication (Washington)*, *50*(1), 46–60.

Hashim, M. J., Alkaabi, M. S. K. M., & Bharwani, S. (2014). Interpretation of way-finding healthcare symbols by a multicultural population: Navigation signage design for global health. *Applied Ergonomics*, *45*(3), 503–509. doi:10.1016/j.apergo.2013.07.002 PMID:23932379

Hortin, J. (1994). Theoretical Foundations of Visual Learning. In D. Moore, & F. M. Dwyer (Eds.), *Visual Literacy: A Spectrum of Visual Learning*. Englewood Cliffs, NJ: Educational Technology Publications.

Hyler, S. E., & Moore, J. (1996). Teaching Psychiatry? Let Hollywood Help! *Academic Psychiatry*, *20*(4), 212–219. doi:10.1007/BF03341883 PMID:24442743

Jung, H. C. (2012). Death education for medical personnel utilizing cinema. *The Korean Journal of Gastroenterology*, *60*(3), 140–148. doi:10.4166/kjg.2012.60.3.140 PMID:23018534

Kalra, G. (2012). Talking about stigma towards mental health professionals with psychiatry trainees: A movie club approach. *Asian Journal of Psychiatry*, *5*(3), 266–268. doi:10.1016/j.ajp.2012.06.005 PMID:22981056

Karenberg, A. (2008). Multiple sclerosis on-screen: From disaster to coping. *Multiple Sclerosis Journal*, *14*(4), 530–540. doi:10.1177/1352458507084587 PMID:18208879

Kelly, B. D. (2006). Psychiatry in contemporary Irish cinema: A qualitative study. *Irish Journal of Psychological Medicine*, *23*(2), 74–79. doi:10.1017/S0790966700009617 PMID:30290482

Kember, J. (2004). David Lynch and the Mug Shot: Facework. In E. Sheen, & A. Davison (Eds.), *The Elephant Man and The Straight Story. The Cinema of David Lynch: American Dreams, Nightmare Visions* (pp. 19–34). London, UK: Wallflower Press.

Knox, S. L. (2006). Death, afterlife, and the eschatology of consciousness: Themes in contemporary cinema. *Mortality, 11*(3), 233–252. doi:10.1080/13576270600775007

Koch, T. (2011). *Disease maps: epidemics on the ground.* Chicago, IL: University of Chicago Press. doi:10.7208/chicago/9780226449401.001.0001

Koplan, J. P. (2003). Communication during public health emergencies. *Journal of Health Communication, 8*(sup1S1), 144–145. doi:10.1080/713851967 PMID:14692583

Krementsov, N. (2015). Conjoined twins: Scientific cinema and Pavlovian physiology. *Endeavour, 39*(3-4), 168–178. doi:10.1016/j.endeavour.2015.10.001 PMID:26601729

Krieger, J. L., Parrott, R. L., & Nussbaum, J. F. (2010). Metaphor use and health literacy: A pilot study of strategies to explain randomization in cancer clinical trials. *Journal of Health Communication, 16*(1), 3–16. doi:10.1080/10810730.2010.529494 PMID:21128152

Kuiper, J. B. (1961). The Stage Antecedents of the Film Theory of SM Eisenstein. *Educational Theatre Journal, 259-263*. doi:10.2307/3204346

Legendre, C. M., Charpentier-Côté, C., Drouin, R., & Bouffard, C. (2011). Neurofibromatosis type 1 and the “elephant man’s” disease: the confusion persists: an ethnographic study. *PLoS One, 6*(2). doi:10.1371/journal.pone.0016409 PMID:21347399

Little, G. A., Kahn, R., & Green, R. M. (1999). Parental Dreams, Dilemmas, and Decision-Making in Cinéma Vérité. *Journal of Perinatology, 19*(3), 194–196. doi:10.1038j.jp.7200163 PMID:10685221

McDonagh, D., Goggin, N., & Squier, J. (2005). Signs, symbols, and subjectivity: An alternative view of the visual. *Computers and Composition, 22*(1), 79–86. doi:10.1016/j.compcom.2004.12.009

Membrives, M. D., Isern, M. T. I., & Matheu, M. C. L. (2016). Literature review: Use of commercial films as a teaching resource for health sciences students. *Nurse Education Today, 36*, 264–267. doi:10.1016/j.nedt.2015.10.002 PMID:26490325

Menon, K. V., & Ranjith, G. (2009). Malayalam cinema and mental health. *International Review of Psychiatry (Abingdon, England)*, *21*(3), 218–223. doi:10.1080/09540260902748043 PMID:19459097

Messaris, P. (1998). Visual aspects of media literacy. *Journal of Communication*, *48*(1), 70–80. doi:10.1111/j.1460-2466.1998.tb02738.x

Miguel, C. (2016). Visual intimacy on social media: From selfies to the co-construction of intimacies through shared pictures. *Social Media+ Society*, *2*(2), doi:10.1177/2056305116641705

Müller, M. G. (2008). Visual Competence: A new paradigm for studying visuals in the social sciences? *Visual Studies*, *23*(2), 101–112. doi:10.1080/14725860802276248

Niemiec, R. M. (2010). International Cinema: An Abundant Mental Health Resource of Films for Education, Communication, and Transformation. In *The Cinematic Mirror for Psychology and Life Coaching* (pp. 123–153). New York, NY: Springer. doi:10.1007/978-1-4419-1114-8_7

Pati, D., Harvey, T. E. Jr, Willis, D. A., & Pati, S. (2015). Identifying elements of the health care environment that contribute to wayfinding. *HERD: Health Environments Research & Design Journal*, *8*(3), 44–67. doi:10.1177/1937586714568864 PMID:25929471

Pirkis, J., Blood, R. W., Francis, C., & McCallum, K. (2006). On-screen portrayals of mental illness: Extent, nature, and impacts. *Journal of Health Communication*, *11*(5), 523–541. doi:10.1080/10810730600755889 PMID:16846952

Prince, S., & Hensley, W. E. (1992). The Kuleshov effect: Recreating the classic experiment. *Cinema Journal*, *31*(2), 59–75. doi:10.2307/1225144

Reese, V. (1995). Dermatology in the cinema. *Journal of the American Academy of Dermatology*, *33*(6), 1030–1035. doi:10.1016/0190-9622(95)90297-X PMID:7490348

Schulenberg, S. E. (2003). Psychotherapy and movies: On using films in clinical practice. *Journal of Contemporary Psychotherapy*, *33*(1), 35–48. doi:10.1023/A:1021403726961

Scott, N. (2014). The Monstrous Metallic in Medicine and Horror Cinema. *Medicina Nei Secoli*, *26*(1), 312–332. PMID:25702391

Sesonske, A. (1980). Time and tense in Cinema. *The Journal of Aesthetics and Art Criticism*, *38*(4), 419–426. doi:10.2307/430323

Sweeny, R. W. (2004). Lines of sight in the "network society": Simulation, art education, and a digital visual culture. *Studies in Art Education*, *46*(1), 74–87. doi:10.1080/00393541.2004.11650070

Tobia, A., Mintz, J., Rudge, D., Bisen, V., Trenton, A., Draschil, T., & Dobkin, R. (2016). Deconstructing the film sinister through the lens of psychiatry. *African Journal of Psychiatry (South Africa)*, *19*(2). doi:10.4172/2378-5756.1000354

Van Dijck, J. (2002). Medical documentary: Conjoined twins as a mediated spectacle. *Media Culture & Society*, *24*(4), 537–556. doi:10.1177/016344370202400405

Vertov, D. (1984). *Kino-Eye: The Writings of Dziga Vertov*. London, UK: University of California.

Virzi, A., Dipasquale, S., Signorelli, M., Aguglia, E., Bianchini, O., & Palermo, F. (2011). Movie portrayals of physicians and the doctor-patient relationship. *Journal of Cognitive and Behavioral Psychotherapies*, *6*(2), 475–485.

Wakefield, M. A., Loken, B., & Hornik, R. C. (2010). Use of mass media campaigns to change health behaviour. *Lancet*, *376*(9748), 1261–1271. doi:10.1016/S0140-6736(10)60809-4 PMID:20933263

Wilson, N., Heath, D., Heath, T., Gallagher, P., & Huthwaite, M. (2014). Madness at the movies: Prioritised movies for self-directed learning by medical students. *Australasian Psychiatry*, *22*(5), 450–453. doi:10.1177/1039856214545550 PMID:25135436

KEY TERMS AND DEFINITIONS

Accelerated Montage: Process of shortening the video length or duration and increase the speed, in order to transmit the idea of excitement and rhythm.

Close-Ups: Camera shot that frames a person or object very tightly.

Deep Focus: Creating the illusion of depth through the use of a short-focal length lens.

Kuleshov Effect: The viewer's perception towards a certain sequence of shots is changed, in comparison with a single shot.

Montage: Editing technique in which different shots are organized in a sequence to shorten space, time and/or other information.

ENDNOTES

1 The Elephant Man, https://www.imdb.com/title/tt0080678/ (Access date: August 13, 2019)

2 There has been a confusion between Neurofibromatosis type I and Proteus Syndrome as "The Elephant Man" (Biesecker, 2011; Cohen, 1988; Legendre, Charpentier-Côté, & Bouffard, 2011)

3 Lorenzo Oil, https://www.imdb.com/title/tt0104756/ (Access date: August 13, 2019)

4 Adrenoleukodystrophy (ALD) is X-linked recessive genetic disease occurring only in males whose mother is a defective gene carrier. It is often characterized by adrenal insufficiency, abnormalities in blood pressure, attention deficit and progressive loss of vision, cognitive, motor and intellectual capacities.

5 Life According to Sam, https://www.imdb.com/title/tt2558550/ (Access date: August 13, 2019)

6 Progeria Syndrome is characterized by a premature ageing and results from a tiny change in the DNA that causes an abnormal protein – *progerine* to be created.

7 Cuerdas, https://www.imdb.com/title/tt3381028/ (Access date: August 13, 2019)

8 Imagine, https://www.rarediseasefilmfestival.com/work#/imagine/ (Access date: August 13, 2019)

9 Niemann-Pick Type C (NPC) is characterized by the body's inability to transport cholesterol and fatty substances, resulting in the its accumulation in body and brain tissues.

10 In Crystal Skin, https://www.imdb.com/title/tt4947274/ (Access date: August 13, 2019)

11 Epidermolysis bullosa (EB) is characterized by mechanical trauma and blister formation. This also may embody scars, musculoskeletal deformities and affect respiratory, gastrointestinal and genitourinary tracts.

12 Brain on Fire, https://www.imdb.com/title/tt3704700/ (Access date: August 13, 2019)

13 Anti-NMDA receptor encephalitis is characterized by the lack of NMDA receptors that control the brain's electrical impulses, having an impact on reality perception, patients' memory, sleep, speech, vision, hearing, movement and leading to seizures.

14 Ian, https://www.rarediseasefilmfestival.com/new-gallery-2 (Access date: August 13, 2019)

15 Midnight Sun, https://www.imdb.com/title/tt4799066/ (Access date: August 13, 2019)

16 Xeroderma pigmentosum (XP) is characterized by the sensitivity to DNA to ultraviolet radiation, leading to its damage and affect the skin, eyelids, eyes' surface, tip of the tongue and may possibly lead to neurodegeneration and hearing loss.

Chapter 11
How Is the Administrator's Experience in Managing Health Facebook Groups?
The Impact of Social Media in Patients With IBD

Claudia Pernencar
https://orcid.org/0000-0001-8981-2133
Nova Institute of Communication, Portugal

Inga Saboia
https://orcid.org/0000-0002-3635-2927
UFC Virtual, Brazil

ABSTRACT

This decade, patients with chronic conditions take advantage of technological resources to share experiences, look for help, and get together in groups. Social media has become a productive spot of health information for users. This chapter clarifies the administrators' user experience of social media health groups within the context of the Inflammatory Bowel Disease (IBD). Semi-structured interviews with 7 Portuguese and Brazilian managers of Facebook groups were carried out. The authors propose a model of participation in online communities that take into account the variables of Presence–Interconnection between users in daily lives; Relationship–Aspects of experience where users meet; Reputation–Positioning of users related to the status; Groups–Relationship issues between members; Conversations – Extension of the user interaction; Sharing–Represents the exchange, distribution, and reception and Education–The information transmitted. Findings reinforced that administrators' groups use social media to lead patients´ empowerment.

DOI: 10.4018/978-1-7998-2088-8.ch011

INTRODUCTION

Social media, as a phenomenon of the current decade, assemble a group of digital tools under a single term. The use of these media is permeated by the ideology of contribution, in which users take advantage of technological resources not only for sharing, but also to create content (Kaplan, 2013). As a consequence of the factors pointed out, citizens with different goals are using different media while interacting with a multitude of content and people, forming groups, communicating and increasing their network. In some cases, coming together for a common purpose. In fact, it is interesting to recognize that the health topic is actively used with digital media since the beginning of the current decade.

Relative to this fact, a study (Fox & Duggan, 2013) revealed that 72% of Internet users looked for information on the experience of others with the same type of health problems, and 8% posted this type of content. In the same period, Hartley argued (2012) that communication about health in the digital context was a critical issue because citizens were simultaneously positioned as both patients and 'active' participants in healthcare (Erikainen, Pickersgill, Cunningham-Burley, & Chan, 2019).

The profile of participants mentioned before is what some authors (Guo, Reich, Groshek, & Farraye, 2016) announced as 'e-patients.' The term was coined to describe those who are looking for health information in the online environment. They also warned, in their study, that adults were using social media networks to improve their knowledge in this particular field. This means that not only patients were connecting with disease communities but, they were accessing to these and being co-producers of knowledge and information with a linguistic level that can be perceived by most of the patients. Regarding the conception of these communities, they are driven by support and a follow-up of other patients during treatments (Frohlich, 2016; Guo et al., 2016; Reich et al., 2019).

Studies have shown that participation in this type of groups had improved patients' quality of life through sharing experiences with others, and families, promoting the socialization and clinical orientation which means, they, likewise, are also exchanging information about new medical treatments(Szeto et al., 2018). These communities have substantially grown, and about this phenomenon, a different paradigm has emerged, i.e. patients whose quality of life depends on several healthcare services are exploring the advantages of social media to have feedback in real-time. They are also using these tools to help them managing their disease condition (Patel, Chang, Greysen, & Chopra, 2015; Taft & Keefer, 2016).

Social media as tools for disease management in chronic illnesses such as asthma, diabetes and cardiac diseases have been observed before (e.g. Ferguson et al., 2014; Hawn, 2009; Nickels & Dimov, 2012). Regarding patients with Inflammatory Bowel Disease (IBD), they are often using these tools to discuss their disease with peers, obtain educational disease-related information, and communicate with their physicians and patient-related organizations (Frohlich, 2016; Guo et al., 2016; Patel et al., 2015; Reich et al., 2019; Szeto et al., 2018; Taft & Keefer, 2016).The Facebook platform, as a social media tool, has empowered patients with chronic conditions expanding new ways of achieving knowledge, leading discussions, or promoting causes.

Beyond some intangible benefits of this involvement, there are significant tangible profits to the increased use of digital communication by IBD patients. These include low-cost access to crucial information about the disease, new ways of interacting with the community – build relationships, additional opportunities and sources to understand who the healthcare providers of specific customer services are (Carroll & Ramachandran, 2014).

After an introduction elucidating about the context of this chapter, in the following sections a clinical summary about IBD and the evolution of IBD health information in the digital world will be introduced. Secondly, a framework to analyze related Facebook Health Groups information and the theory that will contribute to implementing it will be discussed. Thirdly, the methods used to analyze the object of this study, i.e. the interviews to administrators of IBD Facebook groups coming from two countries, Portugal and Brazil, will be presented. Fourthly, the discussion of the interviews is analyzed, followed, finally, by the concluding remarks. With these, the authors aim to comprehend, mainly, the administrators' user experience in IBD Facebook groups.

Additionally, it is worth noting that other chronic conditions and patients' involvement with communication, technology and design macro fields, in countries like Portugal and Brazil have been previously discussed (Pernencar, 2013; Pernencar, Romão, & Simões, 2016; Pernencar et al., 2018; Saboia, Pisco Almeida, Sousa, & Pernencar, 2018).

IBD COMMUNITIES AND GROUPS

Inflammatory Bowel Disease (IBD) include two related disorders that involve chronic immune-mediated inflammation of the digestive tract of unknown cause, Crohn's Disease (CD) and Ulcerative Colitis (UC) (Lennard-Jones, 1989). Both these conditions are with no known cause or cure (Clinic, n.d.). These inflammatory diseases of the digestive tract are characterized by abdominal pain, severe diarrhea, and fatigue and weight loss. The treatment options include oral or injectable medications and/or surgical interventions (Auyeung, 2014).

Despite both Crohn's disease and ulcerative colitis occur from ongoing inflammation of the gastrointestinal tract (GI), there are important differences between the two diseases. In Crohn's disease any part of the GI tract can be affected, from the mouth to the anus while it mostly affects the end of the small intestine (the ileum). Most notably, the inflammation in Crohn's disease may extend through the entire thickness of the bowel wall and it can affect some areas of the GI tract leaving other areas untouched (in a 'patched' pattern). Ulcerative colitis, however, is limited to the large intestine (colon) and the rectum. Distinguishably, it affects only the innermost layer of the lining of the intestine. It generally begins in the rectum and lower colon, but it can also spread to the rest of the colon. Thus, rectal bleeding is a symptom of this condition. There are cases of IBD that, however, are difficult to determine if Crohn's disease or ulcerative colitis and in these rare cases, clinicians usually attribute the diagnosis of indeterminate colitis (IC).[1]

In spite of the exact known cause remaining unsolved, nowadays researchers think that it involves the interaction between genes, the immune system, microbiota (microorganisms in the gut) and unidentified environmental factors. The environmental factors 'trigger' harmful immune responses in the intestines attacking the body's own intestinal tract cells, which results in inflammation, particularly in people that have inherited genes that make them susceptible to IBD (Loddo & Romano, 2015).

The incidence and prevalence rates of IBD are increasing. For example, in Europe, the highest reported incidence values are located in Norway, with Ulcerative Colitis – 505 cases per 100,000 individuals –, and in Germany, with Crohn's Disease – 322 cases per 100,000 individuals. In the U.S.A. 700,000 Americans are affected with IBD (Rachel, Millie, Suzanne, Christina, Wenli, Christopher, Kristen, Robert, & Michael, 2014).The North America numerical amount is lower than in Europe: Ulcerative Colitis – 286 cases per 100,000 individuals in the USA; and Crohn's Disease – 319 cases per 100,000 individuals in Canada (Ng et al., 2017).

Taft & Keefer, from the Division of Gastroenterology and Hepatology, Northwestern University Feinberg School of Medicine, Chicago argued (2016) from a clinical perspective, that IBD patterns are hard to characterize because this illness presents significant ramifications such as physical, psychological, social, and others. Patients are often stigmatized, and some outsiders view the disease as "gross" or do not understand how it can affect a person's life.

Searching online for IBD related information is not a new paradigm. Cawdron and Issenman (2002), 17 years ago, surveyed by e-mail 162 tertiary-care clinic patients, aged between 8 and 18 years old, in order to identify if this target population was interested in web-based IBD resources:

- 91,2% of the participants revealed curiosity in searching generic illness content available in specific websites;
- 80% in reading online experiences coming from other patients;
- 81% in seeing others' questions;
- and 51% in chatting with peers about the disease.

Five years later, Cima and colleagues (2007) surveyed 169 adult IBD patients, with a median age of 46 years old, to comprehend the importance of the Internet in producing general health and disease-specific information to this target population. The authors discovered that the topic related to the online search was increasingly being recognized as something crucial for IBD patients because, it was improving their compliance with therapy and satisfaction with their healthcare. An interesting analysis from 2010 (Promislow, Walker, Taheri, & Bernstein, 2010) showed, after screening 30 websites with IBD related information, that medical information, treatment and self-management were fields which patients deemed to be essential for them to increase personal disease knowledge.

Switching from search on the web for IBD health information, to explore this content using social media tools was a natural action for patients (Azer, AlOlayan, AlGhamdi, & AlSanea, 2017; Frohlich, 2016; Guo et al., 2016; Plevinsky & Greenley, 2014; Reich et al., 2019; Szeto et al., 2018). This scenario may show for the research community that social media tools are providing a plus to IBD patients such as, increasing the interaction with other patients in real-time, and sharing the experiences and fears in the groups.

Digging deeper into the context of social media as digital tools, Plevinsky & Greenley (2014) studied their impact as a social functioning (i.e., social support and social connectedness) in IBD youth population (21 participants with ages 14 to 17 years old) in a specific scenario, an IBD post-camp. The authors collected pilot data on a Facebook group created by the participants. Both the camp experience and the Facebook group contributed to improvements in youth social functioning. The authors also showed that supplementing the camp experience with membership to a health group from Facebook enhanced the social functioning in adolescents with IBD. Two years later, a relevant study from Frohlich (2016) involved an ethnographic study, in which 14 online communities were followed. The author recognized that the sense of being actively involved with a disease community through a Facebook group was meaningful and tried to understand how many people were using social media technologies to create their meaning about living with the IBD through discussing specific ways of how people with IBD were using new media technologies to redefine the disease. The results of the study showed that these groups are not always in agreement about how the disease should be redefined: Multiple redefinitions of it exist in the same spaces. The quote of community members to use their public written responses were also a topic of discussion.

Later, Azer and coworkers (2017) evaluated the quality and the accuracy of web-based educational content about IBD. With a total number of 84 websites visited, the authors argued, for upcoming works, that the Internet-based patient education should follow an innovative plan to create online educational material for the public and patients with IBD. The content accuracy and readability level should match with the recommended needs of the target audience, i.e., patients, families and other lay people interested in the topic. However, the authors did not present concrete guidelines of what and how to make these changes. One year later, (Szeto et al., 2018), reported, from a sample of 218 survey participants (aged between 12 to 25 years old) that all patients accessed the Internet daily, but only 17% reported looking up information about IBD "always" or "often." Less than half (47%) turned to medical websites (WebMD or Crohn's and Colitis Foundation) for information, and only a small number (16%) connected with other IBD patients. Patients' preferred method of communication with the provider was by e-mail (88%) compared with a phone call to the office (67%) or hospital website/patient portals (52%). Few patients used mobile applications (apps) to monitor symptoms (2%) or for medication reminders (9%), although there was professed interest.

Recently, Reich and colleagues (2019) published a cross-sectional study within the Crohn's and Colitis Foundation's IBD Partners' Internet-based cohort to determine the factors of using social media to obtain IBD-related information. A total of 1960 IBD patients were included. Most of them reported spending between 30 and 60 minutes on social media *per* day. A proportion of 32% of these patients agreed that these tools could be useful for disease management. Most of them also agreed that it should be used to connect patients with IBD-related organizations, and to obtain IBD-related information online. Half of the respondents could not rate the quality of IBD information posted online.

The two last studies, coming from Crohns's Colitis Foundation[2] and published by the Oxford University Press, reinstates the relevance of understanding how a specific social media tool, the Facebook Social Networking Service, may influence patients with IBD through the existing disease groups as a process of online engagement. This encompasses: (a) IBD information gathering in social media; (b) how and whom are the providers of communication; (c) if it exists sense of belonging in the existing IBD Facebook groups; (d) how is the self-expression around IBD, and (e) what is the influence of these communities in individual disease management.

Therefore, a framework to analyze related Facebook Health Groups information was created to be applied, as an empirical research method, to analyze the interviews coming about the administrators of IBD Facebook groups. The following section will explain, from the theoretical perspective, all the themes involved in this framework.

Figure 1. Schematics of the Facebook Health Group Framework. Source: author's original

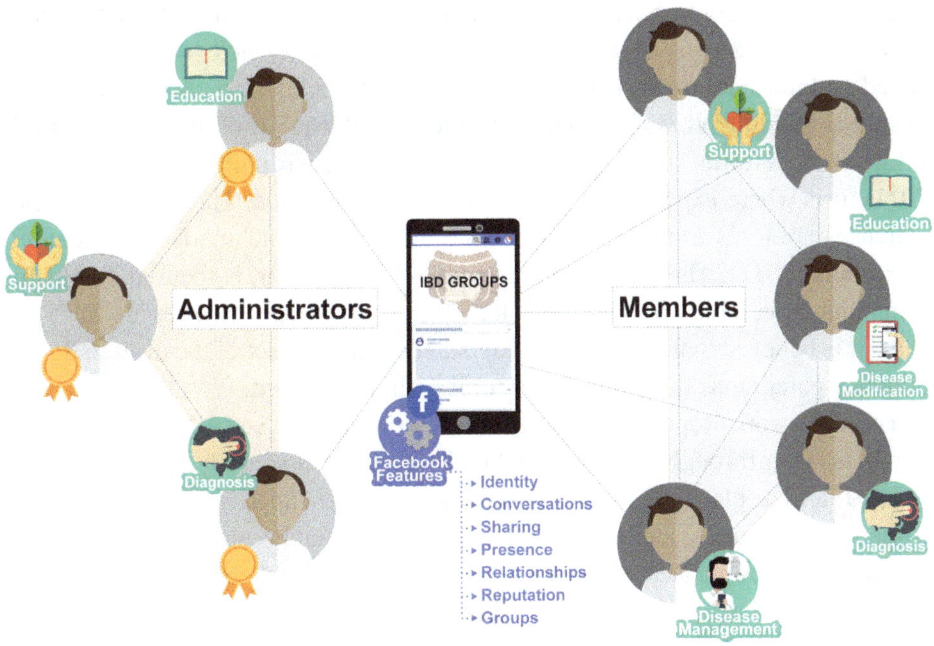

IBD FACEBOOK GROUPS – PROPOSED PROCEDURES OF THE METHODOLOGY

Facebook Health Group Framework

The literature presented above reinforce that the social media tools are being used for patients with IBD, and there is a vast field to be explored as Facebook groups themes. Considering the selected countries to be included in this research - Portugal and Brazil -, it is believed that they are different.[3] Since the purpose of the current study is to understand how Facebook networking may influence, as a process of online engagement, IBD groups, it is believed that working with a holistic analysis model is more relevant. The reason is to bring together inputs from two different worlds, the Information and Communication Technologies (Kietzmann, Hermkens, McCarthy, & Silvestre, 2011) and Health Communication (Frohlich, 2016; Patel et al., 2015). In this context, using an experiential framework may suggest interesting directions about how IBD patients are using social media tools.

The Facebook Health Group Framework proposal from Figure 1 put together two different participants: The Administrators and the Members of the same IBD Facebook group. Content shared between them, which occur during the interaction process, is analyzed using two themes. The first, represented by blue color, is related to Information and Communication Technologies, and shows the "seven functional building blocks", which are technological features of the social network and illustrate relevant role of patients' experience. According to Kietzmann et al. (2011), it is where experiences could occur in social media. The building blocks references are tools from "The honeycomb of social media" model published by the authors (2011). The second, represented by green color, is focused on Health Communication topic. They are selected clinical taxonomy (Patel et al., 2015) in which it is believed that can help in understanding the impact of the disease. In the following paragraphs these two major topics will be detailed.

The framework proposal reflects that the interaction between Administrators and Members occur through the blocks of "Honeycomb of Social Media" (Kietzmann et al., 2011). The blocks aggregate several facets of user experience topics provided by the use of features, and each one can produce different consequences coming from user interaction. Below, the meaning of each block is detailed, following by a description of what is intended to be searched on the administrators IBD Facebook groups interviews:

1. **Identification** is a block that aggregates users' self-presentation experience through features allowing the disclosure of personal data (name, age, profession, etc.) and the identification with any relevant topic (e.g., posts about thoughts, feelings, likes and dislikes). One of the pertinent issues is to understand how members of IBD groups are identified;
2. **Conversations** are an extension that consider the user interaction, which happens through the tools that support the exchange of feedbacks and conversations — Understand what the purposes within the conversations of IBD groups are;
3. **Sharing** functional block represents the exchange, distribution and reception, not only of the digital content but also the experiences among users — Capture what is shared by users in IBD groups;
4. **Presence** block adds the idea that being online on social media provides, among users, the impression that people are accessible and present. It transforms the virtual world and its communities in something "real" — Raise the time spent by the administrators of IBD Facebook groups in following the community and how long it takes them to answer a question;
5. **Relationships** faced with all aspects of the experience already mentioned, and is where the users meet and relate their experiences — Understand how IBD groups foster and assist relations between members;

6. **Reputation** is the facet in which users can display several types of status by setting up a stratified digital environment. The positioning of a user can be improved with effort and their better reputation can generate greater confidence in others — The way the administrators' reputations is perceived by members and how it works considering some management tasks;
7. **Groups** functional block represent the possibility of relationships between members. These social networks can form groups with their own identity and purpose — Understand what is beyond the content of IBD groups and which brings together different user profiles.

After exploring the "seven functional building blocks", and to complete the framework, a clinical taxonomy published in the American Journal of Medicine was included (Patel et al., 2015). The contribute of this axis involves helping with the analysis of social media impact on chronic disease patients' routines and understanding the influence felt by administrators of IBD Facebook groups with the use of social media tools. Regarding the taxonomy referred, the authors present what they call subsequent influences:

- **Support** — Related to user interaction through sharing experiences and emotional support to patients and family members;
- **Education** — Contribute, from the perspective that information transmitted about the diseases and their care, can be learned;
- **Disease modification** — Includes how social media tools are being used for patients' treatment;
- **Diagnosis** — Social media tools contribute to the identification of symptoms and risk factors;
- **Disease management** — Social media can support the decision-making process of the healthcare professional himself.

In summary, the main goal of this study is to comprehend how a specific social media tool, Facebook, may influence patients, through the existing IBD groups, as a process of online engagement. This chapter describes only a part of the study and focus in to understand the administrator's experience in social media IBD Facebook groups. Therefore, other themes from Information and Communications Technologies (Kietzmann et al., 2011) and Health Communication (Patel et al., 2015) were considered in the research, to understand this phenomenon. In the first phase, it was decided to focus only in the groups' directors perspectives, whom are also patients and that are involved with credible content.

Therefore, inside of the main goal other topics should be studied:

1. The purpose of using social media tools;
2. The impact on personal and professional life, namely through care and treatment routines;
3. Knowledge and support achievement.

Besides, it is also relevant to understand how these managers use online resources promoting and facilitating relationships between other members, forming large IBD communities.

In the following section, the methods used during each stage of the analysis for (1) participants settings and (2) interview instruments, and the goals, will be explained.

Participants and Settings

The IBD Facebook groups interviews are the object of the study in this chapter. The analysis includes two phases of research. Below, the process conducted will be detailed. Strategies for describing, defining, or classifying mixed-methods research studies have been designed to be applied, in particular, to the interviews (Cresweel, 2009) but, the present literature limited the discussion of selecting components. Therefore, an empirical research method to analyze the interviews emerged, as aforementioned.

At this phase, the main goal was to identify the sample. This meant to list how many IBD Facebook groups exist in Portugal and Brazil. Before selecting the method of search, the Facebook Research webpage ("Publications," n.d.) [4] was investigated beforehand in order to see if any research method guidelines existed in the Facebook tools. In the Facebook Research webpage, three fields of searching appeared: one, it is an open field where a word or a sentence can be written; the other, a closed field where a Facebook research area is supposed to be selected; and at last, another closed field to choose the year of publication.

The process adopted includes these three fields: the first, an open field where the word "Methods" was written; after that, the "Human-Computer Interaction & UX" item was selected from a closed list; and, in the last field, a range of data was stablished from 2011 to 2019. This process returned a result of eight studies founded. After reading all of the abstracts of the studies found, it was clear to the authors that the Facebook Research webpage ("Publications," n.d.) did not present any guidelines to work with research methods. Based in what was found, another idea emerged – to work with the Preferred Report Items and Meta-Analysis PRISMA flow diagram (as per described by Moher, Liberati, Tetzlaff, Altman, & PRISMA Group, 2009).

Figure 2. Flow diagram of the Facebook group screening, selection and label. Adapted from [PRISMA method- Moher et al., (2009)]]

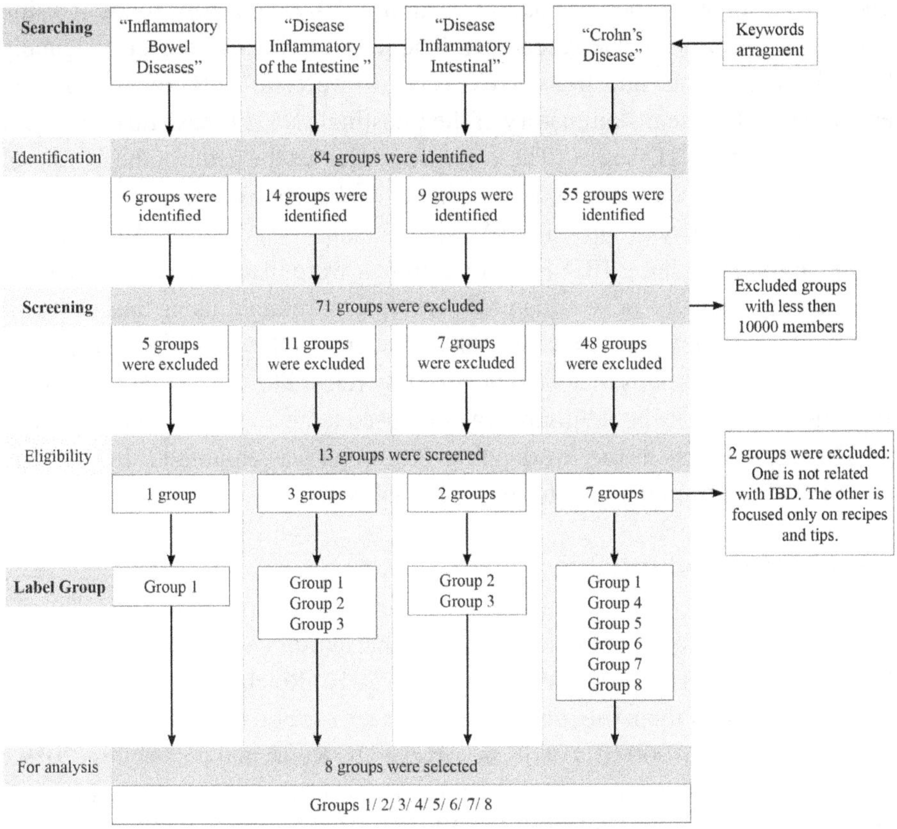

Considering that this methodology is hugely used to report systematic reviews and meta-analyses, any restriction related to adopting this methodology was not found (Selçuk, 2019). So, instead of working with a four-phase flow diagram, a three-phase flow diagram was adopted, with micro-phases inside of each one to filtering and deletion: **Searching** means, looking for IBD through keywords arrangement groups, flowing by their recognition (Identification); **Screening** represents, the phase where all the information collected, about which are the IBD Groups that exit, is inspected following well defined criteria – exclude groups with less than 1000 members – and at the end, only eligible groups are not rejected (Eligibility). **Label Group** is the process of categorizing the eligible groups using different labels that helps with the identification of each group and after that, in the final stage, the closing groups are evaluated (For analysis). In this particular scenario, which includes methods like search, screen, and select only IBD Facebook groups, working with a suggested checklist including a 27-item recommendation list on topics (title, abstract, introduction, methods, results, discussion and financing) was irrelevant.

The **Searching** phase included data collection — IBD Facebook groups — using the Facebook account of one researcher. The keywords arrangement, originally written in Portuguese and later translated to English[5] were: (a) "Inflammatory Bowel Diseases"; (b) "Disease Inflammatory of the Intestine"; (c) "Disease Inflammatory Intestine"; (d) "Crohn's Disease". The keywords reflected the name of the disease of interest. In each of these keywords arrangement, two Facebook filters were checked: (a) "Show only" – "Any group" and (b) "Membership" – "Any group" (Figure 2). After the **Searching** phase, IBD Facebook groups were listed, i.e. **Identification** phase followed. Then, the **Screening** process helped to remove, using the criteria of exclusion, those groups with less than 1000 members. At this phase, the **Eligibility** filter removed those groups that were not directly related to IBD. After this phase, the main list of IBD Facebook groups was supposed to be complete. The last stage, **Label Group**, was where the overlapping of groups was examined. In the final phase, the selected groups were chosen **For Analysis.**

Administrators Interviews

Literature referred before show evidences that some authors worked on the theme of IBD in social media (Frohlich, 2016; Guo et al., 2016; Reich et al., 2019; Szeto et al., 2018) but, most of them use, mainly, surveys as a method of analysis because of the large sample, e.g., 1960 IBD patients surveyed by Reich and colleagues (2019). The only study involving interview to community leaders come from Frohlich (2016). An online ethnographic study of 14 online communities were conducted. This scenario presents a smaller sample of study, close by to what this chapter is working with. This is the reason why interview method was followed.

After selecting the IBD Facebook groups, the administrators of these groups were recruited to participate in semi-structured interviews. Private messages were sent to each manager using Facebook's Messenger tool. The message included a summary with research goals[6] and none of the participants was monetarily compensated. The main argument used to engage external patients with this research was through a short explanation that one researcher involved in this work is a Crohn's Disease patient.

Participants questions from Table 1 were divided into three main topics: (1) Profile description; (2) Personal Impact on IBD knowledge and behaviour; (3) Facebook group creation and manage. The themes are related to what the literature (Guo, Reich, Groshek, & Farraye, 2016) showed as areas of future research about the use of social media for IBD. E.g., patients receiving educational material regarding their illness through social media; the quality of the information posted; assessment of social media preferences and usage in patients with IBD, and others.

Table 1. Questionnaire or survey conducted to IBD Facebook groups' administrators through Google Forms: Free Online Surveys for Personal Use (www.google.com/forms)

Questions Q1-Q5 (Profile description)	
Q1	How long ago was IBD diagnosed?
Q2	What are your age and gender?
Q3	What are your education level and profession?
Q4	Why did you decide to create a specific Facebook group for IBD?
Q5	How much time do you invest per day in the management of the group?
Questions Q6-Q7 (Personal Impact on IBD knowledge and behavior)	
Q6	What impact does the group have in your personal and professional life?
Q7	Does the knowledge gained from other group members influence your disease care routines?
Questions Q8-Q17 (Facebook group creation and manage)	
Q8	What are the formal criteria for approving posts?
Q9	When do you think that it is crucial to intervene in a post?
Q10	As an administrator, can you tell for what "About", "Announcements", and "Description" tabs are used for?
Q11	Are there incentives on the part of group management to accept the participation of specialist doctors and disease associations in interactions with members?
Q12	As an administrator, are you concerned that all the questions are answered quickly?
Q13	When do you consider that it is necessary to contact a group member?
Q14	As an administrator, do you create IBD specific content?
Q15	Are you concerned with creating content for the group on a regular basis?
Q16	As an administrator, what is most relevant in a post, content innovation or credibility?
Q17	As an administrator, did you receive any contact related to healthcare companies to place advertising in the group's page?

Google forms software was used to create the interview model and a link with the questions was shared with each group manager. The results of the process were also collected online.

Considering the author's experience from the patient perspective and, the different perspectives about the countries involved, it was thought that it could be interesting to analyze the interviews from the administrators of IBD Facebook groups following a framework that merged specific categories coming from themes like Social Media Studies and Clinical Studies. As explained before, in the section "Facebook Health Group Framework", an experimental model to analyze the interviews was created matching the theoretical approach from Information and Communications Technologies (Kietzmann et al., 2011) with Health Communication (Patel et al., 2015).

The authors of this chapter started by reading all the interviews. Subsequently, the participants' answers were selected according to the individual experience of each researcher about IBD and the countries involved. After this phase, relevant information to be included in each functional category of the "Honeycomb of Social Media"(Kietzmann et al., 2011) was filtered. Then, all the interviews were screened again, but following different criteria, i.e. clinical taxonomy published in the American Journal of Medicine (Patel et al., 2015) as 'Support and Education'. From the five taxonomies presented, only two categories were selected: Support and Education. This was owing to the direct relationship with patient behavior, not focused on clinical issues (Figure 1). Afterwards, the authors compared and discussed the results.

The most relevant findings will be explained in detail in the later section, following some crucial citations from the administrators of IBD Facebook groups.

RESULTS AND DISCUSSION

Stage 1 – Facebook groups screening and selection

The process, which the task was to search for Facebook groups in the company's webpage – **Searching** phase –, started with choosing the keywords arrangement. The results (Figure 2) showed a total of 84 groups identified — **Identification** phase — "Inflammatory Bowel Diseases" (n=6); "Disease Inflammatory of the Intestine"(n=14); "Disease Inflammatory Intestine" (n=9); "Crohn's Disease" (n=55). After this, IBD Facebook groups with less than 1000 members were excluded, which totaled 71 groups excluded — **Screening** phase —"Inflammatory Bowel Diseases" (n=5); "Disease Inflammatory of the Intestine" (n=11); "Disease Inflammatory Intestine" (n=7); "Crohn's Disease" (n=48). Then, 13 groups were screened considering the **Eligibility** phase — "Inflammatory Bowel Diseases" (n=1); "Disease Inflammatory of the Intestine" (n=3); "Disease Inflammatory Intestine" (n=2); "Crohn's Disease" (n=7). From this list, two groups were excluded because, one was not related to IBD, and the other was related to recipes and tips from another disease. In the final phase, 8 groups were labelled and analyzed – **Label group** and **For Analysis** phases.

Stage 2 – Facebook Groups Administrators Profile Analysis

After concluding the first stage, the researchers sent a private message, as explained before, to each member of the administration of these 8 IBD Facebook groups. To ensure confidentially and privacy about each member, the identification of each participant was changed to an alphanumeric code (Deacon, Pickering, Golding, & Murdock, 1999):

- [Portugal] "Inflammatory Bowel Disease: Starting over needs" — 4 Administrators: **A to D**;
- [Brazil] "Inflammatory Bowel Disease: Starting Over Needs" — 2 Administrators: **E & F**;
- [Brazil] "Diary of an IBD" — 2 Administrators: **G & H**;
- [Brazil] "Crohn's and ulcerative colitis I have I'll win!" — 2 Administrators: **I to K**;
- [Brazil] "Crohn's disease and RCUI" — 2 Administrators: **L & M**;
- [Brazil] "Crohn's Disease and reticulitis: Recipes and tips"—3 Administrators: **G, N and O**;
- [Brazil] "IBD - How to live (*)" — 1 Administrator: **P**;
- [Brazil] Crohn's disease and reticulitis Brazil" — 2 Administrators: **Q to R**.

The study sample included 4 administrators from Portugal and 14 from Brazil. Considering this sample, only eight replies to the message sent by the researchers were obtained. One participant replied arguing that he is a gastroenterology doctor, so he was excluded because it did not make sense to include this profile, even if it represents an IBD Facebook group administrator. In the end, 10 participants did not reply to the researchers contact.

Table 2 presents the demographic characteristics of seven participants that answered the message, following the alphanumeric code attributed to each participant. Although the sample size is small, it is interesting to understand that some indicators may prevail in a larger sample: (1) five participants out of seven have IBD diagnosed over ten years ago, and they may demonstrate experience with the disease; (2) the age frame between 31 and 39 suggests that IBD adult population are interested in social media tools like Reich and colleagues (2019) reported in their study; (3) almost all administrators have a degree, B.S. / B.A. or MSc; and, (3) unfortunately, one female participant lives as a disabled pensioner, which is common in chronic diseases patients.

Stage 3 – Interview Analysis

The seven administrators surveyed shared with the authors relevant contributions, showing that the model of participation in online communities is focused in what Frohlich argued in his article (2016), i.e. social media offers spaces where patients have the freedom to build their narratives reflecting individual/group "health behaviors and illness identities."

Table 2. Demographic analysis of the Administrators of IBD Facebook Groups that replied to the proposed survey

Portugal						
Group code	**Alphanumeric code**	**IBD diagnosed**	**Age**	**Gender**	**Education**	**Profession**
1	A	18 Years	34	Male	B.S.	Civil engineer
	B	12 Years	39	Female	MSc	Policy Coordinator
	C	12 Years	37	Female	Secondary School	Without a profession/ invalidity pensioner
	D	5 Years	31	Female	MSc	Lecture: Portuguese, Latin, Greek, English
Brazil						
2 3	G	4 Years	31	Male	Incomplete B.S. / B.A.	Unemployed
4	L	12 Years	37	Male	B.S.	Systems Analyst Unemployed
	M	10 Years	35	Female	B.S.	Surgical Instrumentation Specialist

This scenario is also recognized in the present body of work. The social media environment acts as "open spaces" of shared IBD experiences and thoughts. The Facebook Health Group Framework presented in Figure 1 gave support such as, guidelines to explore the results of interviews. Each category of the framework was studied in order to explore the interview content. As a result, a summary of the sampling analysis is presented below.

In the **Presence** category, it was found that social media for most of the participants interfered with their lives. All of them demonstrated to be concerned with the idea of always being available to the community. This means being online many times *throughout* the day. As shown by the participants' answers (Q5 and Q6), it is incredible how much time coming from patients' personal lives is dedicated to different tasks related to Facebook group management. It is a large amount of time, but that some administrators considered to be essential. To be online and in the groups constitute part of their "personal life".

Q5 • Participant L – "On average 18 hours."

Q5 • Participant G – "About 7 to 8 hours a day, my time invested in the group."

Q6 • Participant D – "The group is part of my personal life. My husband is almost always aware of events."

The majority of administrators revealed that Presence is shown by the user's availability to find further information and provide support (Q9 and Q12). This means that a fast reply is considered a crucial task, so it was one of the main preoccupations for all administrators. On the other hand, the perception of presence on Facebook is a feature available and easy to see. Some participants said that this task is the responsibility of a specific administrator member.

Q9 • Participant C – "... When it is necessary to inform and support."
Q12 • Participant M – "Yes, there are always members who help with the answers."

After reading the interviews, the idea of self-belong emerged because the patient who has a chronic condition exists and wants to share the experience with other patients (Q4, Q7 and Q8). This shows the purpose of an online group – i.e. to make relationships where experiences are shared and doubts are clarified (Szeto et al., 2018). Another critical issue about this category is that for participants is crucial to help and support others. It is a way to overcome fears and to deal with the disease, together, thus through mutual learning(Q7).

Q4 • Participant B – "There was a lack of a sharing space where patients felt safe to share their experiences."
Q7 • Participant D – "It's a group with such interesting content that, even as a manager, I learn from the experience of many other members."
Q8 • Participant L – "Share doubts, fears and together learn to cope with this disease and help each other like a big family."

Researchers also felt that some managers fully dedicated themselves to their groups without thinking about any exchange or getting anything in return (Q5). Another relevant detail detected during the readings was the relationships between users created by online tools such as Facebook, which may imply decisions about disease management that occur offline. E.g., the answer of a participant to (Q6).

Q5 • Participant G – "We do what we can"
Q6 • Participant M – "It was through the group that I had a doctor's appointment that I treat myself today."

Considering the **Relationship** category, one critical problematic mentioned by some groups was that regularly occurs donation of medications to other patients. One group, from Portugal, adopted an interesting strategy. It defines specific criteria to approve this process online and have shared in the interview how it happens (Q12).

Q12 • Participant B – "And in the case of drug donations to verify that the member actually has the prescribed medication."

For Administrators, online **Relationship** in IBD communities sometimes mean to be strict with other members. They stated that sometimes it is required to manage incorrect verbal treatment, to avoid conflicts, when some problems arise in posts (Q8, Q10 and Q14).

Q8 • Participant L – "Offensive comments to group members will be excluded along with the author."
Q10 • Participant M – "When there are many disagreements and offenses, the post is deleted, and the person banned from the group."
Q14 • Participant D – "When group rules are broken, when there is a lack of respect, or if it jeopardizes the proper functioning of the group."

In addition, one administrator, participant L, from a Brazilian group, reported concerns with privacy.

Q12 • Participant L – "From the moment the member does not follow a certain rule, inbox contact is done to solve the problem and to have everything on record."

After reading all the interviews, researchers agreed that **Reputation** category is the most relevant one, hence it will be detailed in this chapter. In three groups, two from Brazil and one from Portugal, occurred a similar scenario where members are invited to become an administrator member (Q4).

Q4 • Participant M – "I was invited to the group administrator when I joined as a member."
Q4 • Participant L – "Then she published the vacancies for administrator, and I talked to her and started managing the page with her."
Q4 • Participant D – "The group was already created; I was invited by the creator and administrator (at the time) to join the administration."

In two questions, Q4 and Q7, **Relationship** and **Reputation** categories overlapped. In this particular scenario, the **Reputation** of an administrator was for participants something crucial to manage what can happen online between group members in a post, for example. Another interesting point is when members try to overlap their doctor statements during an appointment (that occurs offline), with experiences shared by other patients. Some administrators, one from the Portuguese group and another one from the Brazilian group, referred that they felt an obligation to intervene and to say something.

Q4 • Participant B – "With any assurance that the information shared is based on the best available evidence."

Q7 • Participant L – "Of course the group is a space for sharing experiences, but this space should never overlap with medical knowledge when it comes to treatments as these vary according to each person as well as the response time."

Reputation also involves guaranteeing that the credibility of the contents is considered before being posted. It is a point that most administrators referred to be crucial to follow (Q8). One administrator, from a Brazilian group (Participant L), wrote in the interview all the rules for group members.

Q8 • Participant L – "Any post needs approval from the group administrator or moderator. To belong to the group, the user must submit a request where there is a questionnaire to be answered and the rules of the group. The only ways to participate are by request or invitation by another member and both require a questionnaire response and acceptance of the rules."

Q8 • Participant C – "Related to IBD, not disrespectful, content to be trustworthy."

From a commercial perspective, **Reputation** is a category where several participants shared their preoccupation as administrators. They are meticulous in the management of the group (Q11 and Q17).

Q11 • Participant D – "We do not accept advertising (of whatever kind), denotative content posts, alternative medicines that undermine the science of traditional medicine."

Q17 • Participant L – "NO MONEY DONATIONS ALLOWED. Every day we receive contacts to disclose from companies, health professionals, drug suppliers, websites… but they are refused because this is not the group's goal!"

Groups category can be the most suggestive as a social media functionality presented by Kietzmann et al. (2011). Indeed, creating groups can mean to build an extension of the administrators as patients to other members, improving the sense of community with a common purpose, bringing all together with their experiences and support each other (Q4 and Q8).

Q4 • Participant C – "For the need for a narrower group to share experiences and information with which I identify."

Q8 • Participant L – "Postings of political, sporting or religious content will not be allowed with the author being banned out of the group. There are specific groups for these issues."

Q8 • Participant B – "They have to be related to DII and/or its daily management."

The purpose of online **Conversations** and mutual help reflect the sense of community that other authors reported in IBD patients' environment (Azer et al., 2017; Frohlich, 2016; Plevinsky & Greenley, 2014; Reich et al., 2019). Problems in online conversations always existed, and verbal disrespect is not something new. Administrator consider the group to be an open space that can serve for emotional support (Q4, Q6, and Q8).

Q4 • Participant B – "There was a lack of sharing space where patients felt safe to share their experiences."

Q6 • Participant A – "Acquisition of personal experiences, feeling of help, and more knowledge about IBD."

Q8 • Participant L – "We are here to help in the best way possible and we count on your support!"

Changes in **Conversations** that fall outside of the groups primary purpose do happen. These topics have to be continuous and cannot be left in the open. Quick replies are crucial to create a sense of being online and, to show the idea that conversations are always monitored (Q12).

Q12 • Participant M – "Yes, there are always members who help with the answers."

Q12 • Participant D – "I wish so, but it is impossible given the number of daily posts. We have two managers who are always more on top of the event and effectively try to do so whenever possible."

Sharing experiences consist of "verbalizing" thoughts to help answering questions, and to give information and emotional support. This category is another one that emerges because it involves the main purpose of a Facebook group (Q4, Q6 and Q8).

Q4 • Participant C – "For the need for a narrower group to share experiences and information with which I identify."

Q6 • Participant A – "Acquisition of personal experiences, feeling of help."

Q8 • Participant L – "Share doubts, fears and together learn to cope with this disease and help each other like a big family."

Individual's identity leads who share information in these groups. The authors of this work believe that all patients reveal their identity when they are **Sharing** content with others (Q4, Q6 and Q12).

One category presented in the framework followed is overlapped, the **Education**. Several authors (Kietzmann et al., 2011; Patel et al., 2015) revealed similar importance to the topic but exhibiting different perspectives (See section "Facebook Health Group Framework"). Member education by sharing questions, experience or even information seems to be relevant to all administrators but always considering the accuracy or credibility that exists behind of all information (Q4, Q7 and Q10).

Q4 • Participant B – "With any guarantee that the information shared is based on the best available evidence."
Q7 • Participant C – "In a way, yes, although it filters and only does something after informing the gastroenterologist doctor."
Q10 • Participant D – "When there are comments that could mislead other members, when they give wrong medication and treatment advice."

The results of the interviews also showed that the **Education** of IBD Facebook group members reflect the patients' behavior outside of the online world. Some administrators identified that (Q6 and Q10):

Q6 • Participant M – "Very important, because we clarified many doubts and it was through the group that I had the doctor's appointment that I treat myself today."
Q6 • Participant C – "Positive, because in it I acquired more" baggage "to deal with the pathology, in both contexts."
Q10 • Participant C – "When they break the rules, when it's necessary to inform and support."

Health Communication, where the Emotional category is included (Patel et al., 2015), represents according to the participants, emotional support, group support, and a "safe place" feeling (Q8 and Q10).

Q8. • Participant L – "Share doubts, fears and together learn to cope with this disease and help each other like a big family[...] We are here to help in the best way possible and we count on your support!"
Q10 • Participant C – "When they break the rules, when it's necessary to inform and support."

CONCLUSION

Studies Limitation

This work faced some limitations. The process involving the contact with administrators was difficult because none of the authors / researchers knew any member or administrator of a IBD Facebook group. Several messages were sent but some did not get a reply, even with the help of other members outside of these groups.

Final Remarks

This chapter has described an investigation to a Facebook phenomenon, the administrators' experience in social media IBD Facebook groups, following different criteria of analysis coming from Information and Communications Technologies and Health Communication. Evidences from this study suggest that after understanding the preoccupations of the administrators, it is crucial to analyze the members perspective about using this online tool as an approach of overcome fears and to deal with the disease together.

The findings of this pilot study suggest that the Administrator's Experience in Managing Health Facebook Groups fall under the model of participation in online communities proposed in this Chapter, being subdivided into the following blocks: Presence that refers to the way social media for most of the participants interfered with their lives; Identification that is relative to the users' self-presentation experience; Conversation that considers the user interaction and exchange of feedback; Sharing of the digital content by uses in IBD groups; Relationships that are essential in group and member's assistance towards health; Reputation (i.e. status) and Groups that may reinforce patients' identity and purpose.

The insights gained from this research may be of assistance to policymakers, IBD patients and other stakeholders involved in the decision-making process of healthcare. It lays the groundwork for future research into the use of social media in disease management, its impact on personal and professional life, namely through care and treatment routines; and, finally, health management and support achievement.

REFERENCES

Auyeung, J. (2014, January 31). Inflammatory Bowel Disease: Etiology, Pathogenesis and Current Therapy. Retrieved October 4, 2019, from Current Pharmaceutical Design website: http://www.eurekaselect.com/111540/article

Azer, S. A., AlOlayan, T. I., AlGhamdi, M. A., & AlSanea, M. A. (2017). Inflammatory bowel disease: An evaluation of health information on the internet. *World Journal of Gastroenterology*, *23*(9), 1676–1696. doi:10.3748/wjg.v23.i9.1676 PMID:28321169

Carroll, C. L., & Ramachandran, P. (2014). The Intelligent Use of Digital Tools and Social Media in Practice Management. *Chest*, *145*(4), 896–902. doi:10.1378/chest.13-0251 PMID:24687711

Cawdron, R., & Issenman, R. (2002). Patient Web-Resource Interest and Internet Readiness in Pediatric Inflammatory Bowel Disease. *Journal of Pediatric Gastroenterology and Nutrition*, *35*(4), 518–521. doi:10.1097/00005176-200210000-00011 PMID:12394377

Cima, R. R., Anderson, K. J., Larson, D. W., Dozois, E. J., Hassan, I., Sandborn, W. J., ... Pemberton, J. H. (2007). Internet use by patients in an inflammatory bowel disease specialty clinic. *Inflammatory Bowel Diseases*, *13*(10), 1266–1270. doi:10.1002/ibd.20198 PMID:17567877

Clinic, M. (n.d.). Crohn's disease—Symptoms and causes. Retrieved October 4, 2019, from Mayo Clinic website: https://www.mayoclinic.org/diseases-conditions/crohns-disease/symptoms-causes/syc-20353304

Cresweel, J. (2009). *Research Design: Qualitative, Quantitative, and Mixed Methods Approaches*. Thousand Oaks, CA: SAGE.

Deacon, D., Pickering, M., Golding, P., & Murdock, G. (1999). *Researching Communications: A Practical Guide to Methods in Media and Cultural Analysis*. London, UK: Hodder Education.

Erikainen, S., Pickersgill, M., Cunningham-Burley, S., & Chan, S. (2019). Patienthood and participation in the digital era. *Digital Health*, *5*. doi:10.1177/2055207619845546 PMID:31041112

Ferguson, C., Inglis, S. C., Newton, P. J., Cripps, P. J. S., MacDonald, P. S., & Davidson, P. M. (2014). Social media: A tool to spread information: a case study analysis of twitter conversation at the Cardiac Society of Australia & New Zealand 61st annual scientific meeting 2013. *Collegian (Royal College of Nursing, Australia)*, *21*(2), 89–93. doi:10.1016/j.colegn.2014.03.002 PMID:25109206

Fox, S., & Duggan, M. (2013, January 15). Health Online 2013. Retrieved November 24, 2019, from Pew Research Center: Internet, Science, & Tech website: https://www.pewresearch.org/internet/2013/01/15/health-online-2013/

Frohlich, D. O. (2016). The Social Construction of Inflammatory Bowel Disease Using Social Media Technologies. *Health Communication*, *31*(11), 1412–1420. doi:10.1080/10410236.2015.1077690 PMID:27050670

Guo, L., Reich, J., Groshek, J., & Farraye, F. A. (2016). Social Media Use in Patients with Inflammatory Bowel Disease. *Inflammatory Bowel Diseases*, *22*(5), 1231–1238. doi:10.1097/MIB.0000000000000713 PMID:26894839

Hartley, J. (2012). Designing Easy-to-Read Text. In Writing Health Communication: An Evidence-Based Guide (pp. 7–22). doi:10.4135/9781446288054.n2

Hawn, C. (2009). Take two aspirin and tweet me in the morning: How Twitter, Facebook, and other social media are reshaping health care. *Health Affairs (Project Hope)*, *28*(2), 361–368. doi:10.1377/hlthaff.28.2.361 PMID:19275991

Kaplan, K. (2013, June 31). When and How to Create Customer Journey Maps. Retrieved April 20, 2015, from Nielsen Norman Group website: https://www.nngroup.com/articles/customer-journey-mapping/

Kietzmann, J. H., Hermkens, K., McCarthy, I. P., & Silvestre, B. S. (2011). Social media? Get serious! Understanding the functional building blocks of social media. *Business Horizons*, *54*(3), 241–251. doi:10.1016/j.bushor.2011.01.005

Lennard-Jones, J. E. (1989). Classification of inflammatory bowel disease. *Scandinavian Journal of Gastroenterology. Supplement*, *170*(sup170), 2–6, discussion 16–19. doi:10.3109/00365528909091339 PMID:2617184

Loddo, I., & Romano, C. (2015). Inflammatory Bowel Disease: Genetics, Epigenetics, and Pathogenesis. *Frontiers in Immunology*, *6*, 551. doi:10.3389/fimmu.2015.00551 PMID:26579126

Moher, D., Liberati, A., Tetzlaff, J., & Altman, D. G.PRISMA Group. (2009). Preferred reporting items for systematic reviews and meta-analyses: The PRISMA statement. *PLoS Medicine*, *6*(7). doi:10.1371/journal.pmed.1000097 PMID:19621072

Ng, S. C., Shi, H. Y., Hamidi, N., Underwood, F. E., Tang, W., Benchimol, E. I., ... Kaplan, G. G. (2017). Worldwide incidence and prevalence of inflammatory bowel disease in the 21st century: A systematic review of population-based studies. *Lancet*, *390*(10114), 2769–2778. doi:10.1016/S0140-6736(17)32448-0 PMID:29050646

Nickels, A., & Dimov, V. (2012). Innovations in technology: Social media and mobile technology in the care of adolescents with asthma. *Current Allergy and Asthma Reports*, *12*(6), 607–612. doi:10.100711882-012-0299-7 PMID:22976493

Patel, R., Chang, T., Greysen, S. R., & Chopra, V. (2015). Social Media Use in Chronic Disease: A Systematic Review and Novel Taxonomy. *The American Journal of Medicine*, *128*(12), 1335–1350. doi:10.1016/j.amjmed.2015.06.015 PMID:26159633

Pernencar, C., Romão, T., & Simões, G. (2016). *The Design Process of an e-Health project – Applying the HSI framework for interface analysis.* Presented at the 2016 IEEE 4th International Conference on Serious Games and Applications for Health (SeGAH), Orlando, FL.

Pernencar, C., Sousa, P., Frontini, R., Martinho, R., Runte, D., Mendes, D., & Carvalho, M. (2018). Planning a health promotion program: Mobile app gamification as a tool to engage adolescents. *CENTERIS 2018 - International Conference on ENTERprise Information Systems / ProjMAN 2018 - International Conference on Project MANagement / HCist 2018 - International Conference on Health and Social Care Information Systems and Technologies, CENTERIS/ProjMAN/HCist 2018, 138*, 113–118. 10.1016/j.procs.2018.10.016

Pernencar, C. A. (2013, May). My Crohn's diease on real time information. In *2013 IEEE 2nd International Conference on Serious Games and Applications for Health (SeGAH)* (pp. 1-7). IEEE. 10.1109/SeGAH.2013.6665304

Plevinsky, J. M., & Greenley, R. N. (2014). Exploring Health-related Quality of Life and Social Functioning in Adolescents with Inflammatory Bowel Diseases After Attending Camp Oasis and Participating in a Facebook Group. *Inflammatory Bowel Diseases*, *20*(9), 1611–1617. doi:10.1097/MIB.0000000000000120 PMID:25025714

Promislow, S., Walker, J. R., Taheri, M., & Bernstein, C. N. (2010). How well does the Internet answer patients' questions about inflammatory bowel disease? *Canadian Journal of Gastroenterology*, *24*(11), 671–677. doi:10.1155/2010/957264 PMID:21157582

Publications. (n.d.). Retrieved October 21, 2019, from Facebook Research website: https://research.fb.com/publications/

Randell, R. L., Long, M. D., Cook, S. F., Wrennall, C. E. D., Chen, W., Martin, C. F., ... Kappelman, M. D. (2014, March 1). Validation of an Internet-Based Cohort of Inflammatory Bowel Disease (CCFA Partners). *Inflammatory Bowel Diseases*, *20*(3), 541–544. https://doi.org/10.1097/01.MIB.0000441348.32570.34

Reich, J., Guo, L., Groshek, J., Weinberg, J., Chen, W., Martin, C., ... Farraye, F. A. (2019). Social Media Use and Preferences in Patients With Inflammatory Bowel Disease. *Inflammatory Bowel Diseases*, *25*(3), 587–591. doi:10.1093/ibd/izy280 PMID:30203036

Saboia, I., Pisco Almeida, A. M., Sousa, P., & Pernencar, C. (2018). I am with you: A netnographic analysis of the Instagram opinion leaders on eating behavior change. *CENTERIS 2018 - International Conference on ENTERprise Information Systems / ProjMAN 2018 - International Conference on Project MANagement / HCist 2018 - International Conference on Health and Social Care Information Systems and Technologies, 138*, 97–104. 10.1016/j.procs.2018.10.014

Selçuk, A. A. (2019). A Guide for Systematic Reviews: PRISMA. *Turkish Archives of Otorhinolaryngology*, *57*(1), 57–58. doi:10.5152/tao.2019.4058 PMID:31049257

Szeto, W., van der Bent, A., Petty, C. R., Reich, J., Farraye, F., & Fishman, L. N. (2018). Use of Social Media for Health-Related Tasks by Adolescents With Inflammatory Bowel Disease: A Step in the Pathway of Transition. *Inflammatory Bowel Diseases*, *24*(6), 1114–1122. doi:10.1093/ibd/izy021 PMID:29788360

Taft, T. H., & Keefer, L. (2016). A systematic review of disease-related stigmatization in patients living with inflammatory bowel disease. *Clinical and Experimental Gastroenterology*, *9*, 49–58. doi:10.2147/CEG.S83533 PMID:27022294

ENDNOTES

1. Inflammatory bowel disease (IBD), https://www.cdc.gov/ibd/what-is-IBD.htm (access date: November 9, 2019) ; The Facts About Inflammatory Bowel Diseases. New York, NY: Crohn's and Colitis Foundation of America; 2014 retrieved from https://www.crohnscolitisfoundation.org/sites/default/files/2019-02/Updated%20IBD%20Factbook.pdf (access date: November 9, 2019);
2. "The Crohn's & Colitis Foundation is a non-profit, volunteer-fueled organization dedicated to finding the cures for Crohn's disease and ulcerative colitis, and to improving the quality of life of children and adults affected by these diseases. It was founded in 1967 by Irwin M. and Suzanne Rosenthal, William D. and Shelby Modell, and Henry D. Janowitz, M.D. "https://www.crohnscolitisfoundation.org/" (Access date: November 9, 2019);
3. Related to the sample presented in this chapter, it is important to explain one detail: 1 researcher is an IBD Portuguese Patient with the disease since 2002,

and the other researcher is Brazilian non-patient. Crohn's patient for fifteen years that has undergone several distinct treatments and gone through innovative hospital innovative care, a surgery, and other disease complications;

4 Facebook research is the company repository where anyone has free access to Facebook scientific publications. https://research.fb.com/publications/ (Access date: November 9, 2019);

5 "Doenças Inflamatórias do Intestino"; "Doença Inflamatória do Intestino"; "Doença de Crohn"; "Doença Inflamatória Intestinal";

6 "DII Facebook Group Administrators - Profile and Management Assessment." As part of an investigation in Portugal and Brazil on the management of the Facebook groups dedicated to Inflammatory Bowel Diseases, we now request that you answer the questions in this questionnaire or via voice mail in Messenger by 22 September. This study is to be published in 2020.

Compilation of References

Aartsma-Rus, A., Furlong, P., Vroom, E., van Ommen, G. J., Niks, E., Straathof, C., ... Karcagi, V. (2011). The risks of therapeutic misconception and individual patient (n= 1)"trials" in rare diseases such as Duchenne dystrophy. *Neuromuscular Disorders*, *21*(1), 13–15. doi:10.1016/j.nmd.2010.09.012 PMID:21051233

Abrahamyan, L., Feldman, B. M., Tomlinson, G., Faughnan, M. E., Johnson, S. R., Diamond, I. R., & Gupta, S. (2016, December). Alternative designs for clinical trials in rare diseases. In American Journal of Medical Genetics Part C: Seminars in Medical Genetics, 172(4), pp. 313-331. Doi:10.1002/ajmg.c.31533

Ache, K., & Wallace, L. (2008). Human papillomavirus vaccination coverage on YouTube. American Journal of Preventive Medicine. *American Journal of Preventive Medicine*, *35*(4), 389–392. doi:10.1016/j.amepre.2008.06.029 PMID:18675530

Aetna. (2015). How consumers use social media for health care education. Retrieved from https://news.aetna.com/2015/07/how-consumers-use-social-media-for-healthcare-education/

Aghamohammadi, A., Bahrami, A., Mamishi, S., Mohammadi, B., Abolhassani, H., Parveneh, N., & Razei, N. (2010). Impact of delayed diagnosis in children with primary antibody deficiencies. *Journal of Microbiology, Immunology, and Infection*, *44*(3), 229–234. doi:10.1016/j.jmii.2011.01.026 PMID:21524619

Ahmed, O. H., Sullivan, S. J., Schneiders, A. G., & McCrory, P. (2010). iSupport: Do social networking sites have a role to play in concussion awareness? *Disability and Rehabilitation*, *32*(22), 1877–1883. doi:10.3109/09638281003734409 PMID:20367328

Ainsworth, M. D. S. (1991). Attachments and other affectional bonds across the life cycle. In C. M. Parkes, J. Stevenson-Hinde, & P. Marris (Eds.), *Attachment across the life cycle* (pp. 33–51). New York: Routledge.

Ainsworth, M. D. S., & Bell, S. M. (1969). Some contemporary patterns of mother-infant interaction in the feeding situation. In A. Ambrose (Ed.), *Stimulation in early infancy* (pp. 133–170). San Diego, CA: Academic Press.

Ainsworth, M., Blehar, M., Waters, E., & Wall, S. (1978). *Patterns of attachment: A psychological study of the strange situation*. Hillsdale, NJ: Erlbaum.

Ajzen, I. (1991). The theory of planned behavior. *Organizational Behavior and Human Decision Processes*, *50*(2), 179–211. doi:10.1016/0749-5978(91)90020-T

Ajzen, I. (1992). *Persuasive communication theory in social psychology: A historical perspective* (pp. 1–16). Amherst, MA: University of Massachusetts.

Akli, S., Chomel, J. C., Lacorte, J. M., Bachner, L., Kahn, A., & Poenaru, L. (1993). Ten novel mutations in the HEXA gene in non-Jewish Tay-Sachs patients. *Human Molecular Genetics*, *2*(1), 61–67. doi:10.1093/hmg/2.1.61 PMID:8490625

Akram, A., O'Brien, A., O'Neill, A., & Latham, R. (2009). Crossing the line–learning psychiatry at the movies. *International Review of Psychiatry (Abingdon, England)*, *21*(3), 267–268. doi:10.1080/09540260902746880 PMID:19459104

Albakri, A. (2018). Restrictive cardiomyopathy: A review of literature on clinical status and meta-analysis of diagnosis and clinical management. *Pediatric Dimensions*, *3*(2). doi:10.15761/pd.1000170

Albuquerque, S., Pereira, M., Fonseca, A., & Carnavarro, M. (2015). Resiliência, stresse parental e sobrecarga de pais de crianças com diagnóstico de anomalia congénita. [Resilience, parental stress and overload of parents of children diagnosed with congnital anomaly]. *Psychologica, 58*(2), 7-23. doi: -2_1. doi:10.14195/1647-8606_58

Albus., J.S. (1971). A theory of cerebellar function. *Mathematical Bioscience 10*(1-2), 25-61. (71)90051-4 doi:10.1016/0025-5564

Aledo, L. D. (2007). La representación de la discapacidad en los medios de comunicación. *Comunicación e cidadanía: revista internacional de xornalismo social= Social Journalism International Review*, (1), 289-306.

Al-Falki, Y. H., Alshehri, M. A., Joseph, M. R. P., & Hamid, M. E. (2018). Fungal keratitis caused by a rare ocular pathogen, Gjaerumia minor: A case report. *Saudi Journal of Ophthalmology*, *32*(2), 160–163. doi:10.1016/j.sjopt.2017.09.007 PMID:29942188

Ali, K. (2014). From lecture halls to cinema screens: Learning about the psyche through films. *Medical Humanities*, *40*(1), 69–69. doi:10.1136/medhum-2013-010479 PMID:24298043

Ali, S. R., Bryce, J., Cools, M., Korbonits, M., Beun, J. G., Taruscio, D., ... Ahmed, S. F. (2019). The current landscape of European registries for rare endocrine conditions. *European Journal of Endocrinology*, *180*(1), 89–98. doi:10.1530/EJE-18-0861 PMID:30407922

Almeida, B., & Melgaço, P. (2016). Quando a criança nasce doente: A subjetividade do infante e as relações familiares. *Psicologia em Revista*, *22*(2), 356–373. doi:10.5752/P.1678-9523.2016V22N2P356

ALS. (2019). ALS Ice Bucket Challenge. Retrieved from https://www.als.net/icebucketchallenge/

Altheide, D. L. (2004). Ethnographic content analysis. In M. S. Lewis-Beck, A. Bryman, & T. F. Liao. (Eds.), The Sage encyclopedia of social science research methods, 3 vols. (pp. 325-326). Thousand Oaks, CA: Sage.

Alves, C., & Oliveira, C. S. (2014). Hearing loss among patients with Turner's syndrome: Literature review1. *Revista Brasileira de Otorrinolaringologia (English Ed.)*, *80*(3), 257–263. doi:10.1016/j.bjorl.2013.08.002 PMID:25153112

Amano, M., & Shimizu, T. (2014). Emphysematous cystitis: A review of the literature. *Internal Medicine (Tokyo, Japan)*, *53*(2), 79–82. doi:10.2169/internalmedicine.53.1121 PMID:24429444

Anderson, M., Elliott, E. J., & Zurynski, Y. A. (2013). Australian families living with rare disease: Experiences of diagnosis, health services use and needs for psychosocial support. *Orphanet Journal of Rare Diseases*, *8*(1), 22. doi:10.1186/1750-1172-8-22 PMID:23398775

Andreasen, N. C. (1999). A unitary model of schizophrenia: Bleuler's "fragmented phrene" as schizencephaly. *Archives of General Psychiatry*, *56*(9), 781–787. doi:10.1001/archpsyc.56.9.781 PMID:12884883

Andreasen, N. C., Nopoulos, P., O'Leary, D. S., Miller, D. D., Wassink, T., & Flaum, M. (1999). Defining the phenotype of schizophrenia: Cognitive dysmetria and its neural mechanisms. *Biological Psychiatry*, *46*(7), 908–920. doi:10.1016/S0006-3223(99)00152-3 PMID:10509174

Andreasen, N. C., & Pierson, R. (2008). The role of the cerebellum in schizophrenia. *Biological Psychiatry*, *64*(2), 81–88. doi:10.1016/j.biopsych.2008.01.003 PMID:18395701

Andsager, J. L., Bemker, V., Choi, H. L., & Torwel, V. (2006). Perceived similarity of exemplar traits and behavior. *Communication Research*, *33*(1), 3–18. doi:10.1177/0093650205283099

Annandale, E. C. (2014). *The Sociology of Health and Medicine: A Critical Introduction*. Cambridge, UK: Polity Press.

Antheunis, M. L., Tates, K., & Nieboer, T. E. (2013). Patients' and health professionals' use of social media in health care: Motives, barriers and expectations. *Patient Education and Counseling*, *92*(3), 426–431. doi:10.1016/j.pec.2013.06.020 PMID:23899831

Araújo, Y. B., Collet, N., Moura, F. M., & Nóbrega, R. D. (2009). Conhecimento da família acerca da condição crônica na infância. [Family knowledge about chronic condition in childhood]. *Texto & Contexto Enfermagem*, *18*(3), 498–505. doi:10.1590/S0104-07072009000300013

Arcos, J. M. (2013). El Día Mundial de las enfermedades raras en las noticias de prensa: el ejemplo de Andalucía. *Discurso y Sociedad*, 7(1), 224-247. Recuperado de http://www.dissoc.org/ediciones/v07n01/DS7(1)

Ardigò, A. (1997). *Società e salute*. Milano, Italy: Franco Angeli.

Argov, Z., & Navon, R. (1984). Clinical and genetic variations in the syndrome of adult GM2 gangliodosis resulting from hexosaminidase a deficiency. *Annals of Neurology*, *16*(1), 14–20. doi:10.1002/ana.410160105 PMID:6235771

Aristotle. (IV century BC/2005). Retórica. Lisboa, Portugal: Imprensa Nacional-Casa da Moeda.

Arksey, H. (1994). Expert and lay participation in the construction of medical knowledge. *Sociology of Health & Illness*, *16*(4), 44–468. doi:10.1111/1467-9566.ep11347516

Armayones, M., Requena, S., Gómez-Zuñiga, B., Pousada, M., & Bañón, A. M. (2015). El uso de Facebook en asociaciones españolas de enfermedades raras: ¿cómo e para qué lo utilizan? *Gaceta Sanitaria*, *29*(5), 335–340. doi:10.1016/j.gaceta.2015.05.007 PMID:26145457

Armstrong, D. (2014). Actors, patients and agency: A recent history. *Sociology of Health & Illness*, *36*(2), 163–174. doi:10.1111/1467-9566.12100 PMID:24372176

Asan, O., Young, H. N., Chewning, B., & Montague, E. (2015). How physician electronic health record screen sharing affects patient and doctor non-verbal communication in primary care. *Patient Education and Counseling*, *98*(3), 310–316. doi:10.1016/j.pec.2014.11.024 PMID:25534022

ASHUA – Associación Síndrome Hemolítico Urémico Atípico España. (2018, February). *ASHUA reivindica el papel de los pacientes em la investigación sobre el diagnóstico del SHUa em el Día Mundial de las Enfermedades Raras.* Retrieved from https://www.ashua.es/blog/55

Asociación para la investigación en medios de comunicación. (2015). 'Datos EGM. Resumen General – AIMC'. Retrieved from http://www.aimc.es/-Datos-EGM-Resumen-General-.html. [Access date: 18 May 2016].

Assal, F. (2018). Diogenes Syndrome. *Frontiers of Neurology and Neuroscience*, *41*, 90–97. doi:10.1159/000475688 PMID:29145187

Athanasiou, D., Nafría, B., Vroom, E. (2018). Share4Rare: Social media platform dedicated to rare diseases, using collective intelligence for the generation of awareness and knowledge. *Orphanet Journal of Rare Diseases 2018, 13*(Suppl 2):P2, 167. doi:10.118613023-018-0895-2

Augè, M., & Herzlich, C. (a cura di). (1986). Il senso del male. Antropologia, storia e sociologia della malattia, Milano, Italy: Il Saggiatore.

Aujoulat, I., d'Hoore, W., & Deccache, A. (2007). Patient empowerment in theory and practice: Polysemy or cacophony? *Patient Education and Counseling*, *66*(1), 13–20. doi:10.1016/j.pec.2006.09.008 PMID:17084059

Au, P. Y. B., Innes, A. M., & Kline, A. D. (1993-2019). Au-Kline Syndrome. In M. P. Adam, H. H. Ardinger, R. A. Pagon, S. E. Wallace, L. J. H. Bean, K. Stephens, & A. Amemiya (Eds.), *GeneReviews((R))*. Seattle, WA: University of Washington, Seattle.

Auyeung, J. (2014, January 31). Inflammatory Bowel Disease: Etiology, Pathogenesis and Current Therapy. Retrieved October 4, 2019, from Current Pharmaceutical Design website: http://www.eurekaselect.com/111540/article

Avellaneda, A., Izquierdo, M., Torrent-Farnell, J., & Ramón, J. R. (2007). Enfermedades raras: Enfermedades crónicas que requieren un nuevo enfoque sociosanitario. *Anales del Sistema Sanitario de Navarra*, *30*(2), 177–190. doi:10.4321/S1137-66272007000300002 PMID:17898813

Aymé, S. (2000). *Les injustices de la naissance*. Paris, France: Hachette Littératures.

Aymé, S., Kole, A., & Groft, S. (2008). Empowerment of patients: Lessons from the rare diseases community. *Lancet*, *371*(9629), 2048–2051. doi:10.1016/S0140-6736(08)60875-2 PMID:18555918

Aymé, S., & Schmidtke, J. (2007). Networking for rare diseases: A necessity for Europe. *Bundesgesundheitsblatt, Gesundheitsforschung, Gesundheitsschutz*, *50*(12), 1477–1483. doi:10.100700103-007-0381-9 PMID:18026888

Azer, S. A., AlOlayan, T. I., AlGhamdi, M. A., & AlSanea, M. A. (2017). Inflammatory bowel disease: An evaluation of health information on the internet. *World Journal of Gastroenterology*, *23*(9), 1676–1696. doi:10.3748/wjg.v23.i9.1676 PMID:28321169

Babrow, A. S., Kasch, C. R., & Ford, L. A. (1998). The many meanings of uncertainty in illness: Toward a systematic accounting. *Health Communication*, *10*(1), 1–23. doi:10.120715327027hc1001_1 PMID:16370987

Baddini-Martinez, J., Baldi, B. G., Costa, C. H. d., Jezler, S., Lima, M. S., & Rufino, R. (2015). Update on diagnosis and treatment of idiopathic pulmonary fibrosis. Jornal brasileiro de pneumologia: publicacao oficial da Sociedade Brasileira de Pneumologia e Tisilogia, 41(5), 454-466. doi:10.1590/S1806-37132015000000152

Balsebre, A. (2001). *Historia de la radio en España*. Madrid, Spain: Cátedra.

Bamforth, I. (2010). Stendhal's Syndrome. *The British Journal of General Practice*, *60*(581), 945–946. doi:10.3399/bjgp10X544780

Bañón Hernández, A. M. (2007). Las enfermedades raras y su representación discursiva. Propuestas para un análisis crítico. *Discurso & Sociedad*, *2*(1), 188–229.

Bañón Hernández, A. M., Alcaraz, J. F., Almela, J. S., & Sanchis, I. R. (2011). *Desafíos y estrategias comunicativas de las enfermedades raras: La investigación médica como referente: Estudio cuantitativo-discursivo de la prensa escrita impresa y digital española (2009-2010)*. Valencia, Spain: CIBERER.

Bañón Hernandezy, A. M., & Requena Romero, S. (2014). La representación de las enfermedades poco frecuentes en el discurso periodístico español. Propuestas para el análisis. *Pragmática Sociocultural/Sociocultural Pragmatics*, *8*(2), 180-222. doi:10.1515oprag-2014-0023

Banos, J. E. (2007). How literature and popular movies can help in medical education: Applications for teaching the doctor-patient relationship. *Medical Education*, *41*(9), 918. doi:10.1111/j.1365-2923.2007.02829.x PMID:17727535

Barataud, B. (2001). *Cinq mille maladies rares, le choc de la génétique: constat, perspectives et possibilités d'évolution.* Retrieved from http://www.ladocumentationfrancaise.fr/rapports-publics/014000706/index.shtml

Barnes, J. A. (1954). Class and committees in a Norwegian island parish. *Human Relations*, *7*(1), 39–58. doi:10.1177/001872675400700102

Barritt, A. W., Anderson, S. J., Leigh, P. N., & Ridha, B. H. (2017). Late-onset Tay-Sachs disease. *Practical Neurology*, *17*(5), 396–399. doi:10.1136/practneurol-2017-001665 PMID:28739864

Barroso, R., & Machado, C. (2010). Definições, dimensões e determinantes da parentalidade. [Definitions, dimensions, and determinants of parenting]. *Psychologica*, *1*(52), 211–229. doi:10.14195/1647-8606_52-1_10

Barry, A. (1994). Perceptual Aesthetics and Visual Language. In D. Moore, & F. M. Dwyer (Eds.), *Visual Literacy: A Spectrum of Visual Learning, Englewood Cliffs*. New Jersey: Educational Technology Publications.

Bartholomew, K., & Horowitz, L. M. (1991). Attachment styles among young adults: A test of a four-category model. *Journal of Personality and Social Psychology*, *61*(2), 226–244. doi:10.1037/0022-3514.61.2.226 PMID:1920064

Basagoiti, I., & Fernández-Luque, L. (2011). Compartir información sanitaria: ePacientes: comunicación e interacción. In V. *Traver Salcedo, & L. Fernández Luque (Coords.), El ePaciente y las redes sociales*. Valencia, Spain: Publidisa.

Bates, M. D., Bucuvalas, J. C., Alonso, M. H., & Ryckman, F. C. (1998). Biliary atresia: Pathogenesis and treatment. *Seminars in Liver Disease*, *18*(3), 281–293. doi:10.1055-2007-1007164 PMID:9773428

Batra, R., & Ray, M. L. (1986). Affective responses mediating acceptance of advertising. *The Journal of Consumer Research*, *13*(2), 234–249. doi:10.1086/209063

Baudrillard, J. (1994). *Simulacra and Simulation.* United States of America: The University of Michigan.

Beach, M. C., Keruly, J., & Moore, R. D. (2006). Is the quality of the patient-provider relationship associated with better adherence and health outcomes for patients with HIV? *Journal of General Internal Medicine*, *21*(6), 661. doi:10.1111/j.1525-1497.2006.00399.x PMID:16808754

Becker, M. (1978). Compliance with a medical regimen for asthma. *Public Health Reports*, *93*, 268–277. PMID:652949

Becker, M. H. (1974). The Health Belief Model and Personal Health Behavior. *Health Education Monographs*, *2*(4), 324–508. doi:10.1177/109019817400200407

Begin, P. (2006). Buñuel, Eisenstein, and the 'Montage of Attractions': An Approach to Film in Theory and Practice. *Bulletin of Spanish Studies*, *83*(8), 1113–1132. doi:10.1080/14753820601073613

Bell, D. J., & Gaillard, F. (2019). Mondini malformation. Retrieved from https://radiopaedia.org/articles/mondini-malformation?lang=gb

Bell, S. M., & Ainsworth, M. D. S. (1972). Infant crying and maternal responsiveness. *Child Development*, *43*(4), 1171–1190. doi:10.2307/1127506 PMID:4643768

Beltran-Quintero, M. L., Bascou, N. A., Poe, M. D., Wenger, D. A., Saavedra-Matiz, C. A., Nichols, M. J., & Escolar, M. L. (2019). Early progression of Krabbe disease in patients with symptom onset between 0 and 5 months. *Orphanet Journal of Rare Diseases*, *14*(1), 46. doi:10.118613023-019-1018-4 PMID:30777126

Bennett, P., & Murphy, S. (1997). *Psychology and Health Promotion*. Buckingham, UK: Open University Press.

Bensing, J. (1991). Doctor-patient communication and the quality of care. *Social Science & Medicine*, *32*(11), 1301–1310. doi:10.1016/0277-9536(91)90047-G PMID:2068614

Berman, J. J. (2014). What are the Rare Diseases, and Why do we Care? In Rare Diseases and Orphan Drugs (pp. 3-8). doi:10.1016/B978-0-12-419988-0.00001-8

Bernard, J. A., Orr, J. M., & Mittal, V. A. (2017). Cerebello-thalamo-cortical networks predict positive symptom progression in individuals at ultra-high risk for psychosis. *NeuroImage. Clinical*, *14*, 622–628. doi:10.1016/j.nicl.2017.03.001 PMID:28348953

Bernhardt, J. M. (2004). Communication at the Core of Effective Public Health. *American Journal of Public Health*, *94*(2), 2051–2053. doi:10.2105/AJPH.94.12.2051 PMID:15569948

Biason-Lauber, A. (2003). Disorders of Steroid Synthesis and Metabolism. In Physician's Guide to the Laboratory Diagnosis of Metabolic Diseases. Berlin, Germany: Springer. doi:10.1007/978-3-642-55878-8_35

Biason-Lauber, A., Boscaro, M., Mantero, F., & Balercia, G. (2010). Defects of steroidogenesis. *Journal of Endocrinological Investigation, 33*(10), 756-766. doi:10.3275/6869 10.1007/bf03346683

Bickmore, T. W., Pfeifer, L. M., Byron, D., Forsythe, S., Henault, L. E., Jack, B. W., ... Paasche-Orlow, M. K. (2010). Usability of conversational agents by patients with inadequate health literacy: Evidence from two clinical trials. *Journal of Health Communication*, *15*(sup2S2), 197–210. doi:10.1080/10810730.2010.499991 PMID:20845204

Biehl, J. (2016). Patient-Citizen-Consumers: Judicialization of health and metamorphosis of biopolitics. *Lua Nova: Revista de Cultura e Política*, (98), 77-105. Doi:10.1590/0102-6445077-105/98

Biesecker, L. G. (2001). The multifaceted challenges of Proteus syndrome. *Journal of the American Medical Association*, *285*(17), 2240–2243. doi:10.1001/jama.285.17.2240 PMID:11325326

Black, A. P., & Baker, M. (2011). The impact of parent advocacy groups, the Internet, and social networking on rare diseases: The IDEA League and IDEA League United Kingdom example. *Epilepsia*, *52*(Suppl 2), 102–104. doi:10.1111/j.1528-1167.2011.03013.x PMID:21463291

Black, D. W. (2007). A review of compulsive buying disorder. *World Psychiatry; Official Journal of the World Psychiatric Association (WPA)*, *6*(1), 14–18. Retrieved from https://www.ncbi.nlm.nih.gov/pubmed/17342214 PMID:17342214

Blake, K. D., & Prasad, C. (2006). CHARGE syndrome. *Orphanet Journal of Rare Diseases*, *1*(1), 34. doi:10.1186/1750-1172-1-34 PMID:16959034

Blanch, D. C., Hall, J. A., Roter, D. L., & Frankel, R. M. (2009). Is it good to express uncertainty to a patient? Correlates and consequences for medical students in a standardized patient visit. *Patient Education and Counseling*, *76*(3), 300–306. doi:10.1016/j.pec.2009.06.002 PMID:19604663

Blom, J. D. (2016). Alice in Wonderland syndrome: A systematic review. *Neurology. Clinical Practice*, *6*(3), 259–270. doi:10.1212/CPJ.0000000000000251 PMID:27347442

Blom, R. M., van Wingen, G. A., van der Wal, S. J., Luigjes, J., van Dijk, M. T., Scholte, H. S., & Denys, D. (2016). The Desire for Amputation or Paralyzation: Evidence for Structural Brain Anomalies in Body Integrity Identity Disorder (BIID). *PLoS One*, *11*(11). doi:10.1371/journal.pone.0165789 PMID:27832097

Boat, T. F., & Field, M. J. (Eds.). (2010). *Rare Diseases and Orphan Products: Accelerating Research and Development (Vol. 2)*. Washington, DC: National Academies Press.

Boermans, J., & Egger, J. (2010). Compulsive buying or oniomania: An overview. *Tijdschrift voor Psychiatrie*, *52*, 29–39. PMID:20054795

Bopp, K. D. (2000). Information services that make patients co-producers of quality health care. In *Studies in health technology and informatics* (Vol. 76, pp. 93–106). Information Technology Strategies from the United States and the European Union; doi:10.3233/978-1-60750-920-2-93

Borhani, A. A., Wiant, A., & Heller, M. T. (2014). Cystic Hepatic Lesions: A Review and an Algorithmic Approach. *AJR. American Journal of Roentgenology*, *203*(6), 1192–1204. doi:10.2214/AJR.13.12386 PMID:25415696

Bourget, D., & Whitehurst, L. (2004). Capgras syndrome: A review of the neurophysiological correlates and presenting clinical features in cases involving physical violence. *Canadian Journal of Psychiatry*, *49*(11), 719–725. doi:10.1177/070674370404901102 PMID:15633849

Bouwman, M. G., Teunissen, Q. G. A., Wijburg, F. A., & Linthorst, G. E. (2010). 'Doctor Google' ending the diagnostic odyssey in lysosomal storage disorders: Parents using internet search engines as an efficient diagnostic strategy in rare diseases. *Archives of Disease in Childhood*, *95*(8), 642–U96. doi:10.1136/adc.2009.171827 PMID:20418338

Bowlby, J. (1971). Attachment and loss: Attachment (vol. 1). Harmandsworth: Penguin Books.

Bowlby, J. (1981). Attachment and Loss: Loss, Sadness, and Depression (Vol. 3). Middesex: Penguin Books.

Bowlby, J. (1969). Attachment and loss: Vol. 1. *Attachment*. New York: Basic Books.

Bowlby, J. (1973). *Attachment and loss: Separation, anxiety, and anger* (Vol. 2). New York: Basic Books.

Bowlby, J. (1988). *A secure base: Parent-child attachment and healthy human development*. London, UK: Basic Books.

Braga-Neto, P., Pedroso, J. L., Gadelha, A., Laureano, M. R., de Souza Noto, C., Garrido, G. J., & Barsottini, O. G. (2016). Psychosis in Machado-Joseph Disease: Clinical Correlates, Pathophysiological Discussion, and Functional Brain Imaging. Expanding the Cerebellar Cognitive Affective Syndrome. *Cerebellum 15*(40), 483-490. doi:10.100712311-015-0716-2

Brashers, D. E., Goldsmith, D. J., & Hsieh, E. (2002). Information seeking and avoiding in health contexts. *Human Communication Research*, *28*(2), 258–271. doi:10.1111/j.1468-2958.2002.tb00807.x

Brashers, D. E., Hsieh, E., Neidig, J. L., & Reynolds, N. R. (2006). Managing uncertainty about illness: Health care providers as credible authorities. In R. M. Dailey, & B. A. Le Poire (Eds.), *Applied interpersonal communication matters: Family, health, and community relations* (pp. 219–240). New York: Peter Lang.

Brashers, D. E., Neidig, J. L., & Goldsmith, D. J. (2004). Social support and the management of uncertainty for people living with HIV or AIDS. *Health Communication*, *16*(3), 305–331. doi:10.1207/S15327027HC1603_3 PMID:15265753

Brazil, K., & Krueger, P. (2002). Patterns of family adaptation to childhood asthma. *Journal of Pediatric Nursing*, *17*(3), 167–173. doi:10.1053/jpdn.2002.124110 PMID:12094358

Brismar, J., Brismar, G., Coates, R., Gascon, G., & Ozand, P. (1990). Increased density of the thalamus on CT scans in patients with GM2 gangliosidoses. *AJNR. American Journal of Neuroradiology*, *11*(1), 125–130. PMID:2105593

Brody, H. (1995). Relationship-centered care: Beyond the finishing school. *The Journal of the American Board of Family Practice*, *8*, 416–418. doi:10.3122/jabfm.8.5.416 PMID:7484233

Bronstein, M. G., & Kakkis, E. D. (2016). Patients as key partners in rare disease drug development. *Nature Reviews. Drug Discovery*, *15*(11), 731. doi:10.1038/nrd.2016.133 PMID:27444223

Bruce, J. E., Quirke, S., & Shaw, S. R. (2010). Families of children with genetic disorders. In *P. McCabe, & S. Shaw (Eds.), Genetic and acquired disorders: Current topics and interventions for educators* (pp. 59–67). Thousand Oaks, CA: Corwin.

Brunelle, R., Baradaran, N., & Keeler, S. (2016). Iliac artery endofibrosis: Case study of an elite triathlete. *Canadian Family Physician Medecin de Famille Canadien*, *62*(4), 318–e184. Retrieved from https://www.ncbi.nlm.nih.gov/pubmed/27076542 PMID:27076542

Bruni, S., Lavery, C., & Broomfield, A. (2016). The diagnostic journey of patients with mucopolysaccharidosis I: A real-world survey of patient and physician experiences. *Molecular Genetics and Metabolism Reports*, *8*, 67–73. doi:10.1016/j.ymgmr.2016.07.006 PMID:27536552

Bryman, A. (2012). *Social records methods*. New York: Oxford University Press.

Budych, K., Helms, T. M., & Schultz, C. (2012). How do patients with rare diseases experience the medical encounter? Exploring role behavior and its impact on patient–physician interaction. *Health Policy (Amsterdam)*, *105*(2-3), 154–164. doi:10.1016/j.healthpol.2012.02.018 PMID:22464590

Bull, L. N., Roche, E., Song, E. J., Pedersen, J., Knisely, A. S., van der Hagen, C. B., ... Freimer, N. B. (2000). Mapping of the Locus for Cholestasis-Lymphedema Syndrome (Aagenaes Syndrome) to a 6.6-cM Interval on Chromosome 15q. *American Journal of Human Genetics*, *67*(4), 994–999. doi:10.1086/303080 PMID:10968776

Bulmer, M. (1987). *The Social Basis of Community Care*. London, UK: Routledge.

Buntin, M. B., Jain, S. H., & Blumenthal, D. (2010). Health information technology: Laying the infrastructure for national health reform. *Health Affairs*, *29*(6), 1214–1219. doi:10.1377/hlthaff.2010.0503 PMID:20530358

Burke-Garcia, A., & Scally, G. (2014). Trending now: Future directions in digital media for the public health sector. *J. Public Health*, *36*(4), 527–534. doi:10.1093/pubmed/fdt125 PMID:24468840

Burke, K. (1969). *A rhetoric of motives*. Berkeley, CA: University of California Press.

Bury, M. (1982). Chronic illness as biographical disruption. *Sociology of Health & Illness*, *4*(2), 167–182. doi:10.1111/1467-9566.ep11339939 PMID:10260456

Byrne, P. (2009). Why psychiatrists should watch films (or What has cinema ever done for psychiatry?). *Advances in Psychiatric Treatment*, *15*(4), 286–296. doi:10.1192/apt.bp.107.005306

Cao, H., Chén, O. Y., Chung, Y., Forsyth, J. K., McEwen, S. C., Gee, D. G., & Mirzakhanian, H. (2018). Cerebello-thalamo-cortical hyperconnectivity as a state-independent functional neural signature for psychosis prediction and characterization. *Nature Communications*, *9*(1), 3836. doi:10.103841467-018-06350-7 PMID:30242220

Cape, G. (2009). Movies as a vehicle to teach addiction medicine. *International Review of Psychiatry (Abingdon, England)*, *21*(3), 213–217. doi:10.1080/09540260902747094 PMID:19459096

Cardoso, M. H. C. A. (2000). *A herança arcaica de um modelo: História, Medicina e a síndrome de Down* (Doctoral dissertation). Retrieved from Biblioteca da Saúde da Mulher e da Criança, FIOCRUZ. (000043084)

Cardoso, A., & Silva, A. P. (2010). Representing nursing knowledge on maternal and neonatal health: A study on the cultural suitability of ICNP. *International Nursing Review*, *57*(4), 426–434. doi:10.1111/j.1466-7657.2010.00829.x PMID:21050193

Carpenter, D. M., Blalock, S. J., & DeVellis, R. F. (2012). Patients with rare diseases using pharmacists for medication information. *Journal of the American Pharmaceutical Association*, *52*(6), e175–e182. doi:10.1331/JAPhA.2012.12047 PMID:23942759

Carretón Ballester, M. C., & López Villafranca, P. (2016). The impact of the Ebola Virus and rare diseases in the media and the perception of risk in Spain. *Catalan Journal of Communication & Cultural Studies*, *8*(2), 245–263. doi:10.1386/cjcs.8.2.245_1

Carroll, C. L., & Ramachandran, P. (2014). The Intelligent Use of Digital Tools and Social Media in Practice Management. *Chest*, *145*(4), 896–902. doi:10.1378/chest.13-0251 PMID:24687711

Casasús, J. M., & Núñez Ladèvèze, L. (1991). Estilo y géneros periodísticos. Barcelona, Spain: Ed. Ariel.

Cashman, C. R. (2019). Golden Ages and Silver Screens: The Construction of the Physician Hero in 1930-1940 American Cinema. *The Journal of Medical Humanities*, 1–16. doi:10.100710912-019-09554-0 PMID:30838501

Cassel, J. (1976). The contribution of the social environment to host resistance: The Fourth Wade Hampton Frost Lecture. *American Journal of Epidemiology*, *104*(2), 107–123. doi:10.1093/oxfordjournals.aje.a112281 PMID:782233

Castillo S. (2013) . Las enfermedades raras en la prensa española: una aproximación empírica desde la teoría del framing. Ambitos: *Revista internacional de comunicación*, (22), 71-80.

Castillo Sánchez, S. (2013). Las enfermedades raras en la prensa española: una aproximación empírica desde la teoría del framing. *Ambitos: Revista internacional de comunicación, 22*, 71-80.

Castillo Sánchez, S. (2012). Representación social de las enfermedades raras en la prensa española. Aposta. *Revista de Ciencias Sociales*, *54*, 1.

Castillo, S. (2012b). *Discurso visual de las enfermedades raras: encuadres latentes*. Tonos digital: Revista electrónica de estudios filológicos, 23, 1-24.

Castillo, S. S., & Mercado Sáez, M. T. (2014). El encuadre de las enfermedades raras en la prensa española. *Anuario Electrónico de Estudios en Comunicación Social, 7*(1), 104-128. Recuperado de https:// dialnet.unirioja.es/servlet/articulo?codigo=4800928 (Access date: August 13, 2019)

Castillo-Esparcia, A., & López-Villafranca, P. (2016). Communication strategies employed by rare disease patient organizations in Spain. *Ciência & Saúde Coletiva, 21*(8). Retrieved from http://www.scielo.br/scielo.php?pid=S1413-81232016000802423&script=sci_arttext&tlng=en (Access date: August 25, 2019)

Castillo-Esparcia, A., & López-Villafranca, P. (2016). Las estrategias de comunicación de las organizaciones de pacientes con enfermedades raras (ER) en España. *Ciencia & Saude Coletiva*, *21*(8), 2423–2436. doi:10.1590/1413-81232015218.19852015 PMID:27557016

Castillo, S. S. (2012a). Representación social de las enfermedades raras en la prensa española. Aposta. *Revista de Ciencias Sociales*, (54): 1–31.

Cawdron, R., & Issenman, R. (2002). Patient Web-Resource Interest and Internet Readiness in Pediatric Inflammatory Bowel Disease. *Journal of Pediatric Gastroenterology and Nutrition*, *35*(4), 518–521. doi:10.1097/00005176-200210000-00011 PMID:12394377

CDC. (2019). Hearing Loss in Children - Data & Statistics. Retrieved from https://www.cdc.gov/ncbddd/hearingloss/data.html

Center for Disease Control and Prevention - CDC. (2009). Social media at CDC. Retrieved from www.cdc.gov/socialmedia/campaigns/h1n1/#Microblogs

Centers for Disease Control and Prevention. (2019). *Health Communication. Gateway to Health Communication & Social Marketing Practice*, Centers for Disease Control and Prevention; 2019. Available at http://www.cdc.gov/healthcommunication/healthbasics/whatishc.html (Accessed August 7th 2019).

Chasset, F., Richez, C., Martin, T., Belot, A., Korganow, A.-S., & Arnaud, L. (2019). Rare diseases that mimic Systemic Lupus Erythematosus (Lupus mimickers). *Joint, Bone, Spine*, *86*(2), 165–171. doi:10.1016/j.jbspin.2018.10.007 PMID:30837156

Cho, H. (2012). *Health Communication Message Design: Theory and Practice*. Thousand Oaks, CA: Sage.

Cima, R. R., Anderson, K. J., Larson, D. W., Dozois, E. J., Hassan, I., Sandborn, W. J., ... Pemberton, J. H. (2007). Internet use by patients in an inflammatory bowel disease specialty clinic. *Inflammatory Bowel Diseases*, *13*(10), 1266–1270. doi:10.1002/ibd.20198 PMID:17567877

Cipriani, G., Lucetti, C., Vedovello, M., & Nuti, A. (2012). Diogenes syndrome in patients suffering from dementia. *Dialogues in Clinical Neuroscience*, *14*(4), 455–460. PMID:23393422

Cirlot, J. E. (2013). *A dictionary of symbols*. New York: Philosophical Library.

Clayton, M. F., Dudley, W. N., & Musters, A. (2008). Communication with breast cancer survivors. *Health Communication*, *23*(3), 207–221. doi:10.1080/10410230701808376 PMID:18569050

Cline, R. J., & Haynes, K. M. (2001). Consumer health information seeking on the Internet: The state of the art. *Health Education Research*, *16*(6), 671–692. doi:10.1093/her/16.6.671 PMID:11780707

Clinic, M. (n.d.). Crohn's disease—Symptoms and causes. Retrieved October 4, 2019, from Mayo Clinic website: https://www.mayoclinic.org/diseases-conditions/crohns-disease/symptoms-causes/syc-20353304

Cohen, J. M. (1988). Understanding Proteus syndrome, unmasking the elephant man, and stemming elephant fever. *Neurofibromatosis*, *1*(5-6), 260–280. PMID:3152479

Cohen, J. S., & Biesecker, B. B. (2010). Quality of life in rare genetic conditions: A systematic review of the literature. *American Journal of Medical Genetics. Part A*, *152*(5), 1136–1156. doi:10.1002/ajmg.a.33380 PMID:20425818

Collins, R., Finn, A., McFadyen, S., & Hoskins, C. (2001). Public service broadcasting beyond 2000: Is there a future for public service broadcasting? *Canadian Journal of Communication*, *26*(1). doi:10.22230/cjc.2001v26n1a1192

Cooper, C. P., & Roter, D. L. (2000). If it bleeds it leads"? Attributes of TV health news stories that drive viewer attention. *Public Health Reports*, *115*(4), 331–338. doi:10.1093/phr/115.4.331 PMID:11059426

Coopman, S. J. (2003). Communicating Disability: Metaphors of Oppression, *Metaphors of Empowerment. Annals of the International Communication Association*, *27*(1), 337–394. doi:10.1080/23808985.2003.11679030

Corbett, E. (2004). Classical Rhetoric. In J. Rivkin, & M. Ryan (Eds.), Literary theory, an anthology (pp. 142-161). Malden, MA: Blackwell Publishing.

Coren, S., & Girgus, J. S. (1980). Principles of perceptual organization and spatial distortion: The gestalt illusions. *Journal of Experimental Psychology. Human Perception and Performance*, *6*(3), 404–412. doi:10.1037/0096-1523.6.3.404 PMID:6447756

Coulson, N. S., Buchanan, H., & Aubeeluck, A. (2007). Social support in cyberspace: A content analysis of communication within a Huntington's disease online support group. *Patient Education and Counseling*, *68*(2), 173–178. doi:10.1016/j.pec.2007.06.002 PMID:17629440

Crawford, R. (1980). Healthism and the medicalization of everyday life. *International Journal of Health Services*, *10*(3), 365–388. doi:10.2190/3H2H-3XJN-3KAY-G9NY PMID:7419309

Cresweel, J. (2009). *Research Design: Qualitative, Quantitative, and Mixed Methods Approaches*. Thousand Oaks, CA: SAGE.

Crum-Cianflone, N. F. (2008). Bacterial, fungal, parasitic, and viral myositis. *Clinical Microbiology Reviews*, *21*(3), 473–494. doi:10.1128/CMR.00001-08 PMID:18625683

Cruz Moya, O., & Requena Romero, S. (2013). El día de las enfermedades raras en las noticias televisivas. análisis crítico de su representación audiovisual. *Discurso & Sociedad*, *7*(1), 200–223.

Cruz, O. (2005). *Parentalidade* [Parenting]. Coimbra, Portugal: Quarteto.

Czaja, A. J. (2016). Diagnosis and Management of Autoimmune Hepatitis: Current Status and Future Directions. *Gut and Liver*, *10*(2), 177–203. doi:10.5009/gnl15352 PMID:26934884

D'haeneens, L., Sousa, H., & Hultén, O. (2011). From Public Service Broadcasting to Public Service Media, In T. Josef, M. Werner, & D. Leen (Eds.), Media in Europe today, Bristol, UK: Intellect, pp. 187-197.

Da Costa, L., O'Donohue, M.-F., van Dooijeweert, B., Albrecht, K., Unal, S., Ramenghi, U., ... MacInnes, A. W. (2018). Molecular approaches to diagnose Diamond-Blackfan anemia: The EuroDBA experience. *European Journal of Medical Genetics*, *61*(11), 664–673. doi:10.1016/j.ejmg.2017.10.017 PMID:29081386

Dagli, A. I., Mueller, J., & Williams, C. A. Angelman Syndrome. (2017). In: M. P. Adam, H. H. Ardinger, R. A. Pagon, & S. E. Wallace (Eds.), *GeneReviews*. Retrieved from https://www.ncbi.nlm.nih.gov/books/NBK1144/

Damjanović, A., Vuković, O., Jovanović, A. A., & Jašović-Gašić, M. (2009). Psychiatry and movies. *Psychiatria Danubina, 21*(2), 230–235. PMID:19556954

Darwin, E., Hirt, P. A., Fertig, R., Doliner, B., Delcanto, G., & Jimenez, J. J. (2018). Alopecia Areata: Review of Epidemiology, Clinical Features, Pathogenesis, and New Treatment Options. *International Journal of Trichology, 10*(2), 51–60. doi:10.4103/ijt.ijt_99_17 PMID:29769777

Datta, V. (2009). Madness and the movies: An undergraduate module for medical students. *International Review of Psychiatry (Abingdon, England), 21*(3), 261–266. doi:10.1080/09540260902748001 PMID:19459103

Dave, S., & Tandon, K. (2011). Cinemeducation in psychiatry. *Advances in Psychiatric Treatment, 17*(4), 301–308. doi:10.1192/apt.bp.107.004945

Davies, W. (2016). Insights into rare diseases from social media surveys. *Orphanet Journal of Rare Diseases, 11*(151). doi:10.118613023-016-0532-x PMID:27829465

Davis, R. E., & Resnicow, K. (2012). The Cultural Variance Framework for Tailoring Health Messages. In H. Cho (Ed.), *Health Communication Message Design: Theory and Practice* (pp. 115–135). Thousand Oaks, CA: Sage.

Dawkins, H. J. S., Draghia-Akli, R., Lasko, P., Lau, L. P. L., Jonker, A. H., Cutillo, C. M., ... Austin, C. P. (2018). Progress in Rare Diseases Research 2010-2016: An IRDiRC Perspective. *Clinical and Translational Science, 11*(1), 11–20. doi:10.1111/cts.12501 PMID:28796411

De Fiore, L., Costantini, A., Di, M. M., Gori, S., Lorusso, D., Rosti, G., & Pinto, C. (2014). Cancer on the big screen. How and when movies deal with oncological diseases. *Recenti Progressi in Medicina, 105*(5), 198–209. doi:10.1701/1493.16455 PMID:24873943

De la Torre-Díez, I., Díaz-Pernas, F. J., & Antón-Rodríguez, M. (2012). A content analysis of chronic diseases social groups on Facebook and Twitter. *Telemedicine Journal and e-Health, 18*(6), 404–408. doi:10.1089/tmj.2011.0227 PMID:22650380

Deacon, D., Pickering, M., Golding, P., & Murdock, G. (1999). *Researching Communications: A Practical Guide to Methods in Media and Cultural Analysis*. London, UK: Hodder Education.

Debra Austria. (2013). Schmetterlingskinder. Retrieved from https://www.debra-austria.org/schmetterlingskinder/

Debra International. (2013). Epidermolysis bullosa. Retrieved from http://www.debra-international.org/what-is-eb.html

Debra International. (2016). EB awareness campaign images. Retrieved from http://www.debra-international.org/news-and-events/media-center/eb-awareness-campaign-images.html

Deik, A., & Saunders-Pullman, R. (2014). Atypical presentation of late-onset Tay-Sachs disease. *Muscle & Nerve, 49*(5), 768–771. doi:10.1002/mus.24146 PMID:24327357

Delbaere, M., McQuarrie, E. F., & Phillips, B. J. (2011). Personification in advertising. *Journal of Advertising*, *40*(1), 121–130. doi:10.2753/JOA0091-3367400108

DeLeve, L. D. (2003). Vascular liver diseases. *Current Gastroenterology Reports*, *5*(1), 63–70. doi:10.100711894-003-0011-0 PMID:12530950

DeLeve, L. D., Valla, D. C., & Garcia-Tsao, G. (2009). Vascular disorders of the liver. *Hepatology (Baltimore, Md.)*, *49*(5), 1729–1764. doi:10.1002/hep.22772 PMID:19399912

Dellve, L., Samuelsson, L., Tallborn, A., Fasth, A., & Hallberg, L. (2006). Stress and well-being among parents of children with rare diseases: A prospective intervention study. *Journal of Advanced Nursing*, *53*(4), 392–402. doi:10.1111/j.1365-2648.2006.03736.x PMID:16448482

Demakakos, P., Pillas, D., Marmot, M., & Steptoe, A. (2016). Parenting style in childhood and mortality risk at older ages: A longitudinal cohort study. *The British Journal of Psychiatry*, *211*(6), 1–7. doi:10.1192/bjp.bp.115.163543 PMID:26941265

Demily, C., & Sedel, F. (2014). Psychiatric manifestations of treatable hereditary metabolic disorders in adults. *Annals of General Psychiatry*, *13*(1), 27. doi:10.118612991-014-0027-x PMID:25478001

Denis, A., Mergaert, L., Fostier, C., Cleemput, I., & Simoens, S. (2010). A comparative study of European rare disease and orphan drug markets. *Health Policy (Amsterdam)*, *97*(2-3), 173–179. doi:10.1016/j.healthpol.2010.05.017 PMID:20800761

Derzon, J. H., & Lipsey, M. W. (2002). A Meta-Analysis of the Effectiveness of Mass-Communication for Changing Substance-use: Knowledge, Attitudes, and Behavior. In W. D. Crano, & M. Burgoon (Eds.), *Mass Media and Drug Prevention: Classic and Contemporary Theories and Research* (pp. 231–258). London, UK: Lawrence Erlbaum Associates.

Devlin, A. (2014). Wayfinding in healthcare facilities: Contributions from environmental psychology. *Behavioral Science*, *4*(4), 423–436. doi:10.3390/bs4040423 PMID:25431446

DeVrieze, B. W., & Hurley, J. A. (2019). Goodpasture Syndrome (Anti-glomerular Basement Membrane Antibody Disease). In *StatPearls*. Treasure Island, FL: StatPearls Publishing.

Dew, K., & Jutel, A. G. (2014). I am not a doctor, but…: The lay-professional relationship in diagnosis. In A. G. Jutel, & K. Dew (Eds.), *Social issues in diagnosis. Baltimore*, MD: Johns Hopkins University Press.

Díaz, E. J. (2004). La radio y el multimedia, dos alternativas para la divulgación científica. *Quark: Ciencia, medicina, comunicación y cultura*, 34, 40-49.

Diezhandino, M. P. (2002). Periodismo de Servicio. Madrid, Spain: Bosch Ed.

Dobrenova, F. V., Grabner-Kräuter, S., Diehl, S., & Terlutter, R. (2019). The use of advertising appeals in breast cancer detection messages: A web content analysis. *Women & Health*, *59*(8), 867–882. doi:10.1080/03630242.2019.1565904 PMID:30714487

Donelle, L., & Booth, R. G. (2012). Health Tweets: An Exploration of Health Promotion on Twitter. *Online Journal of Issues in Nursing*, *17*(3). doi:10.3912/OJIN.Vol17No03Man04 PMID:23036060

Donovan-Kicken, E., & Bute, J. J. (2008). Uncertainty of social network members in the case of communication-debilitating illness or injury. *Qualitative Health Research*, *18*(1), 5–18. doi:10.1177/1049732307309005 PMID:18174531

Dooms, M. M. (2016). Orphan devices: yesterday is history; tomorrow is mystery: towards a European orphan device directive? *Orphanet Journal of Rare Diseases*, *11*(1), 22. doi:10.118613023-016-0393-3 PMID:26939863

Doucet, A. (2001). You see the need perhaps more clearly than I have. *Journal of Family Issues*, *22*(3), 328–357. doi:10.1177/019251301022003004

Doyle, M. (2015). Peer support and mentorship in a US rare disease community: Findings from the cystinosis in emerging adulthood study. *The Patient-Patient-Centered Outcomes Research*, *8*(1), 65–73. doi:10.100740271-014-0085-9 PMID:25231828

Dragojlovic, N., & Lynd, L. D. (2014). Crowdfunding drug development: The state of play in oncology and rare diseases. *Drug Discovery Today*, *19*(11), 1775–1780. doi:10.1016/j.drudis.2014.06.019 PMID:24973645

Dulac, G. (2001). Les stéréotypes sociaux sur les rôles et l'implication des pères dans les services à la famille. *Défi Jeunesse*, *7*(2), 26–32.

Dutta, M. J. (2008). *Communicating Health: A Culture-Centered Approach*. Malden, MA: Policy.

Dwyer, A. A., Quinton, R., Morin, D., & Pitteloud, N. (2014). Identifying the unmet health needs of patients with congenital hypogonadotropic hypogonadism using a web-based needs assessment: Implications for online interventions and peer-to-peer support. *Orphanet Journal of Rare Diseases*, *9*(1), 83. doi:10.1186/1750-1172-9-83 PMID:24915927

Dykens, E. M. (2013). Aging in rare intellectual disability syndromes. *Developmental Disabilities Research Reviews*, *18*(1), 75–83. doi:10.1002/ddrr.1130 PMID:23949831

Dysart-Gale, D. (2010). Techne, technology, and disenchantment in the wind in The Wind in the Willows. In J. C. Horne, & D. R. White (Eds.), *Kenneth Grahame's the wind in the willows: A children's classic at 100*. Lanham, MD: Scarecrow Press.

Eagly, A. H., & Chaiken, S. (1993). *The Psychology of Attitudes*. Orlando, FL: Harcourt Brace Jovanovich College Publishers.

EASL Clinical Practice Guidelines. (2012). EASL Clinical Practice Guidelines: Wilson's disease. *Journal of Hepatology*, *56*(3), 671–685. doi:10.1016/j.jhep.2011.11.007 PMID:22340672

EASL Clinical Practice Guidelines. (2015). EASL Clinical Practice Guidelines: Autoimmune hepatitis. *Journal of Hepatology*, *63*(4), 971–1004. doi:10.1016/j.jhep.2015.06.030 PMID:26341719

EASL Clinical Practice Guidelines. (2016). Vascular diseases of the liver. *Journal of Hepatology*, *64*(1), 179–202. doi:10.1016/j.jhep.2015.07.040 PMID:26516032

Eggly, S., Penner, L. A., Greene, M., Harper, F. W. K., Ruckdeschel, J. C., & Albrecht, T. L. (2006). Information seeking during "bad news" oncology interactions: Question asking by patients and their companions. *Social Science & Medicine*, *63*(11), 2974–2985. doi:10.1016/j.socscimed.2006.07.012 PMID:16962218

Eleftheriou-Smith, L.-M. (2014). Rankin's blurred photos show what it's like to suffer from Ataxia. Retrieved from https://www.campaignlive.co.uk/article/rankins-blurred-photos-show-its-suffer-ataxia/1289566

Emerich, T. B., Cavaca, A. G., Santos-Neto, E. T., Gentilli, V. I., & Oliveira, A. E. (2017). Media valuations of health journalism and health dynamics in brazilian print media. *International Journal of Social Science Studies*, *5*(1), 31–42. doi:10.11114/ijsss.v5i1.1997

Engel, P. A., Bagal, S., Broback, M., & Boice, N. (2013). Physician and patient perceptions regarding training in rare diseases: The need for stronger educational initiatives for physicians. *The Journal of Rare Disorders*, *1*(2), 1–15. Retrieved from http://www.journalofraredisorders.com/Interface/errors/404.html?aspxerrorpath=/pub/IssuePDFs/Engel.pdf

Epstein, S. (1995). The construction of lay expertise: AIDS activism and the forging of credibility in the reform of clinical trials. *Science, Technology, & Human Values*, *20*(4), 408–437. doi:10.1177/016224399502000402 PMID:11653331

Epstein, S. (1996). *Impure science. AIDS, activism, and the politics of knowledge*. Berkley, CA: University of California Press.

Erikainen, S., Pickersgill, M., Cunningham-Burley, S., & Chan, S. (2019). Patienthood and participation in the digital era. *Digital Health*, *5*. doi:10.1177/2055207619845546 PMID:31041112

ESB. (2019). On Thursday, February 28, 2019, The Empire State Building will be lit Green, Pink, Light Blue, and Purple in honor of Rocket Pharm & Rare Disease Day. Retrieved from https://www.esbnyc.com/tower-lighting-2019-02-28-000000

Escobar Pérez, L., Ávalos Sandoval, P., & Medeiros, M. (2018). Espacios digitales y enfermedades raras. *Revista Digital Universitaria*, 19(5).

Espinosa, P. S., Smith, C. D., & Berger, J. R. (2006). Alien hand syndrome. *Neurology*, *67*(12), E21. doi:10.1212/01.wnl.0000249303.88754.48 PMID:17190927

Essex-Lopresti, M. (1998). The medical film 1897-1997: Part I. The first half-century. *The Journal of Audiovisual Media in Medicine*, *21*(1), 7–12. doi:10.3109/17453059609063115 PMID:9764516

Estevez Jimenez, P., & Terrón Blanco, J. L. (2011). El diseño de campañas sobre el ictus y su evaluación. Una revisión de 10 años de literatura científica (1999-2009). *Observatorio (OBS*)*, *5*(1), 123- 156. doi:10.15847/obsOBS512011410

Eurodis. (2017). What is a rare disease – Fact Sheet. Retrieved from https://www.eurordis.org/sites/default/files/publications/Fact_Sheet_RD.pdf

European Commission. (2011). Media Use in The European Union [Report]. Standard Eurobarometer 76/Autumn 2011. Retrieved from https://ec.europa.eu/commfrontoffice/publicopinion/archives/eb/eb76/eb76_media_en.pdf [Access date: Aug 20th, 2019]

EURORDIS - *European Organization for Rare Diseases.* (2018). *The voice of RARE DISEASE PATIENTS in Europe* [PDF file]. Retrieved from https://www.eurordis.org/publication/eurordis-leaflet

EURORDIS. (2005). Rare Diseases: Understanding this Public Health Priority.

EURORDIS. (2019). Rare Diseases Europe - The Voice of Rare Disease Patients in Europe. Retrieved from https://www.eurordis.org/about-rare-diseases

Eysenbach, G. (2008). *Credibility of health information and digital media: New perspectives and implications for youth.* Digital media, youth, and credibility, 123-154.

Eysenbach, G. (2001). What is e-health? *Journal of Medical Internet Research, 3*(2), e20. doi:10.2196/jmir.3.2.e20 PMID:11720962

Eysenbach, G. (2008). Medicine 2.0: Social networking, collaboration, participation, apomediation, and openness. *Journal of Medical Internet Research, 10*(3), e22. doi:10.2196/jmir.1030 PMID:18725354

Fahy, T. A. (1989). Lycanthropy: A review. *Journal of the Royal Society of Medicine, 82*(1), 37–39. doi:10.1177/014107688908200115 PMID:2647981

Farmer, A. D., Bruckner Holt, C. E., Cook, M. J., & Hearing, S. D. (2009). Social networking sites: A novel portal for communication. *Postgraduate Medical Journal, 85*(1007), 455–459. doi:10.1136/pgmj.2008.074674 PMID:19734511

Farmer, J., Marien, W., Clark, M., Sherman, A., & Selva, T. (2004). Primary care supports for children with chronic health conditions: Identifying and predicting unmet family needs. *Journal of Pediatric Psychology, 29*(5), 355–367. doi:10.1093/jpepsy/jsh039 PMID:15187174

FEDER – Federacíon Española de Enfermedades Raras. (2018). ¿Qué son las enfermedades raras o poco frecuentes? Retrieved from https://enfermedades-raras.org/index.php/enfermedades-raras (Access date: August 13, 2019)

FEDER – Federacíon Española de Enfermedades Raras. (2018, March). *ASHUA se suma al Día Mundual de las ER.* Retrieved from https://enfermedades-raras.org/index.php?option=com_content&view=article&id=10200 (Access date: August 13, 2019)

FEDER – Federacíon Española de Enfermedades Raras. (2018a). *¿Qué son las enfermedades raras o poco frecuentes?* Retrieved from https://enfermedades-raras.org/index.php/enfermedades-raras (Access date: August 13, 2019)

FEDER – Federacíon Española de Enfermedades Raras. (2018b). *Las Enfermedades Raras em cifras*. Retrieved from https://enfermedades-raras.org/index.php/enfermedades-raras/enfermedades-raras-en-cifras (Access date: August 13, 2019)

Fei, V. L. (2007). The visual semantics stratum: making meaning in sequential images. In T. D. Royce, & W. L. Bowcher (Eds.), *New directions in the analysis of multimodal discourse* (pp. 195–213). Mahwah, NJ: Lawrence Erlbaum.

Ferguson, C., Inglis, S. C., Newton, P. J., Cripps, P. J. S., MacDonald, P. S., & Davidson, P. M. (2014). Social media: A tool to spread information: a case study analysis of twitter conversation at the Cardiac Society of Australia & New Zealand 61st annual scientific meeting 2013. *Collegian (Royal College of Nursing, Australia)*, *21*(2), 89–93. doi:10.1016/j.colegn.2014.03.002 PMID:25109206

Fernandes Filho, J. A., & Shapiro, B. E. (2004). Tay - Sachs disease. *Archives of Neurology*, *61*(9), 1466. doi:10.1001/archneur.61.9.1466 PMID:15364698

Fernandes, I. (2011*). The Elephant Man (1980) by David Lynch: from 'freak' and clinical case to allegory. Cine Qua Non - Bilingual Arts Magazine, #9*. Lisboa, Portugal: CEAUL. 2015. 54-75. Retrieved from http://hdl.handle.net/10451/29473 (Access date: August 13, 2019)

Fernández-Alonso, I., & Fernández-Viso, A. (2012). Internal pluralism in the governance of public service broadcasters in Spain and the role of social groups and professionals. The case of RTVE. Vol XXV, Nr. 2, 203-230.

Ferreira, C. R., & Gah, W. A. (2017). Lysosomal storage diseases. Translational science of rare diseases. 2(1-2): 1-71. doi:. doi:10.3233/TRD-160005

Ferreira, C., & Mota, C. P. (2018). *Vinculação aos pais, parentalidade e estratégias de coping na vivência de pais de filhos com doenças raras*. [Parental attachment, parenting and coping strategies in the experience of parents of children with rare diseases]. Poster presented at *4.º Congresso da Ordem dos Psicólogos Portugueses*, September 12-15, 2018, Braga, Portugal.

Ferreira, C., & Mota, C. P. (2019). *Parentalidade e coping na vivência de pais com filhos com doenças raras: papel mediador da regulação emocional.* [Parenting and coping in the experience of parents with children with rare diseases: Mediating role of emotional regulation]. Oral Communication at table #8 "Intervenção em situações de doença crónica e hospitalização" at the X Congresso Internacional de Psicologia da Criança e do Adolescente - "Psicoterapia e outras abordagens terapêuticas", April 10-11, 2019 at Universidade Lusíada de Lisboa, Portugal.

Fiordelli, M., Diviani, N., & Schulz, P. J. (2013). Mapping mHealth research: A decade of evolution. *Journal of Medical Internet Research*, *15*(5), e95. doi:10.2196/jmir.2430 PMID:23697600

Fishbein, M., & Ajzen, I. (1975). *Belief, Attitude, Intention, and Behavior: An Introduction to Theory and Research*. Longman: Addison Wesley.

Fonseca, R. V. G. (2014). *A construção de uma Política Pública para doenças raras no Brasil* (Undergraduate degree dissertation). Retrieved from Biblioteca Digital da Produção Intelectual Discente. Retrieved from http://bdm.unb.br/handle/10483/8182

Forman, J., Taruscio, D., Llera, V. A., Barrera, L. A., Coté, T. R., Edfjäll, C., ... Tambuyzer, E. (2012). The need for worldwide policy and action plans for rare diseases. *Acta Paediatrica (Oslo, Norway)*, *101*(8), 805–807. doi:10.1111/j.1651-2227.2012.02705.x PMID:22519914

Fornieles, J., & Bañón, A. M. (2011). Análisis del discurso multimodal: las fotografías en la información sobre Enfermedades Raras. In A. M. Bañón & ... (Eds.), *Desafíos y estrategias comunicativas de las enfermedades raras: la investigación médica como referente* (pp. 189–200). Valencia, Spain: CIBERER.

Fotaki, M. (2011). Towards developing new partnerships in public services: Users as consumers, citizens and/or co-producers in health and social care in England and Sweden. *Public Administration*, *89*(3), 933–955. doi:10.1111/j.1467-9299.2010.01879.x PMID:22165151

Fox, S., & Duggan, M. (2013, January 15). Health Online 2013. Retrieved November 24, 2019, from Pew Research Center: Internet, Science, & Tech website: https://www.pewresearch.org/internet/2013/01/15/health-online-2013/

Fox, S., & Jones, S. (2009). The social life of health information. Retrieved from www.pewinternet.org/Reports/2009/8-The-Social-Life-of-Health-Information.aspx

Francescutti, L. P., Martínez Nicolás, M., & Tucho Fernández, F. (2012). *La información sanitaria en los telediarios*. Madrid, Spain: Almud Ediciones.

Frank, A. (1998). *The Wounded Storyteller: Body, Illness, and Ethics*. Chicago, IL: University of Chicago Press.

Freeman, B., & Chapman, S. (2007). Is YouTube telling or selling you something? Tobacco content on the video-sharing website YouTube. *Tobacco Control*, *16*(3), 207–210. doi:10.1136/tc.2007.020024 PMID:17565142

Freidson, E. (1960). Client Control and Medical Practice. *American Journal of Sociology*, *65*, 374–382. doi:10.1086/222726

Freimuth, V., Linnan, H. W., & Potter, P. (2000). Communicating the Threat of Emerging Infections to the Public. *Emerging Infectious Diseases*, *6*(4), 337–374. doi:10.3201/eid0604.000403 PMID:10905966

Fricker, Z. P., & Lichtenstein, D. R. (2019). Primary Sclerosing Cholangitis: A Concise Review of Diagnosis and Management. *Digestive Diseases and Sciences*, *64*(3), 632–642. doi:10.100710620-019-05484-y PMID:30725292

Frohlich, D. O. (2016). The Social Construction of Inflammatory Bowel Disease Using Social Media Technologies. *Health Communication*, *31*(11), 1412–1420. doi:10.1080/10410236.2015.1077690 PMID:27050670

Frossard, V. C., & Dias, M. C. M. (2016). O impacto da internet na interação entre pacientes: Novos cenários em saúde. *Interface (Botucatu)*, *20*(57), 349–361. doi:10.1590/1807-57622014.1334

Fumeo, M., Manfredi, S., & Volta, A. (2019). Emphysematous cystitis: review of current literature, diagnosis and management challenges. Veterinary medicine (Auckland, NZ), 10, 77-83. doi:10.2147/VMRR.S210463

Gabbard, G. (2001). Psychotherapy in Hollywood cinema. *Australasian Psychiatry*, *9*(4), 365–369. doi:10.1046/j.1440-1665.2001.00365.x

Gabbard, G., & Gabbard, K. (1999). *Psychiatry and the Cinema* (2nd ed.). Washington, DC: American Psychiatric Press.

Gaither, R., Bingen, K., & Hopkins, J. (2000). When the bough breaks: The relationship between chronic illness in children and couple functioning. In K. Schmaling, & T. Sher (Eds.), *The Psychology of Couples and Illness: Theory, Research, & Practice* (pp. 337–365). Washington, DC: American Psychological Association. doi:10.1037/10360-012

Gajaria, A., Yeung, E., Goodale, T., & Charach, A. (2011). Beliefs about attention-deficit/hyperactivity disorder and response to stereotypes: Youth postings in Facebook groups. *The Journal of Adolescent Health*, *49*(1), 15–20. doi:10.1016/j.jadohealth.2010.09.004 PMID:21700151

Gao, X., Li, B., Chu, W., Sun, X., & Sun, C. (2016). Alien hand syndrome following corpus callosum infarction: A case report and review of the literature. *Experimental and Therapeutic Medicine*, *12*(4), 2129–2135. doi:10.3892/etm.2016.3608 PMID:27698701

Gass, R. H., & Seiter, J. S. (2010). *Persuasion, social influence, and compliance gaining*. Boston, MA: Allyn & Bacon.

Gates, G. A. (2006). Ménière's Disease Review 2005. *Journal of the American Academy of Audiology*, *17*(1), 16–26. doi:10.3766/jaaa.17.1.3 PMID:16640057

Gaucher Disease News. (2019). Patients, Family and Friends to Take Part in Variety of Rare Disease Day Events Worldwide. Retrieved from https://gaucherdiseasenews.com/2019/02/11/rare-disease-day-marked-by-events-worldwde/

Genetics Home Reference, N. (2019a). Alport syndrome. Retrieved from https://ghr.nlm.nih.gov/condition/alport-syndrome#sourcesforpage

Genetics Home Reference, N. (2019b). Donnai-Barrow syndrome. Retrieved from https://ghr.nlm.nih.gov/condition/donnai-barrow-syndrome

Genetics Home Reference, N. (2019c). Keratitis-ichthyosis-deafness syndrome. Retrieved from https://ghr.nlm.nih.gov/condition/keratitis-ichthyosis-deafness-syndrome

Germain, D. P. (2010). Fabry disease. *Orphanet Journal of Rare Diseases*, *5*(1), 30. doi:10.1186/1750-1172-5-30 PMID:21092187

Giarelli, G., & Venneri, E. (2009). *Sociologia della salute e della medicina*. Milano, Italy: Franco Angeli.

Gilbert, A. C. B. (2012). *Vértice do Impensável. Um estudo de narrativas em síndrome de Down*. Rio de Janeiro, Brazil: Editora Fiocruz. doi:10.7476/9788575415726

Gilbert, W. (1978). Why genes in pieces? *Nature*, *271*(5645), 501. doi:10.1038/271501a0 PMID:622185

Gill, P., Arlitt, M., Li, Z., & Mahanti, A. (2007). YouTube Traffic Characterization: A View from the Edge. IMC of the 7th ACM SIGCOMM Conference on Internet Measurement; Oct. 24–26, 2007, San Diego, CA. Retrieved from https://pages.cpsc.ucalgary.ca/~zongpeng/publications/imc07.pdf

Gilman, S. L. (1988). *Disease and representation: Images of illness from madness to AIDS*. Ithaca, NY: Cornell University Press.

Giugliani, R., Vairo, F. P., Riegel, M., de Souza, C. F., Schwartz, I. V., & Pena, S. D. (2016). Rare disease landscape in Brazil: Report of a successful experience in inborn errors of metabolism. *Orphanet Journal of Rare Diseases*, *11*(1), 76. doi:10.118613023-016-0458-3 PMID:27282290

Gkiouzepas, L., & Hogg, M. K. (2011). Articulating a new framework for visual metaphors in advertising. *Journal of Advertising*, *40*(1), 103–120. doi:10.2753/JOA0091-3367400107

Glanz, K., Rimer, B. K., & Viswanath, K. (Eds.). (2002). *Health Behavior and Health Education: Theory, Research, and Practice* (3rd ed.). San Francisco, CA: John Wiley & Sons.

Glenn, A. D. (2015). Using online health communication to manage chronic sorrow: Mothers of children with rare diseases speak. *Journal of Pediatric Nursing*, *30*(1), 17–24. doi:10.1016/j.pedn.2014.09.013 PMID:25316198

Góes, F. A. D. B. (2006). Um encontro inesperado: Os pais e seu filho com deficiência mental. [An unexpected encounter: Parents and their mentally disabled child]. *Psicologia: Ciência e Profissão*, *26*(3), 450–461. doi:10.1590/S1414-98932006000300009

Gohn, M. G. (2011). Movimentos sociais na contemporaneidade. *Revista Brasileira de Educação*, *16*(47), 333–361. doi:10.1590/S1413-24782011000200005

González-Blasco, P., Delgado-Marroquín, M. T., Moreto, G., & Altisent, R. (2019). Vocación y profesionalismo: Reflexiones de los estudiantes catalizadas por el cine de Spielberg. *Educación Médica*, *20*(4), 249–255. doi:10.1016/j.edumed.2018.10.001

González-Lamuño, D., & García, M. F. (2008). Enfermedades raras en pediatría. [Gobierno de Navarra: Departamento de Salud.]. *Anales del Sistema Sanitario de Navarra*, *31*, 21–29. doi:10.4321/S1137-66272008000400003 PMID:18953370

González-Pacanowski, T., & Medina-Aguerrebere, P. (2011). Blogs para pacientes como nueva fuente de información de salud. *El Profesional de la Información*, *20*(6), 652–658. doi:10.3145/epi.2011.nov.08

Goodwin, J., Jasper, J. M., & Polletta, F. (2001). Introduction: why emotions matter. In J. Goodwin, J. M. Jasper, & F. Polletta (Eds.), *Passionate Politics. Emotions and social movements* (pp. 1–24). Chicago, IL: The University of Chicago Press. doi:10.7208/chicago/9780226304007.003.0001

Gordon, G. H., Joos, S. K., & Byrne, J. (2000). Physician expressions of uncertainty during patient encounters. *Patient Education and Counseling*, *40*(1), 59–65. doi:10.1016/S0738-3991(99)00069-5 PMID:10705065

Graham, H. (1991). The concept of caring in feminist research: The case of domestic service. *Sociology*, *25*(1), 61–78. doi:10.1177/0038038591025001004

Gravholt, C. H., Andersen, N. H., Conway, G. S., Dekkers, O. M., Geffner, M. E., Klein, K. O., ... International Turner Syndrome Consensus, G. (2007a). Clinical Practice Guidelines for the Care of Girls and Women with Turner Syndrome [TS]: Brief Synopsis for Turner Syndrome Girls and Women and for their Parents/Caregivers/Families. *European Journal of Endocrinology, 177*, G1-G70. Retrieved from http://www.eje-online.org/content/177/3/G1.full.pdf+html

Gravholt, C. H., Andersen, N. H., Conway, G. S., Dekkers, O. M., Geffner, M. E., Klein, K. O., ... International Turner Syndrome Consensus, G. (2007b). Clinical practice guidelines for the care of girls and women with Turner syndrome: Proceedings from the 2016 Cincinnati International Turner Syndrome Meeting. *European Journal of Endocrinology, 177*(3), G1-G70. doi:10.1530/EJE-17-0430

Gray, C. (2011). Social media: A guide for researchers. Research Information Network. Retrieved from www.rin.ac.uk/our-work/communicating-and-disseminating-research/social-media-guide-researchers

Gray, D. E. (2003). Gender and coping: The parents of children with high functioning autism. *Social Science & Medicine*, *56*(3), 631–642. doi:10.1016/S0277-9536(02)00059-X PMID:12570979

Greene, J. A., Choudhry, N. K., Kilabuk, E., & Shrank, W. H. (2011). Online social networking by patients with diabetes: A qualitative evaluation of communication with Facebook. *Journal of General Internal Medicine*, *26*(3), 287–292. doi:10.100711606-010-1526-3 PMID:20945113

Greene, J. A., & Podolsky, S. H. (2012). Reform, regulation, and pharmaceuticals – the Kefauver-Harris Amendments at 50. *The New England Journal of Medicine*, *367*(16), 1481–1482. doi:10.1056/NEJMp1210007 PMID:23075174

Greenfield, S., Kaplan, S., & Ware, J. E. (1985). Expanding patient involvement in care. Effects on patient outcomes. *Annals of Internal Medicine*, *102*(4), 520–528. doi:10.7326/0003-4819-102-4-520 PMID:3977198

Griffith, G. M., Hastings, R. P., Nash, S., Petalas, M., Oliver, C., Howlin, P., ... Tunnicliffe, P. (2011). "You have to sit and explain it all, and explain yourself." Mothers' experiences of support services for their offspring with a rare genetic intellectual disability syndrome. *Journal of Genetic Counseling*, *20*(2), 165–177. doi:10.100710897-010-9339-4 PMID:21203808

Grunig, J., & Hunt, T. (1984). *Managing public relations*. New York, NY: CBS College Publishing.

Grushka, K. (2009). Meaning and identities: A visual performative pedagogy for socio-cultural learning. *Curriculum Journal, 20*(3), 237–251. doi:10.1080/09585170903195860

Gumpert, G., & Cathcart, R. (1985). Media grammars, generations, and media gaps. *Critical Studies in Media Communication, 2*(1), 23–35. doi:10.1080/15295038509360059

Gundersen, T. (2011). 'One wants to know what a chromosome is': The internet as a coping resource when adjusting to life parenting a child with a rare genetic disorder. *Sociology of Health & Illness, 33*(1), 81–95. doi:10.1111/j.1467-9566.2010.01277.x PMID:20937053

Guo, L., Reich, J., Groshek, J., & Farraye, F. A. (2016). Social Media Use in Patients with Inflammatory Bowel Disease. *Inflammatory Bowel Diseases, 22*(5), 1231–1238. doi:10.1097/MIB.0000000000000713 PMID:26894839

Gupta, S., & Riis, J. (2011). *Patientslikeme: An online community of patients.* Harvard Business School Marketing Unit Case, (511-093).

Hacking, I. (1999). *The social construction of what?* Cambridge, MA: Harvard University Press.

Hackworth, B. A., & Kunz, M. B. (2011). Health care and social media: Building relationships via social networks. *Academy of Health Care Management Journal, 7*(2), 1.

Hale, J. L., & Dillard, J. P. (1995). Fear Appeals in Health Promotion Campaigns: Too Much, Too Little, or Just Right? In E. Maibach, & R. L. Parrott (Eds.), *Designing Health Messages: Approaches from Communication Theory and Public Health Practice* (pp. 65–80). Thousand Oaks, CA: Sage. doi:10.4135/9781452233451.n4

Hallin, D., & Mancini, P. (2004). *Comparing media systems: Three models of media and politics.* Cambridge, UK: Cambridge University Press. doi:10.1017/CBO9780511790867

Hall, S. (1973). *Encoding and decoding in the media discourse. Stencilled Paper 7.* Birmingham: CCCS.

Hall, S. (1980). Encoding/decoding. In D. Hobson, A. Lowe, & P. Willis (Eds.), *Culture, media, language* (pp. 128–138). London, UK: Hutchinson.

Han, B. (2017). *Sociedade da transparência* (E. P. Giachini, Trans.). Petrópolis, Brazil: Editora Vozes. (Original work published 2012)

Hand, S. S. (2010). *Finishing the mysteries of gods and symbols* (Vol. 0, p. II). Lawrence, W.

Harrison, C. (2003). Visual social semiotics: Understanding how still images make meaning. *Technical Communication (Washington), 50*(1), 46–60.

Harrison, J., & Woods, L. M. (2001). Defining European public service broadcasting. *European Journal of Communication, 16*(4), 477–504. doi:10.1177/0267323101016004003

Hartley, J. (2012). Designing Easy-to-Read Text. In Writing Health Communication: An Evidence-Based Guide (pp. 7–22). doi:10.4135/9781446288054.n2

Harwood, J., & Giles, H. (2005). *Intergroup Communication: Multiple Perspectives*. New York: Peter Lang.

Hashim, M. J., Alkaabi, M. S. K. M., & Bharwani, S. (2014). Interpretation of way-finding healthcare symbols by a multicultural population: Navigation signage design for global health. *Applied Ergonomics*, *45*(3), 503–509. doi:10.1016/j.apergo.2013.07.002 PMID:23932379

Hass, B. H. (2006). Content Management – Inhalte für Neue Medien strategisch nutzen. In C. Scholz (Ed.), *Handbuch Medienmanagement* (pp. 375–391). Berlin, Germany: Springer. doi:10.1007/3-540-32879-3_18

Hawkins, J. D., Brown, E. C., Oesterle, S., Arthur, M. W., Abbott, R. D., & Catalano, R. F. (2008). Early Effects of Communities That Care on targeted risks and intention of delinquent behavior and substance use. *The Journal of Adolescent Health*, *43*(1), 15–22. doi:10.1016/j.jadohealth.2008.01.022 PMID:18565433

Hawn, C. (2009). Take two aspirin and tweet me in the morning: How Twitter, Facebook, and other social media are reshaping health care. *Health Affairs*, *28*(2), 361–368. doi:10.1377/hlthaff.28.2.361 PMID:19275991

Hazan, C., & Shaver, P. (1987). Romantic love conceptualized as an attachment process. *Journal of Personality and Social Psychology*, *52*(3), 511–524. doi:10.1037/0022-3514.52.3.511 PMID:3572722

Heath, R., Franklin, D., & Strasberg, D. (1979). Gross pathology of the cerebellum in patients diagnosed and treated as functional psychiatric disorders. *The Journal of Nervous and Mental Disease*, *167*(1), 585–592. doi:10.1097/00005053-197910000-00001 PMID:573778

Hechtman, P., & Kaplan, F. (1993). Tay–Sachs Disease Screening and Diagnosis: Evolving Technologies. *DNA and Cell Biology*, *12*(8), 651–665. doi:10.1089/dna.1993.12.651 PMID:8397824

Helman, C. G. (2009). *Cultura, Saúde e Doença* (5th ed.). (A. B. Bolner, Trans.). Porto Alegre, Brazil: Artmed. (Original work published 2007)

Hendy, D. (2013). *Public service broadcasting*. Hampshire: Andrew Crisell. doi:10.1007/978-1-137-32898-4

Héon-Klin, V. (2017). European Reference networks for rare diseases: What is the conceptual framework? *Orphanet Journal of Rare Diseases*, *12*(1), 137. doi:10.118613023-017-0676-3 PMID:28784158

Hernández, A. M., Fornieles Alcaraz, J., Solves Almela, J. A., & Rius Sanchis, I. (2012). (Coords.) Desafíos y estrategias comunicativas de las enfermedades raras: la investigación médica como referente: estudio cuantitativo-discursivo de la prensa escrita impresa y digital española (2009-2010). Valencia, Spain: Centro de Investigación Biomédica em Red de Enfermedades Raras (CIBERER).

Hernandez, B. A. (2018). Neurophysiological and Images Studies in a Case of Foreign Accent Syndrome Secondary to Multiple Sclerosis. *Journal of Neurology and Neuroscience, 09*(01). doi:10.21767/2171-6625.1000240

Hesse, B. W., Nelson, D. E., Kreps, G. L., Croyle, R. T., Arora, N. K., Rimer, B. K., & Viswanath, K. (2005). Trust and Sources of Health Information: The Impact of the Internet and Its Implications for Health Care Providers – Findings from the First Health Information National Trends Survey. *JAMA Internal Medicine, 165*(22), 2618–2624. doi:10.1001/archinte.165.22.2618 PMID:16344419

Hesselgrave, B. L. (2003). Helping to manage the high cost of rare diseases. *Managed Care Quarterly, 11*(1), 1–6. PMID:12790059

Hilton-Kamm, D., Sklansky, M., & Chang, R. K. (2014). How not to tell parents about their child's new diagnosis of congenital heart disease: An internet survey of 841 parents. *Pediatric Cardiology, 35*(2), 239–252. doi:10.100700246-013-0765-6 PMID:23925415

Hodgkin, P. (1985). Medicine is war: And other medical metaphors. *British Medical Journal, 291*(6511), 1820–1821. doi:10.1136/bmj.291.6511.1820 PMID:3936590

Hoghughi, M. (2004). Parenting: an introduction. In M. Hoghughi, & N. Long (Eds.), *Theory and research for practice* (pp. 1–18). Handbook of parenting London, UK: Sage.

Hollenbach, J. A., & Oksenberg, J. R. (2015). The immunogenetics of multiple sclerosis: A comprehensive review. *Journal of Autoimmunity, 64*, 13–25. doi:10.1016/j.jaut.2015.06.010 PMID:26142251

Holmström, I., & Röing, M. (2010). The relation between patient-centeredness and patient empowerment: A discussion on concepts. *Patient Education and Counseling, 79*(2), 167–172. doi:10.1016/j.pec.2009.08.008 PMID:19748203

Holtzman, N. A., Bernhardt, B. A., Mountcastle-Shah, E., Rodgers, J. E., Tambor, E., & Geller, G. (2005). The quality of media reports on discoveries related to human genetic diseases. *Public Health Genomics, 8*(3), 133–144. doi:10.1159/000086756 PMID:16113530

Hortin, J. (1994). Theoretical Foundations of Visual Learning. In D. Moore, & F. M. Dwyer (Eds.), *Visual Literacy: A Spectrum of Visual Learning*. Englewood Cliffs, NJ: Educational Technology Publications.

Hou, J., & Shim, M. (2010). The role of provider–patient communication and trust in online sources in Internet use for health-related activities. *Journal of Health Communication, 15*(sup3), 186-199. Doi:10.1080/10810730.2010.522691

House, J. S. (1981). *Work stress and social support*. Reading, MA: Addison-Wesley.

Hovland, C. I., Janis, I. L., & Kelley, H. H. (1953). *Communication and Persuasion: Psychological studies of opinion change. Yale.* Yale University Press.

Hrastelj, J., & Robertson, N. P. (2016). Ice bucket challenge bears fruit for amyotrophic lateral sclerosis. *Journal of Neurology*, *263*(11), 2355–2357. doi:10.100700415-016-8297-7 PMID:27734164

Huck, J. H. J., Verhoeven, N. M., Struys, E. A., Salomons, G. S., Jakobs, C., & van der Knaap, M. S. (2004). Ribose-5-Phosphate Isomerase Deficiency: New Inborn Error in the Pentose Phosphate Pathway Associated with a Slowly Progressive Leukoencephalopathy. *American Journal of Human Genetics*, *74*(4), 745–751. doi:10.1086/383204 PMID:14988808

Hunter, D. J. (2005). Gene–environment interactions in human diseases. *Nature Reviews. Genetics*, *6*(4), 287–298. doi:10.1038/nrg1578 PMID:15803198

Huyard, C. (2009). What, if anything, is specific about having a rare disorder? Patients' judgements on being ill and being rare. *Health Expectations*, *12*(4), 361–370. doi:10.1111/j.1369-7625.2009.00552.x PMID:19840131

Huyard, C. (2009). Who rules rare disease associations? A framework to understand their action. *Sociology of Health & Illness*, *31*(7), 979–993. doi:10.1111/j.1467-9566.2009.01177.x PMID:19619152

Huyard, C. (2009a). How did uncommon disorders become 'rare diseases'? History of a boundary object. *Sociology of Health & Illness*, *31*(4), 463–477. doi:10.1111/j.1467-9566.2008.01143.x PMID:19397760

Huyard, C. (2011a). Quand la puissance publique fait surgir et équipe une mobilisation protestaire. *Revue Francaise de Science Politique*, *61*(2), 183–200. doi:10.3917/rfsp.612.0183

Huyard, C. (2011b). Porquoi s'associer? Quatre motifs d'entrée dans um collectif dans les associations de maladies rares. *Revue Francaise de Sociologie*, *52*(4), 719–745. doi:10.3917/rfs.524.0719

Hyler, S. E., & Moore, J. (1996). Teaching Psychiatry? Let Hollywood Help! *Academic Psychiatry*, *20*(4), 212–219. doi:10.1007/BF03341883 PMID:24442743

Impicciatore, P., Pandolfini, C., Casella, N., & Bonati, M. (1997). Reliability of health information for the public on the World Wide Web: Systematic survey of advice on managing fever in children at home. *BMJ (Clinical Research Ed.)*, *314*(7098), 1875. doi:10.1136/bmj.314.7098.1875 PMID:9224132

Ingelfinger, J. R., & Drazen, J. M. (2011). Patient organizations and research on rare diseases. *The New England Journal of Medicine*, *364*(17), 1670–1671. doi:10.1056/NEJMe1102290 PMID:21410388

Isles, R. (2015). Dundee Scientists on road to cure for "Butterfly Children" condition. Retrieved from http://app.dundee.ac.uk/pressreleases/prmay05/butterfly.html

Iulini, B., Costassa, E. V., Corona, C., Meloni, D., Favole, A., Mazza, M., . . . Casalone, C. (2017). Classical and Atypical Bovine Spongiform Encephalopathy: Epidemiology, Pathogenesis and Diagnosis. In Prion - An Overview. Edited by Yusuf Tutar. doi: . Retrieved from https://www.intechopen.com/books/prion-an-overview/classical-and-atypical-bovine-spongiform-encephalopathy-epidemiology-pathogenesis-and-diagnosis doi:10.5772/67332

Jacobs, R., Boyd, L., Brennan, K., Sinha, C. K., & Giuliani, S. (2016). The importance of social media for patients and families affected by congenital anomalies: A Facebook cross-sectional analysis and user survey. *Journal of Pediatric Surgery*, *51*(11), 1766–1771. doi:10.1016/j.jpedsurg.2016.07.008 PMID:27522307

Jahnová, H., Poupětová, H., Jirečková, J., Vlášková, H., Košťálová, E., Mazanec, R., & Magner, M. (2019). Amyotrophy, cerebellar impairment and psychiatric disease are the main symptoms in a cohort of 14 Czech patients with the late-onset form of Tay-Sachs disease. *Journal ofNeurology*, *266*(8), 1953–1959. doi:10.100700415-019-09364-3 PMID:31076878

Jhaveri K. D., Schrier P. B., Mattana J. (2013). Paging Doctor Google!. *Heuristics vs. technology, 2*, 90. doi:10.12688/f1000research.2-90.v2

Johnson, D., Deterding, S., Kuhn, K. A., Staneva, A., Stoyanov, S., & Hides, L. (2016). Gamification for health and wellbeing: A systematic review of the literature. *Internet interventions, 6,* 89-106. Doi:10.1016/j.invent.2016.10.002

Johnson, W. G. (1981). The clinical spectrum of hexosaminidase deficiency diseases. *Neurology*, *31*(11), 1453–1456. doi:10.1212/WNL.31.11.1453 PMID:7198192

Johnston, C., Hessl, D., Blasey, C., Eliez, S., Erba, H., Dyer-Friedman, J., ... Reiss, A. (2003). Factors associated with parenting stress in mothers of children with Fragile X syndrome. *Developmental and Behavioral Pediatrics*, *24*(4), 267–275. doi:10.1097/00004703-200308000-00008 PMID:12915799

Johnston, S. L., Lock, R. J., & Gompels, M. M. (2002). Takayasu arteritis: A review. *Journal of Clinical Pathology*, *55*(7), 481–486. doi:10.1136/jcp.55.7.481 PMID:12101189

Jones, S. C., & Owen, N. (2006). Using fear appeals to promote cancer screening—are we scaring the wrong people? *International Journal of Nonprofit and Voluntary Sector Marketing*, *11*(2), 93–103. doi:10.1002/nvsm.48

Josephs, K. A. (2007). Capgras Syndrome and Its Relationship to Neurodegenerative Disease. *JAMA Neurology*, *64*(12), 1762–1766. doi:10.1001/archneur.64.12.1762 PMID:18071040

Jung, H. C. (2012). Death education for medical personnel utilizing cinema. *The Korean Journal of Gastroenterology*, *60*(3), 140–148. doi:10.4166/kjg.2012.60.3.140 PMID:23018534

Kaback, M., Lim-Steele, J., Dabholkar, D., Brown, D., Levy, N., & Zeiger, K. (1993). Tay-Sachs disease—carrier screening, prenatal diagnosis, and the molecular era: An international perspective, 1970 to 1993. *Journal of the American Medical Association*, *270*(19), 2307–2315. doi:10.1001/jama.1993.03510190063028 PMID:8230592

Kahn, J. G., Yang, J. S., & Kahn, J. S. (2010). 'Mobile' health needs and opportunities in developing countries. *Health Affairs, 29*(2), 252–258. doi:10.1377/hlthaff.2009.0965 PMID:20348069

Kalra, G. (2012). Talking about stigma towards mental health professionals with psychiatry trainees: A movie club approach. *Asian Journal of Psychiatry, 5*(3), 266–268. doi:10.1016/j.ajp.2012.06.005 PMID:22981056

Kamel Boulos, M. N., & Wheeler, S. (2007). The emerging Web 2.0 social software: An enabling suite of sociable technologies in health and health care education 1. *Health Information and Libraries Journal, 24*(1), 2–23. doi:10.1111/j.1471-1842.2007.00701.x PMID:17331140

Kaplan, K. (2013, June 31). When and How to Create Customer Journey Maps. Retrieved April 20, 2015, from Nielsen Norman Group website: https://www.nngroup.com/articles/customer-journey-mapping/

Kaplan, B. H., Cassel, J. C., & Gore, S. (1977). Social support and health. *Medical Care, 15*(5), 47–58. PMID:853781

Karenberg, A. (2008). Multiple sclerosis on-screen: From disaster to coping. *Multiple Sclerosis Journal, 14*(4), 530–540. doi:10.1177/1352458507084587 PMID:18208879

Karlsen, T. H., Folseraas, T., Thorburn, D., & Vesterhus, M. (2017). Primary sclerosing cholangitis - a comprehensive review. *Journal of Hepatology, 67*(6), 1298–1323. doi:10.1016/j.jhep.2017.07.022 PMID:28802875

Katz, M. S., Utengen, A., Anderson, P. F., Thompson, M. A., Attai, D. J., Johnston, C., & Dizon, D. S. (2016). Disease-specific hashtags for online communication about cancer care. *JAMA Oncology, 2*(3), 392–394. doi:10.1001/jamaoncol.2015.3960 PMID:26539640

Katz, S. (2002). Gender differences in adapting to a child's chronic illness: A causal model. *Journal of Pediatric Nursing, 17*(4), 257–269. doi:10.1053/jpdn.2002.126709 PMID:12219325

Keelan, J., Pavri-Garcia, V., Tomlinson, G., & Wilson, K. (2007). YouTube as a source of information on immunization: A Content Analysis. *Journal of the American Medical Association, 298*(21), 2482–2484. doi:10.1001/jama.298.21.2482 PMID:18056901

Keller, D., & Honig, A. S. (2004). Maternal and paternal stress in families with schoolaged children with disabilities. *The American Journal of Orthopsychiatry, 74*(3), 337–348. doi:10.1037/0002-9432.74.3.337 PMID:15291710

Kelly, B. D. (2006). Psychiatry in contemporary Irish cinema: A qualitative study. *Irish Journal of Psychological Medicine, 23*(2), 74–79. doi:10.1017/S0790966700009617 PMID:30290482

Kember, J. (2004). David Lynch and the Mug Shot: Facework. In E. Sheen, & A. Davison (Eds.), *The Elephant Man and The Straight Story. The Cinema of David Lynch: American Dreams, Nightmare Visions* (pp. 19–34). London, UK: Wallflower Press.

Kersh, J., Hedvat, T. T., Hauser-Cram, P., & Warfield, M. E. (2006). The contribution of marital quality to the wellbeing of parents of children with developmental disabilities. *Journal of Intellectual Disability Research, 50*, 883-893. doi: /. doi:10.1111/j.1365-2788.2006.00906.x

Kietzmann, J. H., Hermkens, K., McCarthy, I. P., & Silvestre, B. S. (2011). Social media? Get serious! Understanding the functional building blocks of social media. *Business Horizons, 54*(3), 241–251. doi:10.1016/j.bushor.2011.01.005

Kilbride, M. K., & Joffe, S. (2018). The new age of patient autonomy: Implications for the patient-physician relationship. *Journal of the American Medical Association, 320*(19), 1973–1974. doi:10.1001/jama.2018.14382 PMID:30326026

Kilic, S., Altintas, S. H., Yilmaz Altintas, N., Ozkaynak, O., Bayram, M., Kusgoz, A., & Taskesen, F. (2017). Six-Year Survival of a Mini Dental Implant-Retained Overdenture in a Child with Ectodermal Dysplasia. *Journal of Prosthodontics, 26*(1), 70–74. doi:10.1111/jopr.12366 PMID:26418841

Kim, W., Kreps, G. L., & Shin, C. N. (2015). The role of social support and social networks in health information–seeking behavior among Korean Americans: A qualitative study. *International Journal for Equity in Health, 14*(40). doi:10.118612939-015-0169-8 PMID:25927546

Kliegman, R. M., Bordini, B. J., Basel, D., & Nocton, J. J. (2017). How Doctors Think. *Pediatric Clinics of North America, 64*(1), 1–15. doi:10.1016/j.pcl.2016.08.002 PMID:27894438

Knight, A. W., & Senior, T. P. (2006). The common problem of rare disease in general practice. *The Medical Journal of Australia, 185*(2), 82–83. doi:10.5694/j.1326-5377.2006.tb00477.x PMID:16842062

Knox, S. L. (2006). Death, afterlife, and the eschatology of consciousness: Themes in contemporary cinema. *Mortality, 11*(3), 233–252. doi:10.1080/13576270600775007

Koch, T. (2011). *Disease maps: epidemics on the ground.* Chicago, IL: University of Chicago Press. doi:10.7208/chicago/9780226449401.001.0001

Kofinas, J. D., Varrey, A., Sapra, K. J., Kanj, R. V., Chervenak, F. A., & Asfaw, T. (2014). Adjunctive social media for more effective contraceptive counseling. *Obstetrics and Gynecology, 123*(4), 763–770. doi:10.1097/AOG.0000000000000172 PMID:24785602

Kontoghiorghe, C. N., Andreou, N., Constantinou, K., & Kontoghiorghes, G. J. (2014). World health dilemmas: Orphan and rare diseases, orphan drugs and orphan patients. *World Journal of Methodology, 4*(3), 163. doi:10.5662/wjm.v4.i3.163 PMID:25332915

Koohy, H., & Koohy, B. (2014). A lesson from the ice bucket challenge: Using social networks to publicize science. *Frontiers in Genetics, 5*, 430. doi:10.3389/fgene.2014.00430 PMID:25566317

Koplan, J. P. (2003). Communication during public health emergencies. *Journal of Health Communication, 8*(sup1S1), 144–145. doi:10.1080/713851967 PMID:14692583

Korompilias, V. (2018). *Relational awareness: Experience architecture manuals*. Copyrighted material.

Kostkova, P. (2015). Grand challenges in digital health. *Frontiers in Public Health, 3*, 134. doi:10.3389/fpubh.2015.00134 PMID:26000272

Kothari, S. (2001). Takayasu's arteritis in children - a review. *Images in Paediatric Cardiology, 3*(4), 4–23. Retrieved from https://www.ncbi.nlm.nih.gov/pubmed/22368604 PMID:22368604

Kowalski, C., Kahana, E., Kuhr, K., Ansmann, L., & Pfaff, H. (2014). Changes over time in the utilization of disease-related Internet information in newly diagnosed breast cancer patients 2007 to 2013. *Journal of Medical Internet Research, 16*(8), e195. doi:10.2196/jmir.3289 PMID:25158744

Kozinets, R. V. (2005). *Netnography: redefined* (2nd ed.). London, UK: Sage.

Krementsov, N. (2015). Conjoined twins: Scientific cinema and Pavlovian physiology. *Endeavour, 39*(3-4), 168–178. doi:10.1016/j.endeavour.2015.10.001 PMID:26601729

Krieger, J. L., Parrott, R. L., & Nussbaum, J. F. (2010). Metaphor use and health literacy: A pilot study of strategies to explain randomization in cancer clinical trials. *Journal of Health Communication, 16*(1), 3–16. doi:10.1080/10810730.2010.529494 PMID:21128152

Kruegel, J., Rubel, D., & Gross, O. (2013). Alport syndrome—insights from basic and clinical research. *Nature Reviews. Nephrology, 9*(3), 170–178. doi:10.1038/nrneph.2012.259 PMID:23165304

Kruse-Jarres, R., Kempton, C. L., Baudo, F., Collins, P. W., Knoebl, P., Leissinger, C. A., ... Kessler, C. M. (2017). Acquired hemophilia A: Updated review of evidence and treatment guidance. *American Journal of Hematology, 92*(7), 695–705. doi:10.1002/ajh.24777 PMID:28470674

Kuehn, B. M. (2011). Patients go online seeking support, practical advice on health conditions. *Journal of the American Medical Association, 305*(16), 1644–1645. doi:10.1001/jama.2011.509 PMID:21521841

Kuiper, J. B. (1961). The Stage Antecedents of the Film Theory of SM Eisenstein. *Educational Theatre Journal, 259-263*. doi:10.2307/3204346

Lakoff, G., & Johnsen, M. (2003). *Metaphors we live by* (2nd ed.). London, UK: The University Chicago Press. doi:10.7208/chicago/9780226470993.001.0001

Lambert, H., & McKevitt, C. (2002). Anthropology in health research: From qualitative methods to multidisciplinarity. *BMJ (Clinical Research Ed.), 325*(7357), 210–213. doi:10.1136/bmj.325.7357.210 PMID:12142313

Lambert, S. D., & Loiselle, C. G. (2007). Health information—seeking behavior. *Qualitative Health Research, 17*(8), 1006–1019. doi:10.1177/1049732307305199 PMID:17928475

Landry, L. G., Ali, N., Williams, D. R., Rehm, H. L., & Bonham, V. L. (2018). Lack Of Diversity In Genomic Databases Is A Barrier To Translating Precision Medicine Research Into Practice. *Health Affairs (Project Hope)*, *37*(5), 780–785. doi:10.1377/hlthaff.2017.1595 PMID:29733732

Lang, P. J. (1995). The emotion probe: Studies of motivation and attention. *The American Psychologist*, *50*(5), 372–385. doi:10.1037/0003-066X.50.5.372 PMID:7762889

Laranjeira, C. (2007). Do vulnerável ser ao resiliente envelhecer: Revisão de literatura. [From vulnerable being to resilient aging: literature review]. *Psicologia: Teoria e Pesquisa (Brasília)*, *23*(3), 327–332. doi:10.1590/S0102-37722007000300012

Lasker, J. N., Sogolow, E. D., & Sharim, R. R. (2005). The role of an online community for people with a rare disease: Content analysis of messages posted on a primary biliary cirrhosis mailing list. *Journal of Medical Internet Research*, *7*(1), e10. doi:10.2196/jmir.7.1.e10 PMID:15829472

Lasswell, H. D., Lerner, D., & Pool, I. D. S. (1952). *Comparative study of symbols: An introduction*. Palo Alto, CA: Stanford University Press.

Laurindo, E. E., & Barros Filho, I. R. (2017). Encefalopatia espongiforme bovina atípica: Uma revisão. *Arquivos do Instituto Biológico*, *84*(0). doi:10.1590/1808-1657000392015

Lautenschlager, S., Kemp, M., Christensen, J. J., Mayans, M. V., & Moi, H. (2017). 2017 European guideline for the management of chancroid. *International Journal of STD & AIDS*, *28*(4), 324–329. doi:10.1177/0956462416687913 PMID:28081686

Lavigne, B., Hamdan, M., Faure, B., Merveille, H., Pareaud, M., Tallon, E., ... Calvet, B. (2016). Syndrome de Diogène et Hoarding disorder: Une même entité? *L'Encéphale*, *42*(5), 421–425. doi:10.1016/j.encep.2016.02.010 PMID:27017316

Lawthom, R., & Chataika, T. (2012). Leave and Wenger, Communities of Practice and Disability. In D. Goodley, B. Hughes, & L. Davis (Eds.), *Disability and social theory. New developments and Directions* (pp. 233–251). New York, NY: Palgrave MacMillan. doi:10.1057/9781137023001_14

Lazard, A. J., Bamgbade, B. A., Sontag, J. M., & Brown, C. (2016). Using visual metaphors in health messages: A strategy to increase effectiveness for mental illness communication. *Journal of Health Communication*, *21*(12), 1260–1268. doi:10.1080/10810730.2016.1245374 PMID:27869576

Leask, J., Hooker, C., & King, C. (2010). Media coverage of health issues and how to work more effectively with journalists: a qualitative study. *BMC public health, 10*(1), 535, 1-7. doi:10.1186/1471-2458-10-535

Lee, R. H. (2018). Acute fatty liver of pregnancy. Retrieved from https://www.uptodate.com/contents/acute-fatty-liver-of-pregnancy

Lee, S. M., Lee, M. J., Lee, J. S., Kim, H. D., Lee, J. S., Kim, J., ... Lee, Y. M. (2008). Newly observed thalamic involvement and mutations of the HEXA gene in a Korean patient with juvenile GM2 gangliosidosis. *Metabolic Brain Disease*, *23*(3), 235–242. doi:10.100711011-008-9090-9 PMID:18648917

Legendre, C. M., Charpentier-Côté, C., Drouin, R., & Bouffard, C. (2011). Neurofibromatosis type 1 and the "elephant man's" disease: the confusion persists: an ethnographic study. *PLoS One*, *6*(2). doi:10.1371/journal.pone.0016409 PMID:21347399

Legroux, L., & Arbour, N. (2015). Multiple Sclerosis and T Lymphocytes: An Entangled Story. *Journal of Neuroimmune Pharmacology*, *10*(4), 528–546. doi:10.100711481-015-9614-0 PMID:25946987

Lemieux, M. J., Mark, B. L., Cherney, M. M., Withers, S. G., Mahuran, D. J., & James, M. N. G. (2006). Crystallographic Structure of Human β-Hexosaminidase A: Interpretation of Tay-Sachs Mutations and Loss of GM2 Ganglioside Hydrolysis. *Journal of Molecular Biology*, *359*(4), 913–929. doi:10.1016/j.jmb.2006.04.004 PMID:16698036

Lennard-Jones, J. E. (1989). Classification of inflammatory bowel disease. *Scandinavian Journal of Gastroenterology. Supplement*, *170*(sup170), 2–6, discussion 16–19. doi:10.3109/00365528909091339 PMID:2617184

León, B. (2010). Spanish public service media on the verge of a new era. In P. Iosifidis (Ed.), *Reinventing Public Service Communication* (pp. 197–208). London, UK: Palgrave Macmillan; doi:10.1057/9780230277113_16

Lewis, N., Gray, S. W., Freres, D. R., & Hornik, R. C. (2009). Examining Cross-Source Engagement With Cancer-Related Information and Its Impact on Doctor–Patient Relations. *Health Communication*, *24*(8), 723–734. doi:10.1080/10410230903264030 PMID:20183381

Liao, P. C., Wei, C. J., & Chen, P. H. (2018). Onset of psychosis following strokes to the cerebellum and thalamus. *Psychosomatics*, *59*(4), 413–414. doi:10.1016/j.psym.2017.09.001 PMID:29054750

Liberal, R., Vergani, D., & Mieli-Vergani, G. (2015). Update on Autoimmune Hepatitis. *Journal of Clinical and Translational Hepatology, 3*(1), 42-52. doi:10.14218/JCTH.2014.00032

Lindor, K. D., & Lee, R. H. (2019). Intrahepatic cholestasis of pregnancy. Retrieved from https://www.uptodate.com/contents/intrahepatic-cholestasis-of-pregnancy

Lin, S., Zhou, Y., Fang, Q., Wu, J., Zhang, Z., Ji, Y., & Luo, Y. (2016). Chromosome 10q26 deletion syndrome: Two new cases and a review of the literature. *Molecular Medicine Reports*, *14*(6), 5134–5140. doi:10.3892/mmr.2016.5864 PMID:27779662

Lippert-Gruener, M., Weinert, U., Greisbach, T., & Wedekind, C. (2005). Foreign accent syndrome following traumatic brain injury. *Brain Injury: [BI]*, *19*(11), 955–958. doi:10.1080/02699050500109506 PMID:16243750

Little Black Book Online. (2014). TBWA\London Teams with Rankin to Raise Awareness of Ataxia. Retrieved from https://lbbonline.com/news/tbwalondon-teams-with-rankin-to-raise-awareness-of-ataxia/

Little, G. A., Kahn, R., & Green, R. M. (1999). Parental Dreams, Dilemmas, and Decision-Making in Cinéma Vérité. *Journal of Perinatology*, *19*(3), 194–196. doi:10.1038j.jp.7200163 PMID:10685221

Liuccio, M. (2018). Le malattie rare: informazione e comunicazione nel patient journey, *Sociologia della comunicazione*, 58, 30-47. Doi:10.3280/SC2018-055003

Liuccio, M., Belotti, R., Comune, A., Zambito, V., & Schulz, J. (2015). Communication in Rare Diseases: A Literature Review. *Journal of Communications Research*, *7*(3), 1–9.

Liuccio, M., Belotti, R., Comune, A., Zambito, V., & Schulz, P. J. (2015). Communication in rare diseases: A literature review. *Journal of Communication Research*, *7*(3), 2–10.

Liuccio, M., & Giorgino, F. (2019). *La sanità medi@ta, Salute, società e comunicazione nell'era delle fake news*. Milan, Italy: Mondadori Università.

Loddo, I., & Romano, C. (2015). Inflammatory Bowel Disease: Genetics, Epigenetics, and Pathogenesis. *Frontiers in Immunology*, *6*(551). doi:10.3389/fimmu.2015.00551 PMID:26579126

López Villafranca, P. (2015a). "La representación de las asociaciones de pacientes en el ente público RTVE. El caso de las Enfermedades Raras". En Peñafiel, C y Echegaray, L. (2015). Estudios de Comunicación y Salud: innovaciones e información científica para el progreso social. Cuadernos Artesanos de Latina, 84. Tenerife: Sociedad Latina de Comunicación Social, 157- 174.

López Villafranca, P. (2015b). Análisis de las campañas de comunicación de pacientes con enfermedades raras en España. *Opción*, *31*(1), 1039–1055.

López Villafranca, P. (2016). Estudio de la presencia de los gabinetes de comunicación en las organizaciones de pacientes con enfermedades raras en España. *Revista Internacional de Relaciones Públicas*, *11*(6), 27–46. doi:10.5783/RIRP-11-2016-03-27-46

López Villafranca, P. (2018). Análisis de estafas de pacientes en la prensa española. El caso de Paco Sanz, el hombre de los 2.000 tumores y el caso de Nadia, la niña con tricodistrofia. *Revista Española de Comunicación en Salud*, *9*(1), 5–13. doi:10.20318/recs.2018.4256

López Villafranca, P., & Castillo Esparcia, A. (2014). El papel del vídeo online en la promoción y difusión de las Enfermedades Raras. In *González, J. E., y Valderrama, M. (2014). Comunicación actual: Redes sociales y lo 2.0 y 3.0* (pp. 127–137). Madrid, Spain: Editorial McGraw Hill.

López-Bastida, J., Oliva-Moreno, J., Linertová, R., & Serrano-Aguilar, P. (2016). Social/economic costs and health-related quality of life in patients with rare diseases in Europe. *The European Journal of Health Economics*, *17*(S1), 1–5. doi:10.100710198-016-0780-7 PMID:27023708

López-Bastida, J., Perestelo-Pérez, L., Montón-álvarez, F., & Serrano-Aguilar, P. (2008). Social economic costs and health-related quality of life in patients with degenerative cerebellar ataxia in Spain. *Movement Disorders*, *23*(2), 212–217. doi:10.1002/mds.21798 PMID:17999424

López-Villafranca, P., & Castillo-Esparcia, A. (2018). El encuadre de las enfermedades raras en los medios de comunicación españoles. *Observatorio (OBS*)*, *12*(2), 136-155. doi:10.15847/obsOBS12220181074

Lucca, S. A. D., & Petean, E. B. L. (2016). Fatherhood: Experiences of fathers of boys diagnosed with Duchenne Muscular Dystrophy. *Ciencia & Saude Coletiva*, *21*(10), 3081–3089. doi:10.1590/1413-812320152110.20302016 PMID:27783781

Lüchmann, L. H. H. (2014). Abordagens teóricas sobre o associativismo e seus efeitos democráticos. *Revista Brasileira de Ciências Sociais*, *29*(85), 159–178. doi:10.1590/S0102-69092014000200011

Lupton, D. (1993). The construction of patienthood in medical advertising. *International Journal of Health Services*, *23*(4), 805–819. doi:10.2190/FPDH-CXKD-RJH3-8REJ PMID:7506237

Lupton, D. (2012). *Medicine as Culture: Illness, Disease and the Body*. London, UK: Sage.

Lupton, D., & Jutel, A. (2015). 'It's like having a physician in your pocket!' A critical analysis of self-diagnosis smartphone apps. *Social Science & Medicine*, *133*, 128–135. doi:10.1016/j.socscimed.2015.04.004 PMID:25864149

Luther, S. (2007). Resilience in development: a synthesis of research across 5 decades. Developmental Psychopathology Vol. 3: Risk, Disorder, and Adaptation (2nd ed.) (Eds. D. Cicchetti, & D. J. Cohen), pp. 739–95. Hoboken, NJ: John Wiley & Sons.

Luz, G., Carvalho, M., & Silva, M. (2011). O significado de uma organização de apoio aos portadores e familiares de fibrose cística na perspectiva das famílias. [The meaning of a support organization for cystic fibrosis patients and families from the perspective of families]. *Texto & Contexto Enfermagem*, *20*(1), 127–134. doi:10.1590/S0104-07072011000100015

Luz, G., Silva, M. R. S., & DeMontigny, F. (2015). Doenças raras: Itinerário diagnóstico e terapêutico das famílias de pessoas afetadas. [Rare diseases: diagnostic and therapeutic itinerary of families of affected people]. *Acta Paulista de Enfermagem*, *28*(5), 395–400. doi:10.1590/1982-0194201500067

Mackenzie, G., & Will, R. (2017). Creutzfeldt-Jakob disease: Recent developments. *F1000 Research*, *6*, 2053–2053. doi:10.12688/f1000research.12681.1 PMID:29225787

MacQueen, G. M., Rosebush, P. I., & Mazurek, M. F. (1998). Neuropsychiatric Aspects of the Adult Variant of Tay - Sachs disease. *The Journal of Neuropsychiatry and Clinical Neurosciences*, *10*(1), 10–19. doi:10.1176/jnp.10.1.10 PMID:9547461

Macri, A., Wilson, A. M., Shafaat, O., & Sharma, S. (2019). Osler-Weber-Rendu Disease (Hereditary Hemorrhagic Telangiectasia, HHT). In *StatPearls*. Treasure Island, FL: StatPearls Publishing.

Maddalena, A., Bale, S., Das, S., Grody, W., & Richards, S. (2005). Technical Standards and Guidelines: Molecular Genetic Testing for Ultra-Rare Disorders. *Genetics in Medicine*, *7*(8), 571–583. doi:10.1097/01.GIM.0000182738.95726.ca PMID:16247296

Maegawa, G. H., Stockley, T., Tropak, M., Banwell, B., Blaser, S., Kok, F., & Clarke, J. T. (2006). The natural history of juvenile or subacute GM2 gangliosidosis: 21 new cases and literature review of 134 previously reported. *Pediatrics*, *118*(5), e1550–e1562. doi:10.1542/peds.2006-0588 PMID:17015493

Maibach, E., & Holtgrave, D. R. (1995). Advances in public health communication. *Annual Review of Public Health, 16*(1), 219–238. doi:10.1146/annurev.pu.16.050195.001251 PMID:7639871

Maier, S., Bajko, Z., Moţăţăianu, A., Stoian, A., Şchiopu, B., & Bălaşa, R. (2017). Late Onset Tay - Sachs disease in a Non-Jewish Patient: Case Report. *Acta Medica Marisiensis, 63*(4), 199–203. doi:10.1515/amma-2017-0034

Majumder, S., & Chari, S. T. (2016). Chronic pancreatitis. *Lancet, 387*(10031), 1957–1966. doi:10.1016/S0140-6736(16)00097-0 PMID:26948434

Maloney, W. J. (2009). Hutchinson-Gilford Progeria syndrome: Its presentation in F. Scott Fitzgerald's short story 'The Curious Case of Benjamin Button' and its oral manifestations. *Journal of Dental Research, 88*(10), 873–876. doi:10.1177/0022034509348765 PMID:19783794

Maltby, H. J., Kristjanson, L., & Coleman, M. E. (2003). The parenting competency framework: Learning to be a parent of a child with asthma. *International Journal of Nursing Practice, 9*(6), 368–373. doi:10.1046/j.1440-172X.2003.00445.x PMID:14984073

Manix, M., Kalakoti, P., Henry, M., Thakur, J., Menger, R., Guthikonda, B., & Nanda, A. (2015). Creutzfeldt-Jakob disease: Updated diagnostic criteria, treatment algorithm, and the utility of brain biopsy. *Neurosurgical Focus, 39*(5), E2. doi:10.3171/2015.8.FOCUS15328 PMID:26646926

Manohar, M., Verma, A. K., Venkateshaiah, S. U., Sanders, N. L., & Mishra, A. (2017). Pathogenic mechanisms of pancreatitis. *World Journal of Gastrointestinal Pharmacology and Therapeutics, 8*(1), 10–25. doi:10.4292/wjgpt.v8.i1.10 PMID:28217371

Marcucci, G., Cianferotti, L., Beck-Peccoz, P., Capezzone, M., Cetani, F., Colao, A., ... Brandi, M. L. (2015). Rare diseases in clinical endocrinology: A taxonomic classification system. *Journal of Endocrinological Investigation, 38*(2), 193–259. doi:10.100740618-014-0202-6 PMID:25376364

Martin, S. C., Stone, A. M., Scott, A. M., & Brashers, D. E. (2010). Medical, personal, and social forms of uncertainty across the transplantation trajectory. *Qualitative Health Research, 20*(2), 182–196. doi:10.1177/1049732309356284 PMID:19955227

Martins, T. C., Moreira, H., & Canavarro, M. C. (2016). Adult attachment and dyadic adjustment: The mediating role of shame. *The Journal of Psychology, 150*(5), 560–575. doi:10.1080/00223980.2015.1114461 PMID:26759960

Masten, A. S., & Powell, J. L. (2003). A resilience framework for research, policy, and practice: Contributions from project competence. In S. S. Luthar (Ed.), Resilience and vulnerability: Adaptation in the context of childhood adversities (pp. 1-25). New York.

Matteucci, I. (2015). Social determinants of health inequalities: Moving toward a socio-constructivist model supported by information and communication technologies. *Global Bioethics, 26*(3-4), 206–217. doi:10.1080/11287462.2015.1101213

Mavilia, M. G., Pakala, T., Molina, M., & Wu, G. Y. (2018). Differentiating Cystic Liver Lesions: A Review of Imaging Modalities, Diagnosis and Management. *Journal of Clinical and Translational Hepatology, 6*(2), 208–216. doi:10.14218/JCTH.2017.00069 PMID:29951366

Mavris, M., & Le Cam, Y. (2012). Involvement of patient organisations in research and development of orphan drugs for rare diseases in Europe. *Molecular Syndromology*, *3*(5), 237–243. doi:10.1159/000342758 PMID:23293582

McAdoo, S. P., & Pusey, C. D. (2017). Anti-Glomerular Basement Membrane Disease. *Clinical Journal of the American Society of Nephrology; CJASN*, *12*(7), 1162–1172. doi:10.2215/CJN.01380217 PMID:28515156

McDivitt, J. A., Zimicki, S., & Hornik, R. C. (1997). Explaining the Impact of Communication Campaigns to Change Vaccination Knowledge and Coverage in the Philippines. *Health Communication*, *9*(2), 95–118. doi:10.120715327027hc0902_1

McDonagh, D., Goggin, N., & Squier, J. (2005). Signs, symbols, and subjectivity: An alternative view of the visual. *Computers and Composition*, *22*(1), 79–86. doi:10.1016/j.compcom.2004.12.009

McKinstry, B. (1992). Paternalism and the doctor-patient relationship in general practice. *The British Journal of General Practice*, *42*(361), 340–342. PMID:1457157

McMullan, M. (2006). Patients using the Internet to obtain health information: How this affects the patient–health professional relationship. *Patient Education and Counseling*, *63*(1-2), 24–28. doi:10.1016/j.pec.2005.10.006 PMID:16406474

McNab, C. (2009). What social media offers to health professionals and citizens. Retrieved from https://www.who.int/bulletin/volumes/87/8/09-066712/en/

Meleis, A. I., Sawyer, L. M., Im, E. O., Messias, D. K. H., & Schumacher, K. (2000). Experiencing transitions: An emerging middle-range theory. *Advances in Nursing Science*, *23*(1), 12–28. doi:10.1097/00012272-200009000-00006 PMID:10970036

Melnyk, B. M., Feinstein, N. F., Moldenhouer, Z., & Small, L. (2001). Coping in parents of children who are chronically ill: Strategies for assessment and intervention. *Pediatric Nursing*, *27*(6), 547–557. PMID:12024526

Melo, D. G., de Paula, P. K., de Araujo Rodrigues, S., de Avó, L. R. D. S., Germano, C. M. R., & Demarzo, M. M. P. (2015). Genetics in primary health care and the National Policy on Comprehensive Care for People with Rare Diseases in Brazil: Opportunities and challenges for professional education. *Journal of Community Genetics*, *6*(3), 231–240. doi:10.100712687-015-0224-6 PMID:25893505

Membrives, M. D., Isern, M. T. I., & Matheu, M. C. L. (2016). Literature review: Use of commercial films as a teaching resource for health sciences students. *Nurse Education Today*, *36*, 264–267. doi:10.1016/j.nedt.2015.10.002 PMID:26490325

Menon, K. V., & Ranjith, G. (2009). Malayalam cinema and mental health. *International Review of Psychiatry (Abingdon, England)*, *21*(3), 218–223. doi:10.1080/09540260902748043 PMID:19459097

Meseguer, J. A. P. (2011). La realidad en un# hashtag. Ponencia presentada en Congreso Aecpa, Sevilla, España.

Messaris, P. (1997). *Visual Persuasion: The role of images in advertising*. Thousand Oaks, CA: Sage.

Messaris, P. (1998). Visual aspects of media literacy. *Journal of Communication*, *48*(1), 70–80. doi:10.1111/j.1460-2466.1998.tb02738.x

Miguel, C. (2016). Visual intimacy on social media: From selfies to the co-construction of intimacies through shared pictures. *Social Media+ Society*, *2*(2), doi:10.1177/2056305116641705

Mikolasevic, I., Filipec-Kanizaj, T., Jakopcic, I., Majurec, I., Brncic-Fischer, A., Sobocan, N., ... Milic, S. (2018). Liver Disease During Pregnancy: A Challenging Clinical Issue. *Medical Science Monitor*, *24*, 4080–4090. doi:10.12659/MSM.907723 PMID:29905165

Mikulincer, M., & Shaver, P. R. (2014). Attachment bonds in romantic relationships. In M. Mikulincer, & P. R. Shaver (Eds.), *Mechanisms of social connection: from brain to group* (pp. 273–290). Washington, DC: American Psychological Association. doi:10.1037/14250-000

Milbrath, V. M., Motta, M. D. G. C., Gabatz, R. I. B., & Freitag, V. L. (2017). O nascimento de um filho com paralisia cerebral: Um tempo presente inesperado. [The birth of a child with cerebral palsy: An unexpected present tense]. *Revista Interdisciplinar em Cultura e Sociedade*, *3*, 47–60.

Ministério da Saúde. (2014). *Portaria n° 199, de 30 de janeiro de 2014. Institui a Política Nacional de Atenção Integral às Pessoas com Doenças Raras, aprova Diretrizes para Atenção Integral às Pessoas com Doenças Raras no âmbito do Sistema Único de Saúde (SUS) e institui incentivos financeiros de custeio*. Brasília: Diário Oficial da União.

Ministerio de Sanidad y Política Social. (2009). *Estrategia em Enfermedades Raras del Sistema de Salud*, Valencia, SP: CIBER de Enfermedades Raras (CIBERER). Instituto de Salud Carlos III w Instituto de Biomedicina de Valencia, CSIC. Ministerio de Sanidad y Política Social (03/032016). *La investigación y la atención sociosanitaria, claves de la estrategia de Sanidad frente a las enfermedades raras* [Press release], Retrieved from https://www.mscbs.gob.es/gabinete/notasPrensa.do?id=3916

Mishel, M. H. (1988). Uncertainty in illness. *Image--the Journal of Nursing Scholarship*, *20*(4), 225–232. doi:10.1188/17.ONF.645-649 PMID:3203947

Mjoseth, J. (2018). Genomic databases weakened by lack of non-European populations. Retrieved from https://www.genome.gov/news/news-release/Genomic-databases-weakened-by-lack-of-non-European-populations

Moberget, T., Alnæs, D., Kaufmann, T., Doan, N. T., Córdova-Palomera, A., Norbom, L. B., ... Westlye, L. T. (2019). Cerebellar Gray Matter Volume Is Associated with Cognitive Function and Psychopathology in Adolescence. *Biological Psychiatry*, *86*(1), 65–75. doi:10.1016/j.biopsych.2019.01.019 PMID:30850129

Moher, D., Liberati, A., Tetzlaff, J., & Altman, D. G.PRISMA Group. (2009). Preferred reporting items for systematic reviews and meta-analyses: The PRISMA statement. *PLoS Medicine*, *6*(7). doi:10.1371/journal.pmed.1000097 PMID:19621072

Montastruc, F., Schwarz, N., Schmitt, L., & Bui, E. (2012). An Overview of the Symptoms and Typical Disorders Associated with Alice in Wonderland Syndrome. *Neuropsychiatry*, *2*(4), 281–289. doi:10.2217/npy.12.37

Monteiro, M., Matos, A. P., & Coelho, R. (2002). A adaptação psicológica de mães cujos filhos apresentam paralisia cerebral: Revisão da literatura. [Psychological adaptation of mothers whose children have cerebral palsy: literature review]. *Revista Portuguesa de Psicossomática*, *4*(2), 149–178.

Mooney-Doyle, K., Deatrick, J. A., & Horowitz, J. A. (2015). Tasks and communication as an avenue to enhance parenting of children birth-5years: An integrative review. *Journal of Pediatric Nursing*, *30*(1), 184–207. doi:10.1016/j.pedn.2014.03.002 PMID:24680918

Moorhead, S. A. (2017). Social media for healthcare communication. *Oxford Research Encyclopedias*. Retrieved from https://oxfordre.com/communication/view/10.1093/acrefore/9780190228613.001.0001/acrefore-9780190228613-e-335 (Access date: August 25, 2019)

Moorhead, S. A., Hazlet, D. E., Harrison, L., Carroll, J. K., Irwin, A., & Hoving, C. (2013). A New Dimension of Health Care: Systematic Review of the Uses, Benefits, and Limitations of Social Media for Health Communication. *Journal of Medical Internet Research*, *15*(4), e85. doi:10.2196/jmir.1933 PMID:23615206

Moreira, P. L., & Angelo, M. (2008). Tornar-se mãe de criança com câncer: Construindo a parentalidade. [Becoming a mother of a child with cancer: Building parenting]. *Revista Latino-Americana de Enfermagem*, *16*(3), 355–361. doi:10.1590/S0104-11692008000300004 PMID:18695806

Morgan, T. (2007). Turner Syndrome. *Diagnosis and Management American Family Physician*, *76*(3), 405–410. PMID:17708142

Morgan, T., Schmidt, J., Haakonsen, C., Lewis, J., Della Rocca, M., Morrison, S., ... Kaphingst, K. A. (2014). Using the internet to seek information about genetic and rare diseases: A case study comparing data from 2006 and 2011. *JMIR Research Protocols*, *3*(1), e10. doi:10.2196/resprot.2916 PMID:24565858

Morris, M. E., Consolvo, S., Munson, S. A., Kramer, A. D. I., Patrick, K., & Tsai, J. (2011). Facebook for Health. Opportunities and Challenges for Driving Behavior Change. CHI'11 Extended Abstracts on Human Factors in Computing Systems. Retrieved from https://dl.acm.org/citation.cfm?id=1979489&dl=ACM&coll=DL

Mortier, K., & Wackens, G. (2004). Ectodermal dysplasia anhidrotic. *Orphanet Encyclopedia*, *3*, 1–6.

Mortimer, N. (2014). Ataxia UK joins forces with Rankin to launch the charity's first campaign. Retrieved from https://www.thedrum.com/news/2014/04/07/ataxia-uk-joins-forces-rankin-launch-charity-s-first-campaign

Mueller, B. (1987). Reflections of culture: An analysis of Japanese and American advertising appeals. *Journal of Advertising Research*, (August): 1–21.

Müller, M. G. (2008). Visual Competence: A new paradigm for studying visuals in the social sciences? *Visual Studies*, *23*(2), 101–112. doi:10.1080/14725860802276248

Mulsow, M., Caldera, Y. M., Pursley, M., Reifman, A., & Huston, A. C. (2002). Multilevel factors influencing maternal stress during the first three years. *Journal of Marriage and the Family*, *64*(4), 944–956. doi:10.1111/j.1741-3737.2002.00944.x

Mursch, K., & Behnke-Mursch, J. (2003). Internet-based interaction among brain tumour patients. Analysis of a medical mailing list. *Zentralblatt fur Neurochirurgie*, *64*(2), 71–75. doi:10.1055-2003-40375 PMID:12838475

Nabi, R. (2002). Anger, fear, uncertainty, and attitudes: A test of the cognitive-functional model. *Communication Monographs*, *69*(3), 204–216. doi:10.1080/03637750216541

Nakash, O., Dargouth, S., Oddo, V., Gao, S., & Alegría, M. (2009). Patient initiation of information: Exploring its role during the mental health intake visit. *Patient Education and Counseling*, *75*(2), 220–226. doi:10.1016/j.pec.2008.10.010 PMID:19062233

Nambisan, P. (2011). Information seeking and social support in online health communities: Impact on patients' perceived empathy. *Journal of the American Medical Informatics Association*, *18*(3), 298–304. doi:10.1136/amiajnl-2010-000058 PMID:21486888

Nanton, V., Docherty, A., Meystre, C., & Dale, J. (2009). Finding a pathway: Information and uncertainty along the prostate cancer patient journey. *British Journal of Health Psychology*, *14*(3), 437–458. doi:10.1348/135910708X342890 PMID:18718111

Nasirian, M., Banazadeh, N., & Kheradmand, A. (2009). Rare variant of lycanthropy and ecstasy. *Addiction & Health*, *1*(1), 53–56. Retrieved from https://www.ncbi.nlm.nih.gov/pubmed/24494083 PMID:24494083

Navon, R., Argov, Z., Frisch, A., Opitz, J. M., & Reynolds, J. F. (1986). Hexosaminidase A deficiency in adults. *American Journal of Medical Genetics*, *24*(1), 179–196. doi:10.1002/ajmg.1320240123 PMID:2939718

Navon, R., Khosravi, R., Melki, J., Drucker, L., Fontaine, B., Turpin, J. C., & Baumann, N. (1997). Juvenile-onset spinal muscular atrophy caused by compound heterozygosity for mutations in the HEXA gene. *Annals of Neurology*, *41*(5), 631–638. doi:10.1002/ana.410410512 PMID:9153525

Navon, R., & Proia, R. (1989). The mutations in Ashkenazi Jews with adult GM2 gangliosidosis, the adult form of Tay-Sachs disease. *Science*, *243*(4897), 1471–1474. doi:10.1126cience.2522679 PMID:2522679

Nederlandse Omroepprogramma Stichting (NOS). (1999). *Hilversummary. Broadcasting news from the Netherlands*. Hilversum, The Netherlands: NOS.

Nelkin, D. (1996). An uneasy relationship: The tensions between medicine and the media. *Lancet (London, England)*, *347*(9015), 1600–1603. doi:10.1016/S0140-6736(96)91081-8 PMID:8667872

Network, H. H. (2019). Rare Endocrine Genetic Diseases | Hormone Health Network. Retrieved from https://www.hormone.org/your-health-and-hormones/rare-endocrine-genetic-diseases

Neudorfer, O., & Kolodny, E. H. (2004). Late-onset Tay-Sachs disease. *The Israel Medical Association Journal*, *6*(2), 107–111. PMID:14986470

Neudorfer, O., Pastores, G. M., Zeng, B. J., Gianutsos, J., Zaroff, C. M., & Kolodny, E. H. (2005). Late-onset Tay-Sachs disease: Phenotypic characterization and genotypic correlations in 21 affected patients. *Genetics in Medicine*, *7*(2), 119–123. doi:10.1097/01.GIM.0000154300.84107.75 PMID:15714079

Neumann, H. P. H., Young, W. F. Jr, & Eng, C. (2019). Pheochromocytoma and Paraganglioma. *The New England Journal of Medicine*, *381*(6), 552–565. doi:10.1056/NEJMra1806651 PMID:31390501

NGO CRD. (2019). Rare Disease Day Policy Event at the United Nations. Retrieved from https://www.ngocommitteerarediseases.org/rare-disease-day-policy-event-at-the-united-nations/?fbclid=IwAR0XKGVO_zukUfs7juFnb3m1PkOWQrO0cRBqH5PNN2c0148ACcmdCOBpgAA

Ng, S. C., Shi, H. Y., Hamidi, N., Underwood, F. E., Tang, W., Benchimol, E. I., ... Kaplan, G. G. (2017). Worldwide incidence and prevalence of inflammatory bowel disease in the 21st century: A systematic review of population-based studies. *Lancet*, *390*(10114), 2769–2778. doi:10.1016/S0140-6736(17)32448-0 PMID:29050646

NHS. (2019). Idiopathic pulmonary fibrosis. Retrieved from https://www.nhs.uk/conditions/idiopathic-pulmonary-fibrosis/

Nicholson, W. K., Grason, H. A., & Powe, N. R. (2003). The relationship of race to women's use of health information resources. *American Journal of Obstetrics and Gynecology*, *188*(2), 580–585. doi:10.1067/mob.2003.15 PMID:12592275

Nickels, A., & Dimov, V. (2012). Innovations in technology: Social media and mobile technology in the care of adolescents with asthma. *Current Allergy and Asthma Reports*, *12*(6), 607–612. doi:10.100711882-012-0299-7 PMID:22976493

Niebel, K., & Davidson, E. (2012). Raising the Bar for HIV Awareness. *Marketing Health Services*, *32*(4), 5–7. PMID:23356034

Niemiec, R. M. (2010). International Cinema: An Abundant Mental Health Resource of Films for Education, Communication, and Transformation. In *The Cinematic Mirror for Psychology and Life Coaching* (pp. 123–153). New York, NY: Springer. doi:10.1007/978-1-4419-1114-8_7

Nieweglowski, V. H., & More, C. L. O. O. (2008). Comunicação equipe-família em unidade de terapia intensiva pediátrica: Impacto no processo de hospitalização. [Team-family communication in a pediatric intensive care unit: impact on the hospitalization process]. *Estudos de Psicologia*, *25*(1), 111–122. doi:10.1590/S0103-166X2008000100011

NIH, & GARD. (2019). Rare diseases: Endocrine diseases. Retrieved from https://rarediseases.info.nih.gov/diseases/diseases-by-category/8/endocrine-diseases

NIH. (2016). Quick Statistics About Hearing. Retrieved from https://www.nidcd.nih.gov/health/statistics/quick-statistics-hearing

NIH. N. H., Lung, and Blood Institute. (2019). Idiopathic Pulmonary Fibrosis. Retrieved from https://www.nhlbi.nih.gov/health-topics/idiopathic-pulmonary-fibrosis

NINDS. (2018). Creutzfeldt-Jakob Disease Fact Sheet. Retrieved from https://www.ninds.nih.gov/Disorders/Patient-Caregiver-Education/Fact-Sheets/Creutzfeldt-Jakob-Disease-Fact-Sheet

Niraj, J., Färkkilä, A., & D'Andrea, A. D. (2019). The Fanconi Anemia Pathway in Cancer. *Annual Review of Cancer Biology*, *3*(1), 457–478. doi:10.1146/annurev-cancerbio-030617-050422 PMID:30882047

Noar, S. M., Benac, C. N., & Harris, M. S. (2007). Does tailoring matter? Meta-analytic review of tailored print health behavior change interventions. *Psychological Bulletin*, *133*(4), 673–693. doi:10.1037/0033-2909.133.4.673 PMID:17592961

Noar, S. M., Harrington, N. G., Van Stee, S. V., & Aldrich, R. S. (2011). Tailored health communication to change lifestyle behaviours. *American Journal of Lifestyle Medicine*, *5*(5), 112–122. doi:10.1177/1559827610387255

Noticias, P. R. (2015). Prnoticias y TyC presentan el estudio 'Prospectiva del sector de las RRPP', Retrieved from http://prnoticias.com/comunicacion/20141311-relaciones-publicas-estudio-prospectiva?jjj=1489486462614. [Access date: 28 Jun. 2019]

O'Brien, J. S., Okada, S., Fillerup, D. L., Veath, M. L., Adornato, B., Brenner, P. H., & Leroy, J. G. (1971). Tay-Sachs disease: Prenatal diagnosis. *Science*, *172*(3978), 61–64. doi:10.1126cience.172.3978.61 PMID:5546285

O'Donohue, W. (2013). *Clinical psychology and the philosophy of science*. Switzerland: Springer. doi:10.1007/978-3-319-00185-2

O'Farrell, N. (2002). Donovanosis. *Sexually Transmitted Infections*, *78*(6), 452–457. doi:10.1136ti.78.6.452 PMID:12473810

O'Keefe, G. J., Boyd, H. H., & Brown, M. R. (1998). Who Learns Preventive Health Care Information From Where: Cross-Channel and Repertoire Comparisons. *Health Communication*, *10*(1), 25–36. doi:10.120715327027hc1001_2 PMID:16370988

O'Malley, A. S., Kerner, J. F., & Johnson, L. (1999). Are we getting the message out to all?: Health information sources and ethnicity. *American Journal of Preventive Medicine*, *17*(3), 198–202. doi:10.1016/S0749-3797(99)00067-7 PMID:10987635

Oates, C. E., Bosch, P., & Hart, M. N. (1986). Movement disorders associated with chronic GM2 gangliosidosis. *European Neurology*, *25*(2), 154–159. doi:10.1159/000116100 PMID:3081350

Oberman, B. S., Patel, V. A., Cureoglu, S., & Isildak, H. (2017). The aetiopathologies of Ménière's disease: a contemporary review. [L'eziopatogenesi della Sindrome di Ménière: stato dell'arte]. Acta otorhinolaryngologica Italica: organo ufficiale della Societa italiana di otorinolaringologia e chirurgia cervico-facciale, 37(4), 250-263. doi:10.14639/0392-100X-793

OBSER. (2019). *Observatorio Sobre Enfermedades Raras.* Retrieved from https://obser.enfermedades-raras.org (Access date: August 13, 2019)

Okazaki, S., Mueller, B., & Taylor, C. R. (2010). Measuring soft-sell versus hard-sell advertising appeals. *Journal of Advertising*, *39*(2), 5–20. doi:10.2753/JOA0091-3367390201

Oliveira, C. R. O., Guimarães, M. C. S., & Machado, R. (2012). Doenças raras como categoria de classificação emergente: o caso brasileiro. *DataGramaZero, 13*(1), 1-10. Retrieved from http://www.brapci.inf.br/index.php/article/view/0000011723/611097bff4311db520c7ab0c01a792e4/

Ong, L. M., Visser, M. R., Lammes, F. B., & De Haes, J. C. (2000). Doctor–patient communication and cancer patients' quality of life and satisfaction. *Patient Education and Counseling*, *41*(2), 145–156. doi:10.1016/S0738-3991(99)00108-1 PMID:12024540

Ontaneda, D., & Fox, R. J. (2015). Progressive multiple sclerosis. *Current Opinion in Neurology*, *28*(3), 237–243. doi:10.1097/WCO.0000000000000195 PMID:25887766

Orfanella, L. (1998). Radio: The intimate medium. *English Journal*, *87*(1), 53–55. doi:10.2307/822022

Orpha.net. (2012). About Rare Diseases. Retrieved from https://www.orpha.net/consor/cgi-bin/Education_AboutRareDiseases.php?lng=EN

Orsini, J. J., Escolar, M. L., Wasserstein, M. P., & Caggana, M. (1993). Krabbe Disease. In M. P. Adam, H. H. Ardinger, R. A. Pagon, S. E. Wallace, L. J. H. Bean, K. Stephens, & A. Amemiya (Eds.), *GeneReviews((R))*. Seattle, WA: University of Washington, Seattle.

Osakabe, H. (2002). *Argumentação e discurso político* (2nd ed.). São Paulo, Brazil: Martins Fontes.

Osher, E., Fattal-Valevski, A., Sagie, L., Urshanski, N., Amir-Levi, Y., Katzburg, S., & Elstein, D. (2011). Pyrimethamine increases β-hexosaminidase A activity in patients with Late Onset Tay Sachs. *Molecular Genetics and Metabolism*, *102*(3), 356–363. doi:10.1016/j.ymgme.2010.11.163 PMID:21185210

Osher, E., Fattal-Valevski, A., Sagie, L., Urshanski, N., Sagiv, N., Peleg, L., & Stern, N. (2015). Effect of cyclic, low dose pyrimethamine treatment in patients with Late Onset Tay Sachs: An open label, extended pilot study. *Orphanet Journal of Rare Diseases*, *10*(1), 45. doi:10.118613023-015-0260-7 PMID:25896637

Osio, A., Fraitag, S., Hadj-Rabia, S., Bodemer, C., de Prost, Y., & Hamel-Teillac, D. (2010). Clinical Spectrum of Tufted Angiomas in Childhood: A Report of 13 Cases and a Review of the Literature. *JAMA Dermatology*, *146*(7), 758–763. doi:10.1001/archdermatol.2010.135 PMID:20644037

Paek, H.-J., Kim, K., & Hove, T. (2010). Content analysis of anti-smoking videos on YouTube: Message sensation value, message appeals, and their relationships with viewer responses. *Health Education Research*, *25*(6), 1085–1099. doi:10.1093/her/cyq063 PMID:20923913

Paek, H.-J., Kim, K., Hove, T., & Huh, J.-Y. (2014). Reduced Harm or Another Gateway to Smoking? Source, Message, and Information Characteristics of E-Cigarette Videos on YouTube. *Journal of Health Communication*, *19*(5), 545–560. doi:10.1080/10810730.2013.821560 PMID:24117370

Pagoto, S., Schneider, K. L., Evans, M., Waring, M. E., Appelhans, B., Busch, A. M., ... Ziedonis, M. (2014). Tweeting it off: Characteristics of adults who tweet about a weight loss attempt. *Journal of the American Medical Informatics Association*, *21*(6), 1032–1037. doi:10.1136/amiajnl-2014-002652 PMID:24928175

Palmer-Wackerly, A. L., & Krieger, J. L. (2015). Dancing around infertility: The use of metaphors in a complex medical situation. *Health Communication*, *30*(6), 612–623. doi:10.1080/10410236.2014.888386 PMID:25061825

Panageas, A. (2019). Disabled Characters in Movies: The Controversy and Science Behind the Screen. *D. U. Quark*, *3*(2). Retrieved from https://dsc.duq.edu/duquark/vol3/iss2/11

Papatheodorou, F., & Machin, D. (2003). The Umbilical Cord That Was Never Cut: The Post-Dictatorial Intimacy between the Political Elite and the Mass Media in Greece and Spain. *European Journal of Communication*, *18*(1), 31–54. doi:10.1177/0267323103018001225

Parrott, R. (2003). Media Issues. In T. L. Thompson, A. M. Dorsey, K. I. Miller, & R. Parrott, (Eds.), Handbook of Health Communication. (pp. 445-448). London, UK: Lawrence Erlbaum Associates.

Parrott, R. (2009). *Talking about health. Why communication matters*. Chichester, UK: Wiley-Blackwell.

Parsons, T. (1996). *Sistema sociale*. Ed. Comunitá.

Pasculli, G., Resta, F., Guastamacchia, E., Suppressa, P., & Sabbà, C. (2004). Health-related quality of life in a rare disease: Hereditary hemorrhagic telangiectasia (HHT) or Rendu–Osler–Weber Disease. *Quality of Life Research: An International Journal of Quality of Life Aspects of Treatment, Care, and Rehabilitation*, *13*(10), 1715–1723. doi:10.100711136-004-7865-y PMID:15651542

Passos-Bueno, M. R., Bertola, D., Horovitz, D. D. G., Ferraz, V. E. F., & Brito, L. A. (2014). Genetics and genomics in Brazil: A promising future. *Molecular Genetics & Genomic Medicine*, *2*(4), 280–291. doi:10.1002/mgg3.95 PMID:25077170

Patel, R., Chang, T., Greysen, S. R., & Chopra, V. (2015). Social Media Use in Chronic Disease: A Systematic Review and Novel Taxonomy. *The American Journal of Medicine*, *128*(12), 1335–1350. doi:10.1016/j.amjmed.2015.06.015 PMID:26159633

Pati, A. (2010). *Scarce support changes lives.* Nursing Standard (through 2013), 24(48), 18.

Pati, D., Harvey, T. E. Jr, Willis, D. A., & Pati, S. (2015). Identifying elements of the health care environment that contribute to wayfinding. *HERD: Health Environments Research & Design Journal*, *8*(3), 44–67. doi:10.1177/1937586714568864 PMID:25929471

Patientslikeme. (2019). *About us.* Retrieved from https://www.patientslikeme.com/about (Access date: August 13, 2019)

Patsos, M. (2001). The Internet and medicine: Building a community for patients with rare diseases. *Journal of the American Medical Association*, *285*(6), 805–805. doi:10.1001/jama.285.6.805-JMS0214-2-1 PMID:11176922

Paunio, M., Virtanen, M., Poltola, H., Cantell, K., Paunio, P., Valle, M., ... Heinonen, O. P. (1991). Increase of Vaccination Coverage by Mass Media and Individual Approach: Intensified Measles, Mumps and Rubella Prevention Program in Finland. *American Journal of Epidemiology*, *133*(11), 1152–1160. doi:10.1093/oxfordjournals.aje.a115827 PMID:2035518

Pavan, S., Rommel, K., Mateo Marquina, M. E., Höhn, S., Lanneau, V., & Rath, A. (2017). Clinical Practice Guidelines for Rare Diseases: The Orphanet Database. *PLoS One*, *12*(1). doi:10.1371/journal.pone.0170365 PMID:28099516

Pecchioni, L. L., Thompson, T. L., & Anderson, D. J. (2006). Interrelations between family and health communication. In L. H. Turner, & R. West (Eds.), *The family communication sourcebook* (pp. 447–468). Thousand Oaks, CA: Sage.

Pelchat, D., Lefebvre, H., & Perreault, M. (2003). Differences and similarities between mothers and fathers experiences of parenting a child with a disability. *Journal of Child Health Care*, *7*(4), 231–247. doi:10.1177/13674935030074001 PMID:14636429

Pelentsov, L. J., Fielder, A. L., & Esterman, A. J. (2016a). The supportive care needs of parents with a child with a rare disease: A qualitative descriptive study. *Journal of Pediatric Nursing*, *31*(3), 207–218. doi:10.1016/j.pedn.2015.10.022 PMID:26651231

Pelentsov, L. J., Fielder, A. L., Laws, T. A., & Esterman, A. J. (2016b). The supportive care needs of parents with a child with a rare disease: Results of an online survey. *BMC Family Practice*, *17*(1), 207–218. doi:10.118612875-016-0488-x PMID:27439905

Pelentsov, L. J., Laws, T. A., & Esterman, A. J. (2015). The supportive care needs of parents caring for a child with a rare disease: A scoping review. *Disability and Health Journal*, *8*(4), 475–491. doi:10.1016/j.dhjo.2015.03.009 PMID:25959710

Pernencar, C. A. (2013, May). My Crohn's diease on real time information. In *2013 IEEE 2nd International Conference on Serious Games and Applications for Health (SeGAH)* (pp. 1-7). IEEE. 10.1109/SeGAH.2013.6665304

Pernencar, C., Romão, T., & Simões, G. (2016). *The Design Process of an e-Health project – Applying the HSI framework for interface analysis.* Presented at the 2016 IEEE 4th International Conference on Serious Games and Applications for Health (SeGAH), Orlando, FL.

Pernencar, C., Sousa, P., Frontini, R., Martinho, R., Runte, D., Mendes, D., & Carvalho, M. (2018). Planning a health promotion program: Mobile app gamification as a tool to engage adolescents. *CENTERIS 2018 - International Conference on ENTERprise Information Systems / ProjMAN 2018 - International Conference on Project MANagement / HCist 2018 - International Conference on Health and Social Care Information Systems and Technologies, CENTERIS/ProjMAN/HCist 2018, 138*, 113–118. 10.1016/j.procs.2018.10.016

Perse, E. M., Kubey, R., & Csikszentmihalyi, M. (1991). Television and the Quality of Life: How Viewing Shapes Everyday Experience. *Contemporary Sociology*, *20*(2), 284. doi:10.2307/2072983

Petersen, A. (2001). Biofantasies: Genetics and medicine in the print news media. *Social Science & Medicine*, *52*(8), 1255–1268. doi:10.1016/S0277-9536(00)00229-X PMID:11281408

Petric, B. (2007). Rhetorical functions of citations in high- and low-rated master's theses. *Journal of English for Academic Purposes*, *6*(3), 238–253. doi:10.1016/j.jeap.2007.09.002

PEW Internet and American Life Project. (2007). E-Patients with a Disability or Chronic Disease. Retrieved from http://www.pewinternet.org/files/old-media/Files/Reports/2007/EPatients_Chronic_Conditions_2007.pdf.pdf

Phillips, B. J. (2000). The impact of verbal anchoring on consumer response to image ads. *Journal of Advertising*, *29*(1), 15–24. doi:10.1080/00913367.2000.10673600

Piccinini, C. A., Castro, E. K., Alvarenga, P., Vargas, S., & Oliveira, V. Z. (2003). A doença crônica orgânica na infância e as práticas educativas maternas. [Chronic organic disease in childhood and maternal educational practices]. *Estudos de Psicologia*, *8*(1), 75–83. doi:10.1590/S1413-294X2003000100009

Pieterse, A. H., Van Dulmen, A. M., Beemer, F. A., Bensing, J. M., & Ausems, M. G. (2007). Cancer genetic counseling: Communication and counselees' post-visit satisfaction, cognitions, anxiety, and needs fulfillment. *Journal of Genetic Counseling*, *16*(1), 85–96. doi:10.100710897-006-9048-1 PMID:17295054

Pillai, R. K., & Jayasree, K. (2017). Rare cancers: Challenges & issues. *The Indian Journal of Medical Research*, *145*(1), 17–27. doi:10.4103/ijmr.IJMR_915_14 PMID:28574010

Piller, I. (2001). Identity constructions in multilingual advertising. *Language in Society*, *30*(2), 153–186. doi:10.1017/S0047404501002019

Piñeiro-Otero, T., & Ribeiro, F. (2015). Radio mobility in the digital era: Interactivity, participation and content share possibilities in Iberian broadcasters. *Comunicação e Sociedade*, *28*, 291–308. doi:10.17231/comsoc.28(2015).2282

Pinto, D., Martin, D., & Chenhall, R. (2016). The involvement of patient organisations in rare disease research: A mixed methods study in Australia. *Orphanet Journal of Rare Diseases*, *11*(1), 2. doi:10.118613023-016-0382-6 PMID:26754025

Pirkis, J., Blood, R. W., Francis, C., & McCallum, K. (2006). On-screen portrayals of mental illness: Extent, nature, and impacts. *Journal of Health Communication*, *11*(5), 523–541. doi:10.1080/10810730600755889 PMID:16846952

Plevinsky, J. M., & Greenley, R. N. (2014). Exploring Health-related Quality of Life and Social Functioning in Adolescents with Inflammatory Bowel Diseases After Attending Camp Oasis and Participating in a Facebook Group. *Inflammatory Bowel Diseases*, *20*(9), 1611–1617. doi:10.1097/MIB.0000000000000120 PMID:25025714

Podolec, P. (2017). Rare cardiovascular diseases. *European Heart Journal*, *38*(43), 3190–3192. doi:10.1093/eurheartj/ehx611 PMID:29145662

Polich, G. R. (2012). Rare disease patient groups as clinical researchers. *Drug Discovery Today*, *17*(3-4), 167–172. doi:10.1016/j.drudis.2011.09.020 PMID:22016088

Polletta, F., & Jasper, J. M. (2001). Collective identities and social movements. *Annual Review of Sociology*, *27*(1), 283–305. doi:10.1146/annurev.soc.27.1.283

Poon, G. P. (2003). 'Making Money and Serving the Public Interest. Public Broadcasting Can and Should do Both', In M. P. McCaulay, E. E. Peterson, B. L. Artz, & D. Halleck (Eds.), Public Broadcasting and the Public Interest.

Porciuncula, R., Spada, P., & Goulart, K. O. B. (2018). Leukoencephalopathy with Evanescent White Matter: A Case Report. *Revista Paulista de Pediatria: Orgao Oficial da Sociedade de Pediatria de Sao Paulo*, *36*(4), 515–518. doi:10.1590/1984-0462/;2018;36;4;00001 PMID:29995139

Porter, R. W., Steinglass, R., Kaiser, J., Olkhovsky, P., Rasmuson, M., Dzhatdoeva, F. A., ... Bragina, V. (2000). Role of Health Communication in Russia's Diphtheria Immunization. *The Journal of Infectious Diseases*, *181*(s1Supplement 1), 220–227. doi:10.1086/315566

Pricewaterhouse Cooper. (2017). Social media "likes" healthcare: From marketing to social business. Retrieved from https://www.pwc.com/us/en/industries/health-industries/library/health-care-social-media.html

Prihodova, I., Kalincik, T., Poupetova, H., & Nevsimalova, S. (2013). Late-onset Tay–Sachs disease can mimic spinal muscular atrophy type III—two case reports. *Ceská a Slovenská Neurologie a Neurochirurgie*, *76/109*(2), 221–224. Retrieved from https://www.ncbi.nlm.nih.gov/pubmed/27491214

Prince, S., & Hensley, W. E. (1992). The Kuleshov effect: Recreating the classic experiment. *Cinema Journal*, *31*(2), 59–75. doi:10.2307/1225144

Priolo, M. (2009). Ectodermal dysplasias: An overview and update of clinical and molecular-functional mechanisms. *American Journal of Medical Genetics. Part A*, *149*(9), 2003–2013. doi:10.1002/ajmg.a.32804 PMID:19504607

Prior, T. W., & Finanger, E. (2016). Spinal Muscular Atrophy. In M. P. Adam, H. H. Ardinger, R. A. Pagon, & S. E. Wallace (Eds.), *GeneReviews*. Retrieved from https://www.ncbi.nlm.nih.gov/books/NBK1352/

Prior, L. (2003). Belief, knowledge and expertise: The emergence of the lay expert in medical sociology. *Sociology of Health & Illness*, *25*(3), 41–57. doi:10.1111/1467-9566.00339 PMID:14498929

Promislow, S., Walker, J. R., Taheri, M., & Bernstein, C. N. (2010). How well does the Internet answer patients' questions about inflammatory bowel disease? *Canadian Journal of Gastroenterology*, *24*(11), 671–677. doi:10.1155/2010/957264 PMID:21157582

Publications. (n.d.). Retrieved October 21, 2019, from Facebook Research website: https://research.fb.com/publications/

Rabeharisoa, V. (2008). Experience, knowledge and empowerment: the increasing role of patient organizations in staging, weighting and circulating experience and knowledge In M. Akrich, J. Nunes, F. Paterson, & V. Rabeharisoa (Eds.), *The dynamics of patient organizations in Europe*. Retrieved from http://books.openedition.org/pressesmines/1588

Rabeharisoa, V., Callon, M., Filipe, A. M., Nunes, J. A., Paterson, F., & Vergnaud, F. (2014). From 'politics of numbers' to 'politics of singularisation': Patients' activism and engagement in research on rare diseases in France and Portugal. *Biosocieties*, *9*(2), 194–217. doi:10.1057/biosoc.2014.4

Rabinow, P. (1996). Artificiality and enlightenment: From sociobiology to biosociality. In *Essays on the Anthropology of Reason* (pp. 91–111). Princeton, NJ: Princeton University Press.

Rajabi, F., Drake, L. A., Senna, M. M., & Rezaei, N. (2018). Alopecia areata: A review of disease pathogenesis. *British Journal of Dermatology*, *179*(5), 1033–1048. doi:10.1111/bjd.16808 PMID:29791718

Rajasimha, H. K., Shirol, P. B., Ramamoorthy, P., Hegde, M., Barde, S., Chandru, V., ... Babar, I. A. (2014). Organization for rare diseases India (ORDI)–Addressing the challenges and opportunities for the Indian rare diseases' community. *Genetical Research*, *96*, e009. doi:10.1017/S0016672314000111 PMID:25579084

Ramirez, A. G., Villarreal, R., McAlister, A., Gallion, K. J., Suarez, L., & Gomez, P. (1999). Advancing the Role of Participatory Communication in the Diffusion of Cancer Screening Among Hispanics. *Journal of Health Communication*, *4*(1), 31–36. doi:10.1080/108107399127075 PMID:10977276

Rammos, A., Meladinis, V., Vovas, G., & Patsouras, D. (2017). Restrictive Cardiomyopathies: The Importance of Noninvasive Cardiac Imaging Modalities in Diagnosis and Treatment-A Systematic Review. *Radiology Research and Practice*, *2017*. doi:10.1155/2017/2874902 PMID:29270320

Ramoni, R. B., Mulvihill, J. J., Adams, D. R., Allard, P., Ashley, E. A., Bernstein, J. A., & McCray, A. T. (2017). The Undiagnosed Diseases Network: Accelerating Discovery about Health and Disease. *American Journal of Human Genetics*, *100*(2), 185–192. doi:10.1016/j.ajhg.2017.01.006 PMID:28157539

Randell, R. L., Long, M. D., Cook, S. F., Wrennall, C. E. D., Chen, W., Martin, C. F., ... Kappelman, M. D. (2014, March 1). Validation of an Internet-Based Cohort of Inflammatory Bowel Disease (CCFA Partners). *Inflammatory Bowel Diseases*, *20*(3), 541–544. https://doi.org/10.1097/01.MIB.0000441348.32570.34

Rapin, I., Suzuki, K., Suzuki, K., & Valsamis, M. P. (1976). Adult (chronic) GM2 gangliosidosis: Atypical spinocerebellar degeneration in a Jewish sibship. *Archives of Neurology*, *33*(2), 120–130. doi:10.1001/archneur.1976.00500020048008 PMID:175770

Rare chromosome disorder support group, R. C. (Producer). 10q25 and 10q26 deletions. Retrieved from https://www.rarechromo.org/media/information/Chromosome%2010/10q25%20and%2010q26%20deletions%20FTNP.pdf

Rare Disease Day. (2008). Overview of Rare Disease Day 2008. Retrieved from https://www.rarediseaseday.org/article/rare-disease-day-2008

Rare Disease Day. (2019a). What is a rare disease? Retrieved from https://www.rarediseaseday.org/article/what-is-a-rare-disease

Rare Disease Day. (2019b). What is Rare Disease Day? Retrieved from https://www.rarediseaseday.org/article/what-is-rare-disease-day

Rare Disease Day. (2019c). Rare Disease Day 2019 theme announced: Bridging health and social care. Retrieved from https://www.rarediseaseday.org/page/news/theme-2019

Rare Disease Day. (2019d). Overview of past Rare Disease Days. Retrieved from https://www.rarediseaseday.org/article/overview-of-past-rare-disease-days

Rare Disease Day. (2019e). Video out now - #ShowYourRare for Rare Disease Day 2019. Retrieved from https://www.rarediseaseday.org/page/news/video-out-now-showyourrare-for-rare-disease-day

Rare Disease UK. (2016). Acedido a 12 de maio de 2017 em https://www.raredisease.org.uk/what-is-a-rare-disease/

Raríssimas – *Associação nacional de deficiências mentais e raras*. (2018). Acedido a 16 de junho de 2018 em http://www.rarissimas.pt/index.php

Rath, A., Wakap, S. S. N., Demarest, S., & Lanneau, V. (2016). *Orphanet Report Series. Prevalence and incidence of rare diseases: bibliographic data.* Diseases listed by decreasing prevalence, incidence or number of published cases. Retrieved from https://www.orpha.net/consor/cgi-bin/Education_Home.php?lng=EN

Rawla, P., & Limaiem, F. (2019). Lymphogranuloma Venereum. In *StatPearls*. Treasure Island, FL: StatPearls Publishing.

Reese, V. (1995). Dermatology in the cinema. *Journal of the American Academy of Dermatology*, *33*(6), 1030–1035. doi:10.1016/0190-9622(95)90297-X PMID:7490348

Regier, D. S., Proia, R. L., D'Azzo, A., & Tifft, C. J. (2016). The GM1 and GM2 Gangliosidoses: Natural History and Progress toward Therapy. *Periaortic Endocrinology Reviews*, *13*(S1), 663–673. PMID:27491214

Reguera, N. (2017). *Las enfermedades raras en grupos de Facebook: Evaluación de la línea de actuación de FEDER mediante minería de textos* (Master's thesis), Universitat Oberta de Catalunya, Barcelona, Spain.

Reguera, N., Subirats, L., & Armayones, M. (2017, June 22–24). Mining Facebook data of people with rare diseases. In *Proceedings of 2017 IEEE 30th International Symposium on Computer-Based Medical Systems (CBMS)* (pp. 588-593). Thessaloniki, Greece: CBMS. 10.1109/CBMS.2017.124

Reich, J., Guo, L., Groshek, J., Weinberg, J., Chen, W., Martin, C., ... Farraye, F. A. (2019). Social Media Use and Preferences in Patients With Inflammatory Bowel Disease. *Inflammatory Bowel Diseases*, *25*(3), 587–591. doi:10.1093/ibd/izy280 PMID:30203036

Reinarman, C., & Levine, H. G. (1995). The Crack Attack: America's Latest Drug Scare, 1986-1992. In J. Best (Ed.), *Images of Issues. Typifying Contemporary Social Problems* (pp. 147–186). New York: Routledge.

Rekatsinas, T., Ghosh, S., Mekaru, S. R., Nsoesie, E. O., Brownstein, J. S., Getoor, L., & Ramakrishnan, N. (2015, June). SourceSeer: Forecasting rare disease outbreaks using multiple data sources. In *Proceedings of the 2015 SIAM International Conference on Data Mining* (pp. 379-387). Society for Industrial and Applied Mathematics. DOI:10.1137/1.9781611974010.43

Research, P. W. C. (2012). Social media "likes" healthcare: From marketing to social business. Retrieved from https://www.pwc.com/us/en/industries/health-industries/library/health-care-social-media.html

Revuelta, G., & Semir, V. (n.d.). Medicina y salud em la prensa diária, Informe Quiral 1997-2006, *Análisis de 10 años de información sanitária em El País, El Mundo, ABC, La Vanguardia Y El Periódico de Catalunya.* Barcelona, Spain: Observatorio de la Comunicación Científica. *Universitat Pompeu Fabra.*

Rifkin, S. B. (2006). Patient Empowerment: Increased Compliance or Total Transformation? In F. Porzsolt, & R. M. Kaplan (Eds.), *Optimizing health: Improving the value of healthcare delivery* (pp. 66–73). Boston, MA: Springer.

Rihani, F. B. (2013). Cervico-oculo-acoustic (Wildervanck) syndrome: Clinicoradiological findings. *BMJ Case Reports*, *2013*(apr23 1). doi:10.1136/bcr-2013-009065 PMID:23616324

Ringrose, J. L. (2018). *Understanding and treating dissociative identity disorder (or multiple personality disorder)*. Routledge. doi:10.4324/9780429484483

Ritchie, H., & Roser, M. (2019). *Mental Health.* Retrieved from https://ourworldindata.org/mental-health

Riva, G. (2002). Virtual reality for health care: The status of research. *Cyberpsychology & Behavior*, *5*(3), 219–225. doi:10.1089/109493102760147213 PMID:12123244

Roberts, H., Seymour, B., Fish II, S. A., Robinson, E., & Zuckerman, E. (2017). Digital health communication and global public influence: A study of the ebola epidemic. *J. Health Communication, 22*(sup1), 51-58. doi:10.1080/10810730.2016.1209598

Robinson, J. D., & Stivers, T. (2001). Achieving activity transitions in primary-care consultations: From history taking to physical examination. *Human Communication Research*, *27*, 253–298. doi:10.1111/j.1468-2958.2001.tb00782.x

Rodero, E., & Sánchez, C. (2007). 'Radiografía de la radio en España', Revista Latina de Comunicación Social, 62, Retrieved from http://www.ull.es/publicaciones/latina/200714RoderoySanchez.htm. [Access date: 19 June 2019]

Rodrigues, L. O. C. (2014, Dec. 1) *LOR Blog [web logcomment]*. Retrieved from http://lorcartunista.blogspot.com.br/

Rogers, R. W. (1983). Cognitive and physiological processes in fear appeals and attitude change: A revised theory of protection motivation. In J. Cacioppo, & R. Petty (Eds.), Social Psychophysiology. (pp. 153-176). New York: Guilford Press.

Rogers, E. M., & Storey, D. (1988). Communication Campaigns. In C. R. Berger, & S. H. Chaffee (Eds.), *Handbook of Communication Science* (pp. 817–847). Newbury Park, CA: Sage.

Rogers, R. W. (1975). A protection motivation theory of fear appeals and attitude change. *The Journal of Psychology*, *91*(1), 93–114. doi:10.1080/00223980.1975.9915803 PMID:28136248

Rosebush, P. I., MacQueen, G. M., Clarke, J. T. R., Callahan, J. W., Strasberg, P. M., & Mazurek, M. F. (1995). Late-onset Tay-Sachs disease presenting as catatonic schizophrenia: Diagnostic and treatment issues. *The Journal of Clinical Psychiatry*, *56*(8), 347–353. PMID:7635850

Rose, N. (2007). *The Politics of Life Itself*. Princeton, NJ: Princeton University Press. doi:10.1515/9781400827503

Rose, N., & Novas, C. (2003). Biological Citizenship. In A. Ong, & S. J. Collier (Eds.), *Global Assemblages: Technology, Politics, and Ethics as Anthropological Problems* (pp. 439–463). Oxford, UK: Blackwell Publishing.

Rosenstock, I. (1974). Historical Origins of the Health Belief Model. *Health Education Monographs*, *2*(4), 328–335. doi:10.1177/109019817400200403

Rossmann, C., & Ziegler, L. (2013). Gesundheitskommunikation: Medienwirkungen im Gesundheitsbereich. In W. Schweiger, & A. Fahr (Eds.), *Handbuch Medienwirkungsforschung* (pp. 385–400). Wiesbaden, Germany: Springer. doi:10.1007/978-3-531-18967-3_20

Roter, D. L., & Hall, J. A. (2006). *Doctor talking with patients/Patients talking with doctors*, Praeger Publishers, Westport.

Rubinelli, S., Camerini, L., & Schulz, P. (2010). *Comunicazione e salute*. Milano, Italy: Apogeo.

Rucker, J. C., Shapiro, B. E., Han, Y. H., Kumar, A. N., Garbutt, S., Keller, E. L., & Leigh, R. J. (2004). Neuro-ophthalmology of late-onset Tay-Sachs disease (LOTS). *Neurology*, *63*(10), 1918–1926. doi:10.1212/01.WNL.0000144275.76658.F4 PMID:15557512

Ruesch, J. (2006). Values, Communication, and Culture: An Introduction. In J. Ruesch, & G. Bateson (Eds.), *Communication – The Social Matrix of Psychiatry* (pp. 3–20). New York, NY: W. W. Worton & Company.

Saboia, I., Pisco Almeida, A. M., Sousa, P., & Pernencar, C. (2018). I am with you: A netnographic analysis of the Instagram opinion leaders on eating behavior change. *CENTERIS 2018 - International Conference on ENTERprise Information Systems / ProjMAN 2018 - International Conference on Project MANagement / HCist 2018 - International Conference on Health and Social Care Information Systems and Technologies, 138*, 97–104. 10.1016/j.procs.2018.10.014

Salmon, C., & Atkin, C. K. (2003). Media campaigns for health promotion. In T. L. Thompson, A. M. Dorsey, K. I. Miller, & R. Parrott (Eds.), *Handbook of Health Communication* (pp. 449–472). Mahwah, NJ: Lawrence Erlbaum.

Sample Ward, A. (2011). Citizen tech: Social media in disaster response. Retrieved from http://amysampleward.org/2011/02/19/citizen-tech-social-media-in-disaster-response/

Sanchez, S., & Ewton, A. (2006). Essential Thrombocythemia: A Review of Diagnostic and Pathologic Features. *Archives of Pathology & Laboratory Medicine*, *130*(8), 1144–1150. doi:10.1043/1543-2165(2006)130[1144:Et]2.0.Co;2 PMID:16879015

Sandhoff, K., Harzer, K., Wässle, W., & Jatzkewitz, H. (1971). Enzyme Alterations and Lipid Storage in Three Variants of Tay-Sachs Disease. *Journal of Neurochemistry*, *18*(12), 2469–2489. doi:10.1111/j.1471-4159.1971.tb00204.x PMID:5135907

SANE. (2019). Factsheet: Dissociative identity disorder. Retrieved from https://www.sane.org/information-stories/facts-and-guides/dissociative-identity-disorder

Santos, B., & Mota, C. P. (2018). *Parentalidade e resiliência em pais de filhos com doenças raras: O efeito moderador da vinculação amorosa*. [Parenting and resilience in parents of children with rare diseases: The moderating effect of romantic attachment]. Comunicação oral apresentada no 4º Congresso da Ordem dos Psicólogos, de 12 a 15 de setembro, Braga.

Santos, B., & Mota, C. P. (2019). *Personalidade e resiliência em pais de filhos com doenças raras: Efeito mediador da vinculação amorosa.* [Personality and resilience in parents of children with rare diseases: Mediating effect of romantic attachment]. Comunicação oral no âmbito da mesa 8 "Intervenção em situações de doença crónica e hospitalização" no X Congresso Internacional de Psicologia da Criança e do Adolescente - "Psicoterapia e outras abordagens terapêuticas", que se realizou nos dias 10 e 11 de abril de 2019 na Universidade Lusíada de Lisboa.

Santos, G. C., Cagliari, C. I., & Teixeira, M. A. (2010). Rare diseases. Challenges for the public health sector in Brazil. Abstract retrieved from *VI International Conference on Rare Disease and Orphan Drugs*, P06.

Santos, M. T., & Pérez, J. A. (2019). Las enfermedades raras y su representación en la prensa española. *Palabra Clave (La Plata)*, *22*(1), 254–287. doi:10.5294/pacla.2019.22.1.10

Sarasohn-Kahn, J. (2008). The wisdom of patients: health care meets online social media. Retrieved from https://www.chcf.org/wp-content/uploads/2017/12/PDF-HealthCareSocialMedia.pdf

Saxton, G. D., Niyirora, J., Guo, C., & Waters, R. (2015). # AdvocatingForChange: The strategic use of hashtags in social media advocacy. *Advances in Social Work*, *16*(1), 154–169. doi:10.18060/17952

Sayar, G., Kagan, G., & Ozten, E. (2014). Man transforming into wolf: A rare case of clinical lycanthropy. *The Journal of Neurobehavioral Sciences*, *1*(2), 50. doi:10.5455/JNBS.1401371806

Scarpa, M.-G., Grazia, M. D., & Tornese, G. (2017). 46,XY ovotesticular disorders of sex development: A therapeutic challenge. *Pediatric Reports*, *9*(4), 7085–7085. doi:10.4081/pr.2017.7085 PMID:29285340

Scheffer, M., Biancarelli, A., & Cassenote, A. (2018). *Demografia médica no Brasil 2018. São Paulo, Brazil.* SP: Conselho Regional de Medicina do Estado de São Paulo & Conselho Federal de Medicina.

Schiavo, R. (2007). *Health communication: From theory to practice* (2nd ed.). San Francisco, CA: John Wiley & Sons.

Schiavo, R. (2007). *Health Communication: From Theory to Practice*. San Francisco, CA: Wiley and Sons.

Schieppati, A., Henter, J. I., Daina, E., & Aperia, A. (2008). Why rare diseases are an important medical and social issue. *Lancet*, *371*(9629), 2039–2041. doi:10.1016/S0140-6736(08)60872-7 PMID:18555915

Schneck, L., Friedland, J., Valenti, C., Adachi, M., Amsterdam, D., & Volk, B. W. (1970). Prenatal diagnosis of Tay-Sachs disease. *Lancet*, *295*(7647), 582–584. doi:10.1016/S0140-6736(70)91624-7 PMID:4190540

Schneider, S., & Velmans, M. (2007). *The Blackwell Companion to Consciousness*. Victoria, Australia: Blackwell Publishing Asia.

Schulenberg, S. E. (2003). Psychotherapy and movies: On using films in clinical practice. *Journal of Contemporary Psychotherapy*, *33*(1), 35–48. doi:10.1023/A:1021403726961

Schumacher, K. R., Stringer, K. A., Donohue, J. E., Yu, S., Shaver, A., Caruthers, R. L., ... Russell, M. W. (2014). Social media methods for studying rare diseases. *Pediatrics*, *133*(5), e1345–e1353. doi:10.1542/peds.2013-2966 PMID:24733869

Schweiger, W. (2002). Cross-Media zwischen Fernsehen und Web. Versuch einer theoretischen Fundierung des Crossmedia-Konzepts. In H. Theunert, & U. Wagner (Eds.), *Medienkonvergenz: Angebot und Nutzung* (pp. 123–136). Munich, Germany: Verlag Reinhard Fischer.

Sciascia, S., Radin, M., Roccatello, D., Sanna, G., & Bertolaccini, M. (2018). Recent advances in the management of systemic lupus erythematosus. *F1000 Research*, *7*(970). doi:10.12688/f1000research.13941.1 PMID:30026918

Scott, L. M. (1994). Images in Advertising: The Need for a Theory of Visual Rhetoric. *The Journal of Consumer Research*, *21*(September), 252–273. doi:10.1086/209396

Scott, N. (2014). The Monstrous Metallic in Medicine and Horror Cinema. *Medicina Nei Secoli*, *26*(1), 312–332. PMID:25702391

Selçuk, A. A. (2019). A Guide for Systematic Reviews: PRISMA. *Turkish Archives of Otorhinolaryngology*, *57*(1), 57–58. doi:10.5152/tao.2019.4058 PMID:31049257

Sergent, S. C. C., Cagliari, C. I., & Teixeira, M. A. (2010). GEDR – Rare diseases study group – Brazil. Abstract retrieved from *VI International Conference on Rare Disease and Orphan Drugs*, P09.

Sesonske, A. (1980). Time and tense in Cinema. *The Journal of Aesthetics and Art Criticism*, *38*(4), 419–426. doi:10.2307/430323

Shah, M. H., Goldner, W. S., Halfdanarson, T. R., Bergsland, E., Berlin, J. D., Halperin, D., ... Zuccarino-Catania, G. (2018). NCCN Guidelines Insights: Neuroendocrine and Adrenal Tumors, Version 2.2018. *Journal of the National Comprehensive Cancer Network*, *16*(6), 693–702. doi:10.6004/jnccn.2018.0056 PMID:29891520

Shannon, C. E., & Weaver, W. (1998). *The mathematical theory of communication*. Urbana, IL: University of Illinois Press.

Shapiro, B. E., Hatters-Friedman, S., Fernandes-Filho, J. A., Anthony, K., & Natowicz, M. R. (2006). Late-onset Tay–Sachs disease: Adverse effects of medications and implications for treatment. *Neurology*, *67*(5), 875–877. doi:10.1212/01.wnl.0000233847.72349.b6 PMID:16966555

Shapiro, B. E., Logigian, E. L., Kolodny, E. H., & Pastores, G. M. (2008). Late-onset Tay–Sachs disease: The spectrum of peripheral neuropathy in 30 affected patients. *Muscle & Nerve*, *38*(2), 1012–1015. doi:10.1002/mus.21061 PMID:18642377

Shapiro, B. E., Pastores, G. M., Gianutsos, J., Luzy, C., & Kolodny, E. H. (2009). Miglustat in late-onset Tay-Sachs disease: A 12-month, randomized, controlled clinical study with 24 months of extended treatment. *Genetics in Medicine*, *11*(6), 425–433. doi:10.1097/GIM.0b013e3181a1b5c5 PMID:19346952

Sharf, B., & Vanderford, M. (2003). Illness narratives and the social construction of health. In T. Thompson, A. Dorsey, K. Miller, & R. Parrott (Eds.), *Handbook of health communication* (pp. 9–34). New Jersey: Lawrence Erlbaum Associates.

Silva, C. X., Brito, E. D., Sousa, F. S., & França, I. S. X. (2010). Criança com paralisia cerebral: Qual o impacto na vida do cuidador? [Child with cerebral palsy: what is the impact on the caregiver's life?]. *Revista da Rede de Enfermagem do Nordeste*, *11*, 204–214.

Silva, E., & Sousa, T. (2015). Avaliação econômica no âmbito das doenças raras: Isto é possível? *Cadernos de Saude Publica*, *31*(3), 1–11. doi:10.1590/0102-311X00213813 PMID:25859711

Simoens, S., Cassiman, D., Dooms, M., & Picavet, E. (2012). Orphan Drugs for Rare Diseases. *Drugs*, *72*(11), 1437–1443. doi:10.2165/11635320-000000000-00000 PMID:22747423

Simou, E. (2015). Health information sources: Trust and satisfaction. *International Journal of Healthcare*, *2*(1), 38–43. doi:10.5430/ijh.v2n1p38

Sitammagari, K. K., & Masood, W. (2019). Creutzfeldt Jakob Disease. In *StatPearls*. Treasure Island, FL: StatPearls Publishing.

Sjurts, I. (2011). *Strategien in der Medienbranche: Grundlagen und Fallbeispiele*. Wiesbaden, Germany: Springer.

Skrabanek, P. (1994). *The death of human medicine and the rise of coercive healthism*. Suffolk, UK: St. Edmundsbury Press.

Skuse, A. J., Butler, N., Power, F., & Woods, N. (2004). *Radio broadcasting for health: A decision maker's guide* (pp. 1–50). London, UK: Department for International Development.

Smith, D. (2013). Health care consumer's use and trust of health information sources. *Journal of Communication in Healthcare*, *4*(3), 200–210. doi:10.1179/1753807611Y.0000000010

Smith, J., Cheater, F., & Bekker, H. (2013). Parents' experiences of living with a child with a long-term condition: A rapid structured review of the literature. *Health Expectations*, *18*(4), 452–474. doi:10.1111/hex.12040 PMID:23311692

Smith, M. L., Menn, M., & McKyer, E. L. J. (2011). Effectiveness of the radio as a health information source. *Journal of Radio & Audio Media*, *18*(2), 196–211. doi:10.1080/19376529.2011.615776

Smith, R. (2006). Medical journals and the mass media: Moving from love and hate to love. *Journal of the Royal Society of Medicine*, *99*(7), 347–352. doi:10.1177/014107680609900717 PMID:16816264

Smith, T., Coyle, J. R., Lightfoot, E., & Scott, A. (2007). Reconsidering models of influence: The relationship between consumer social networks and word-of-mouth effectiveness. *Journal of Advertising Research*, *47*(4), 387–397. doi:10.2501/S0021849907070407

Snyder, L. B. (2001). Development of Communication Campaigns. In W. B. Gudykunst, & B. Mody (Eds.), *Handbook of International and Intercultural Communication* (2nd ed., pp. 457–478). Thousand Oaks, CA: Sage.

Snyder, L. B., & Hamilton, M. A. (2002). A Meta-Analysis of U.S. Health Campaign Effects on Behavior: Emphasize Enforcement, Exposure, and New Information, and Beware the Secular Trend. In R. C. Hornik (Ed.), *Public Health Communication. Evidence for Behavior Change* (pp. 357–383). London, UK: Lawrence Erlbaum Associates.

Soares, J., Araújo, L., & Bellato, R. (2016). Cuidar na situação de adoecimento raro: Vivência da família e sua busca por amparo dos serviços de saúde. [Caring for a rare illness: Family experience and their search for support from health services]. *Revista Saúde e Sociedade*, *25*(4), 1017–1030. doi:10.1590/S0104-12902016162301

Solanas, A., Patsakis, C., Conti, M., Vlachos, I. S., Ramos, V., Falcone, F., ... Martinez-Balleste, A. (2014). Smart health: A context-aware health paradigm within smart cities. *IEEE Communications Magazine*, *52*(8), 74–81. doi:10.1109/MCOM.2014.6871673

Sontag, S. (2007). *Doença como metáfora. AIDS e suas metáforas* (2nd ed.). (R. Figueiredo, & P. H. Britto, Trans.). São Paulo, Brazil: Companhia das Letras. (Original work published 1989)

Spinner, N. B., Leonard, L. D., & Krantz, I. D. (1993). Alagille Syndrome. In M. P. Adam, H. H. Ardinger, R. A. Pagon, S. E. Wallace, L. J. H. Bean, K. Stephens, & A. Amemiya (Eds.), *GeneReviews((R))*. Seattle, WA: University of Washington, Seattle.

Stakišaitis, D., Špokienė, I., Juškevičius, J., Valuckas, K., & Baiardi, P. (2007). Access to information supporting availability of medicines for patients suffering from rare diseases looking for possible treatments: The EuOrphan Service. *Medicina*, *43*(6), 441. doi:10.3390/medicina43060054 PMID:17637514

Stellefson, M., Chaney, B., Ochipa, K., Chaney, D., Haider, Z., Hanik, B., ... Bernhardt, J. M. (2014). YouTube as a source of chronic obstructive pulmonary disease patient education: A social media content analysis. *Chronic Respiratory Disease*, *11*(2), 61–71. doi:10.1177/1479972314525058 PMID:24659212

Strehle, E., & Middlemiss, P. (2007). Children with 4q-syndrome: The parents' perspective. *Journal of Genetic Counseling*, *18*(2), 189–199. PMID:17710871

Streifler, J., Golomb, M., & Gadoth, N. (1989). Psychiatric Features of Adult GM2. *The British Journal of Psychiatry*, *155*(1), 410–413. doi:10.1192/bjp.155.3.410 PMID:2611559

Streinraths, M., Vallance, H. D., & Davidson, G. F. (2008). Delays in diagnosing cystic fibrosis. Can we find ways to diagnose it earlier? *Canadian Family Physician Medecin de Famille Canadien*, *54*, 877–883. Retrieved from http://www.cfp.ca/content/54/6/877.long PMID:18556497

Subirats, L., Reguera, N., Bañón, A., Gómez-Zúñiga, B., Minguillón, J., & Armayones, M. (2018). Mining Facebook data of people with rare diseases: A content-based and temporal analysis. *International Journal of Environmental Research and Public Health*, *15*(9), 1877. doi:10.3390/ijerph15091877 PMID:30200209

Sulik, G. A. (2009). Managing biomedical uncertainty: The technoscientific illness identity. *Sociology of Health & Illness*, *31*(7), 1059–1076. doi:10.1111/j.1467-9566.2009.01183.x PMID:19619153

Swan, M. (2009). Emerging patient-driven health care models: An examination of health social networks, consumer personalized medicine and quantified self-tracking. *International Journal of Environmental Research and Public Health*, *6*(2), 492–525. doi:10.3390/ijerph6020492 PMID:19440396

Sweeny, R. W. (2004). Lines of sight in the "network society": Simulation, art education, and a digital visual culture. *Studies in Art Education*, *46*(1), 74–87. doi:10.1080/00393541.2004.11650070

Szeto, W., van der Bent, A., Petty, C. R., Reich, J., Farraye, F., & Fishman, L. N. (2018). Use of Social Media for Health-Related Tasks by Adolescents With Inflammatory Bowel Disease: A Step in the Pathway of Transition. *Inflammatory Bowel Diseases*, *24*(6), 1114–1122. doi:10.1093/ibd/izy021 PMID:29788360

Taanila, A., Kokkonen, J., & Jarvelin, M. (1996). The long-term effects of children's early-onset disability on marital relationships. *Developmental Medicine and Child Neurology*, *38*(7), 567–577. doi:10.1111/j.1469-8749.1996.tb12121.x PMID:8674907

Tabet, P., & Saliba, I. (2017). Meniere's Disease and Vestibular Migraine: Updates and Review of the Literature. *Journal of Clinical Medicine Research*, *9*(9), 733–744. doi:10.14740/jocmr3126w PMID:28811849

Taft, T. H., & Keefer, L. (2016). A systematic review of disease-related stigmatization in patients living with inflammatory bowel disease. *Clinical and Experimental Gastroenterology*, *9*, 49–58. doi:10.2147/CEG.S83533 PMID:27022294

Tannenbaum, M. B., Hepler, J., Zimmerman, R. S., Saul, L., Jacobs, S., Wilson, K., & Albarracín, D. (2015). Appealing to fear: A meta-analysis of fear appeal effectiveness and theories. *Psychological Bulletin*, *141*(6), 1178–1204. doi:10.1037/a0039729 PMID:26501228

Tanner, A. H. (2004). Agenda building, source selection, and health news at local television stations: A nationwide survey of local television health reporters. *Science Communication*, *25*(4), 350–363. doi:10.1177/1075547004265127

Taylor, K. (2009). Paternalism, participations and partnership-the evolution of patient centeredness in the consultation. In V. Kalitzkus, & P. L. Twohig (Eds.), *Bordering biomedicine*. Amsterdam, The Netherlands: Rodopi; doi:10.1016/j.pec.2008.08.017

Tejada, P. (2010). *Rare Diseases Day. Report on the 2010 Campaign. 2010.* Krakow, Poland: European Organization for Rare Diseases; Retrieved from https://www.rarediseaseday.org/article/rare-disease-day-2010

The Lancet Diabetes & Endocrinology. (2019). Spotlight on rare diseases. *The Lancet Diabetes & Endocrinology, 7*(2), 75. doi:10.10162213-8587(19)30006-3

Theofanidis, D. (2007). Chronic illness in childhood: Psychosocial adaptation and nursing support for the child and family. *Health Science Journal, 2*, 1–8.

Thompson, T. L. (2000). The nature and language of illness explanations. In B. B. Whaley (Ed.), *Explaining Illness: Research, Theory, and Strategies* (pp. 3–40). Mahwah, NJ: Erlbaum.

Timmermans, S., & Buchbinder, M. (2010). Patients-in-waiting: Living between sickness and health in the genomics era. *Journal of Health and Social Behavior, 51*(4), 408–423. doi:10.1177/0022146510386794 PMID:21131618

Tobia, A., Mintz, J., Rudge, D., Bisen, V., Trenton, A., Draschil, T., & Dobkin, R. (2016). Deconstructing the film sinister through the lens of psychiatry. *African Journal of Psychiatry (South Africa), 19*(2). doi:10.4172/2378-5756.1000354

Tommasetti, A., Troisi, O., & Cosimato, S. (2014). Patient empowerment and health online community: two ways to give the new viability doctor-patient relationship= Cooperación y intercambio de conocimiento en la era de Internet: dos maneras de dar nueva viabilidad a la relación médico-paciente. Comunitania. *Revista Internacional de Trabajo Social y Ciencias Sociales*, (8), 9-23. doi:10.5944/comunitania.8.1

Torrente, E., Escarrabill, J., & Martí, T. (2010). Impacto de las redes sociales de pacientes en la práctica asistencial. *Revista de Innovación Sanitaria y Atención Integrada, 2*(1), 1.

Tozzi, A., Mingarelli, R., Agricola, E., Gonfiantini, M., Pandolfi, E., Carloni, E., ... Dallapiccola, B. (2013). The internet user profile of Italian families of patients with rare diseases: A web survey. *Orphanet Journal of Rare Diseases, 8*(76), 1–8. doi:10.1186/1750-1172-8-76 PMID:23680013

Tran, K. D., Smutzer, G. S., Doty, R. L., & Arnold, S. E. (1998). Reduced Purkinje cell size in the cerebellar vermis of elderly patients with schizophrenia. *The American Journal of Psychiatry, 155*(9), 1288–1290. doi:10.1176/ajp.155.9.1288 PMID:9734558

Tran, T. T., Ahn, J., & Reau, N. S. (2016). ACG Clinical Guideline: Liver Disease and Pregnancy. *The American Journal of Gastroenterology, 111*(2), 176–194, quiz 196. doi:10.1038/ajg.2015.430 PMID:26832651

Trebble, T. M., Hansi, N., Hydes, T., Smith, M. A., & Baker, M. (2010). Process mapping the patient journey: An introduction. *BMJ (Clinical Research Ed.), 341.* doi:10.1136/bmj.c4078 PMID:20709715

Trinidad, B., & Lala, V. (2019). Takayasu Arteritis. In *StatPearls*. Treasure Island, FL: StatPearls Publishing.

Trujillano, D., Oprea, G. E., Schmitz, Y., Bertoli-Avella, A. M., Abou Jamra, R., & Rolfs, A. (2017). A comprehensive global genotype–phenotype database for rare diseases. *Molecular genetics & genomic medicine, 5*(1), 66-75. doi: . eCollection 2017 Jan. doi:10.1002/mgg3.262

Turner, C. E., Drenckhahn, V. V., & Bates, M. W. (1935). Effectiveness of radio in health education. *American Journal of Public Health and the Nation's Health, 25*(5), 589–594. doi:10.2105/AJPH.25.5.589 PMID:18014216

U.S. Department of Health and Human Services. (2000). Healthy People 2010: Understanding and improving health and objectives for improving health. US Department of Health and Human Services. Washington, DC. Retrieved from http://www.cdc.gov/nchs/data/hpdata2010/hp2010_final_review.pdf

U.S. Department of Health and Human Services. (2005). Making Health Communication Programs Work. Retrieved from http://www.cancer.gov/publications/health-communication/pink-book.pdf

U.S. Department of Health and Human Services. (2014). What is health literacy. Retrieved from http://www.health.gov/communication/literacy/

Uhlenbusch, N., Löwe, B., Härter, M., Schramm, C., Weiler-Normann, C., & Depping, M. K. (2019). Depression and anxiety in patients with different rare chronic diseases: A cross-sectional study. *PLoS One, 14*(2). doi:10.1371/journal.pone.0211343 PMID:30785907

United Nations – UN. (2919). Goal 3: Ensure healthy lives and promote well-being for all at all ages. Retrieved from https://www.un.org/sustainabledevelopment/health/

Urrutia, J. M. (2013). El Día Mundial de las Enfermedades Raras en las noticias de prensa. *El ejemplo de Andalucía, Discurso, & Sociedad, 7*(1), 224–247.

Urrutia, J. M. (2013). El Día Mundial de las Enfermedades Raras en las noticias de prensa. El ejemplo de Andalucía. *Discurso & Sociedad, 1*(7), 224–247.

Valenzuela-Rodríguez, G. (2012). Análisis de los casos clínicos presentados en la serie médica televisiva Dr. House. *Rev Soc Peru Med Interna, 25*(2), 65.

Van de Bovenkamp, H. M., & Trappenburg, M. J. (2011). Government influence on patient organizations. *Health Care Analysis, 19*(4), 329–351. doi:10.100710728-010-0155-7 PMID:20803075

Van Dijck, J. (2002). Medical documentary: Conjoined twins as a mediated spectacle. *Media Culture & Society, 24*(4), 537–556. doi:10.1177/016344370202400405

van Dijk, M. T., van Wingen, G. A., van Lammeren, A., Blom, R. M., de Kwaasteniet, B. P., Scholte, H. S., & Denys, D. (2013). Neural basis of limb ownership in individuals with body integrity identity disorder. *PLoS One, 8*(8). doi:10.1371/journal.pone.0072212 PMID:23991064

Vance, K., Howe, W., & Dellavalle, R. P. (2009). Social Internet Sites as a source of Public Health Information. *Dermatologic Clinics, 27*(2), 133–136. doi:10.1016/j.det.2008.11.010 PMID:19254656

Vertov, D. (1984). *Kino-Eye: The Writings of Dziga Vertov*. London, UK: University of California.

Vieira, T., Schwartz, I., Muñoz, V., Pinto, L., Steiner, C., Ribeiro, M., ... Giugliani, R. (2008). Mucopolysaccharidoses in Brazil: What happens from birth to biochemical diagnosis? *American Journal of Medical Genetics*, *146A*(13), 1741–1747. doi:10.1002/ajmg.a.32320 PMID:18546277

Villa, À. À., Llombart, B. E., Solanillo, C. F., Queralt, A. R. & Castillo, S. S. (2014). *Las Enfermedades Raras en los Medios.* Madrid: Observatorio de Enfermedades Raras, OBSER.

Virzi, A., Dipasquale, S., Signorelli, M., Aguglia, E., Bianchini, O., & Palermo, F. (2011). Movie portrayals of physicians and the doctor-patient relationship. *Journal of Cognitive and Behavioral Psychotherapies*, *6*(2), 475–485.

Wadhera, R. (2016). Celebrities and social cause–detailed analysis of importance of choosing a celebrity followed by pulse polio advertisement. *International Journal of Advance Research, Ideas. Innovations in Technology*, *2*(6), 1–9.

Wakefield, M. A., Loken, B., & Hornik, R. C. (2010). Use of mass media campaigns to change health behaviour. *Lancet*, *376*(9748), 1261–1271. doi:10.1016/S0140-6736(10)60809-4 PMID:20933263

Waldboth, V., Patch, C., Mahrer-Imhof, R., & Metcalfe, A. (2016). Living a normal life in an extraordinary way: A systematic review investigating experiences of families of young people's transition into adulthood when affected by a genetic and chronic childhood condition. *International Journal of Nursing Studies*, *62*, 44–59. doi:10.1016/j.ijnurstu.2016.07.007 PMID:27450665

Walker, K. K. (2013). Rare disease-specific social media sites: An opportunity for collaboration. *Journal of Communication in Healthcare*, *6*(1), 71–76. doi:10.1179/1753807612Y.0000000026

Wallack, L., Dorfman, L., Jernigan, D., & Themba-Nixon, M. (1993). *Media advocacy and public health: Power for prevention.* Newbury Park, CA: Sage.

Wamelink, M. M., Gruning, N. M., Jansen, E. E., Bluemlein, K., Lehrach, H., Jakobs, C., & Ralser, M. (2010). The difference between rare and exceptionally rare: Molecular characterization of ribose 5-phosphate isomerase deficiency. *Journal of Molecular Medicine (Berlin, Germany)*, *88*(9), 931–939. doi:10.100700109-010-0634-1 PMID:20499043

Wang, W., Wang, S. A., Medeiros, L. J., & Khoury, J. D. (2017). Pure erythroid leukemia. *American Journal of Hematology*, *92*(3), 292–296. doi:10.1002/ajh.24626 PMID:28006859

Waring, J. J. (2009). Constructing and re-constructing narratives of patient safety. *Social Science & Medicine*, *69*(12), 1722–1731. doi:10.1016/j.socscimed.2009.09.052 PMID:19883965

Warne, T., & McAndrew, S. (2007). Passive patient or engaged expert? Using a Ptolemaic approach to enhance mental health nurse education and practice. *International Journal of Mental Health Nursing*, *16*(4), 224–229. doi:10.1111/j.1447-0349.2007.00471.x PMID:17635621

Watson, L., Richardson, A. R. W., Holt, R. C. L., Jones, C. A., & Beresford, M. W. (2012). Henoch Schonlein Purpura – A 5-Year Review and Proposed Pathway. *PLoS One*, *7*(1). doi:10.1371/journal.pone.0029512 PMID:22235302

Weber Shandwick. (2018). The Great American Search for Healthcare Information. Retrieved from https://www.webershandwick.com/wp-content/uploads/2018/11/Healthcare-Info-Search-Report.pdf

Weiss, M. (1997). Signifying the pandemics: Metaphors of AIDS, cancer, and heart disease. *Medical Anthropology Quarterly*, *11*(4), 456–476. doi:10.1525/maq.1997.11.4.456 PMID:9408901

White, J. J. (1990). An Overview of the Genitourinary System. In H. K. Walker, W. D. Hall, & J. W. Hurst (Eds.), *Clinical Methods: The History, Physical, and Laboratory Examinations*. Boston, MA: Butterworths, Butterworth Publishers.

WHO -World Health Organization. (2012, June). *Coming together to combat rare diseases.* Bulletin of the World Health Organization, 90(6), June 2012, 401-476. Retrieved from https://www.who.int/bulletin/volumes/90/6/12-020612/en/ (Access date: August 13, 2019)

Wicks, P., Massagli, M., Frost, J., Brownstein, C., Okun, S., Vaughan, T., ... Heywood, J. (2010). Sharing health data for better outcomes on PatientsLikeMe. *Journal of Medical Internet Research*, *12*(2), e19. doi:10.2196/jmir.1549 PMID:20542858

Wijnberg-Williams, J., Van de Wiel, M., Kamps, W., & Hoekstra-Weebers, M. (2015). Effects of communication styles on marital satisfaction and distress of parents of pediatric cancer patients: A prospective longitudinal study. *Psycho-Oncology*, *24*(1), 106–112. doi:10.1002/pon.3617 PMID:25045011

Williams, P. H. (2011). Policy framework for rare disease health disparities. *Policy, Politics, & Nursing Practice*, *12*(2), 114–118. doi:10.1177/1527154411404243 PMID:21486874

Williford, A. P., Calkins, S. D., & Keane, S. P. (2007). Predicting change in parenting stress across early childhood: Child and maternal factors. *Journal of Abnormal Child Psychology*, *35*(2), 251–263. doi:10.100710802-006-9082-3 PMID:17186365

Wilson, C. (2013). Orphan drugs and orphan drug legislation. In E. Hernberg-Ståhl, & M. Reljanović (Eds.), *Orphan Drugs Understanding the Rare Disease Market and Its Dynamics, Woodhead Publishing Series in Biomedicine*. Cambridge, UK: Woodhead Publishing. doi:10.1533/9781908818393.9

Wilson, N., Heath, D., Heath, T., Gallagher, P., & Huthwaite, M. (2014). Madness at the movies: Prioritised movies for self-directed learning by medical students. *Australasian Psychiatry*, *22*(5), 450–453. doi:10.1177/1039856214545550 PMID:25135436

Winston, E. R., Dawn Medlin, B., & Adriana Romaniello, B. (2012). An e-patient's end-user community (EUCY): The value added of social network applications. *Computers in Human Behavior*, *28*(3), 951–957. doi:10.1016/j.chb.2011.12.016

Witte, K. (1992). Putting the fear back into fear appeals: The extended parallel process model. *Communication Monographs*, *59*(4), 329–349. doi:10.1080/03637759209376276

Witte, K. (1998). Fear as motivator, fear as inhibitor: Using the extended parallel process model to explain fear appeal successes and failures. In P. A. Andersen, & L. K. Guerrero (Eds.), *Handbook of communication and emotion: Research, theory, applications, and contexts* (pp. 423–450). San Diego, CA: Academic Press.

Woerndl, M., Papagiannidis, S. S., Bourlakis, M., & Li, F. (2008). Internet-induced marketing techniques: Critical factors in viral marketing campaigns. *International Journal of Business Science and Applied Management, 3*, 33–45.

World Economic Forum. (2017). The future of treating rare diseases. Retrieved from https://www.weforum.org/agenda/2017/01/the-future-of-treating-rare-diseases/

World Health Organization - WHO. (2018). Statement for Rare Disease Day. Retrieved from https://www.who.int/mediacentre/news/statements/2018/rare-disease-day/en/

Wright, C. R. (1960). Functional analysis and mass communication. *Public Opinion Quarterly, 24*(4), 605–620. doi:10.1086/266976

Wright, K. B., Bell, S. B., Wright, K. B., & Bell, S. B. (2003). Health-related support groups on the Internet: Linking empirical findings to social support and computer-mediated communication theory. *Journal of Health Psychology, 8*(1), 39–54. doi:10.1177/1359105303008001429 PMID:22113899

Wright, K. B., Sparks, L., & O'Hair, H. D. (2008). *Health Communication in the 21st century*. Oxford, UK: Blackwell.

Xu, W. W., Chiu, I. H., Chen, Y., & Mukherjee, T. (2015). Twitter hashtags for health: Applying network and content analyses to understand the health knowledge sharing in a Twitter-based community of practice. *Quality & Quantity, 49*(4), 1361–1380. doi:10.100711135-014-0051-6

Yaffe, M. G., Kaback, M. M., Goldberg, M., Miles, J., Itabashi, H., McIntyre, H., & Mohandas, T. (1979). An amyotrophic lateral sclerosis-like syndrome with hexosaminidase - A deficiency: A new type of GM2 ganglisidosis [Abstract]. *Neurology, 29*(1), 611.

Yeh, C. H., Lee, T. T., Chen, M. L., & Li, W. (2000). Adaptational process of parents of pediatric oncology patients. *Pediatric Hematology and Oncology, 17*(2), 119–131. doi:10.1080/088800100276479 PMID:10734654

Yılmaz, E., Afşarlar, Ç. E., Karaman, İ., Özgüner, İ. F., Karaman, A., & Hızlı, F. (2013). Congenital hemiscrotal agenesis: Report of a rare entity. *Journal of Pediatric Urology, 9*(1), e76–e77. doi:10.1016/j.jpurol.2012.09.005 PMID:23044375

Yokoyama, T., Nakamura, S., Horiuchi, E., Ishiyama, M., Kawashima, R., Nakamura, K., & Yagishita, S. (2014). Late onset GM2 gangliosidosis presenting with motor neuron disease: An autopsy case. *Neuropathology, 34*(3), 304–308. doi:10.1111/neup.12088 PMID:24354582

Yoon, P. W., Bresee, J. S., Olney, R. S., James, L. M., & Khoury, M. J. (1997). Epidemiology of biliary atresia: A population-based study. *Pediatrics, 99*(3), 376–382. doi:10.1542/peds.99.3.376 PMID:9041292

Yzer, M. (2012). The integrative model of behavioral prediction as a tool for designing health messages. In H. Cho (Ed.), *Health communication message design: Theory and practice* (pp. 21–40). London, UK: Sage.

Zagalo-Cardoso, J. A. (2001). Doenças genéticas: Impacto psicológico e representações sociais. [Genetic diseases: Psychological impact and social representations] In *M. C. Canavarro (Org.), Psicologia da Gravidez e da Maternidade* (pp. 211–235). Coimbra, Portugal: Quarteto Editora.

Zaid, T., Burzawa, J., Basen-Engquist, K., Bodurka, D. C., Ramondetta, L. M., Brown, J., & Frumovitz, M. (2014). Use of social media to conduct a cross-sectional epidemiologic and quality of life survey of patients with neuroendocrine carcinoma of the cervix: A feasibility study. *Gynecologic Oncology*, *132*(1), 149–153. doi:10.1016/j.ygyno.2013.10.015 PMID:24145111

Zamel, R., Khan, R., Pollex, R. L., & Hegele, R. A. (2008). Abetalipoproteinemia: Two case reports and literature review. *Orphanet Journal of Rare Diseases*, *3*(1), 19–19. doi:10.1186/1750-1172-3-19 PMID:18611256

Zaroff, C. M., Neudorfer, O., Morrison, C., Pastores, G. M., Rubin, H., & Kolodny, E. H. (2004). Neuropsychological assessment of patients with late onset GM2 gangliosidosis. *Neurology*, *62*(12), 2283–2286. doi:10.1212/01.WNL.0000130498.19019.02 PMID:15210895

Zelnik, N., Khazanov, V., Sheinkman, A., Karpati, A. M., & Peleg, L. (2000). Clinical Manifestations of Psychiatric Patients Who Are Carriers of Tay - Sachs disease. *Neuropsychobiology*, *41*(3), 127–131. doi:10.1159/000026644 PMID:10754426

Zhao, D., & Rosson, M. B. (2009). How and why people Twitter. In *Proceedings of the ACM 2009 international conference on Supporting group work - GROUP '09* (p. 243). New York, NY: ACM Press. 10.1145/1531674.1531710

Zuo, Z., Polski, J. M., Kasyan, A., & Medeiros, L. J. (2010). Acute erythroid leukemia. *Archives of Pathology & Laboratory Medicine*, *134*(9), 1261–1270. doi:10.1043/2009-0350-ra.1 PMID:20807044

Zurynski, Y., Deverell, M., Dalkeith, T., Johnson, S., Christodoulou, J., Leonard, H., & Elliott, E. J. (2017). Australian children living with rare diseases: Experiences of diagnosis and perceived consequences of diagnostic delays. *Orphanet Journal of Rare Diseases*, *12*(1), 68. doi:10.118613023-017-0622-4 PMID:28399928

Zurynski, Y., Frith, K., Leonard, H., & Elliott, E. (2008). Rare childhood diseases: How should we respond? *Archives of Disease in Childhood*, *93*(12), 1071–1074. doi:10.1136/adc.2007.134940 PMID:18684747

About the Contributors

Liliana Vale Costa is a researcher at Digimedia - Digital Media and Interaction Research Centre and invited lecturer in Editorial Media, at the University of Aveiro (Portugal). She holds a European Ph.D. in Information and Communication in Digital Platforms at the University of Aveiro and University of Porto (with internship at the Disruptive Media Learning Lab, Coventry University); a M.A degree in Multimedia Communication and a B.Sc. in New Technologies of Communication, both at the University of Aveiro. Her research interests are universal design, digital games, virtual communities, three-dimensional environments, ageing studies, learning, human-computer interaction, computer-mediated communication, natural interfaces, eHealth, mobile apps and digital inclusion.

Sonia Oliveira is member of HMRI (Hunter Medical Research Institute) and HCRA (Hunter Cancer Research Alliance) (Australia) and CICECO - Aveiro Institute of Materials (Portugal). She received her PhD in Human Physiology from the University of Newcastle, Australia, and also holds a Master in Cellular and Molecular Biology from the University of Aveiro, Portugal. During her PhD, she explored the Nerve-Cancer connection in tumors. She also worked in the genetic and molecular control of the mammalian male meiosis and in the anatomical and physiologic effects of compounds present in herbal extracts. She has broad research interests namely in pathology, regenerative medicine and in neurophysiology. She is interested in using biotechnology and biomimetic systems to cure mammalian disorders, namely through the application of stem cells to correct mammalian tissues defects.

* * *

Celia Belim has a Ph.D. in Social Sciences, specialty of Communication Sciences (2016). She is an Assistant Professor at the School of Social and Political Sciences from the University of Lisboa (Portugal). She has worked in various communication sub-fields, such as journalism, organizational communication and media advisory. She has been publishing and participating in international conferences on her focus of interest, which are media representations, filmic analysis, semiotics, political image and communication, media, political and public agenda, and health communication.

Yolanda Berdasco-Gancedo is a journalist and a Spanish philologist with a Ph.D. and thesis on the language of specialized media. She has spent most of her career around specialized journalism. She has worked for media and government institutions and currently teaches at Madrid Open University (UDIMA, Spain), while covering some public interest issues in public media.

Sandra Diehl (PhD, Saarland University, Germany) is an Associate Professor at the Department for Media and Communication at the University of Klagenfurt, Austria. Her research interests include intercultural advertising and CSR and (m- and e-) health communication. She has published in several journals (e.g., International Journal of Advertising, Journal of Business Research, Media and Psychology, International Marketing Review) and authored and edited several books. She is board member of the European Advertising Academy.

Cátia Filipa da Silva Ferreira recently earned her master's in Clinical Psychology from the University of Trás-Os-Montes and Alto Douro (Portugal) where she focused in the psychological aspects of parental attachment and parenthood in the coping and management processes of having a child with a rare disorder.

Nathan Gadoth is the chairman of the Department of Neurology at the Maynei Hayeshuah Medical Center, Bnei-Brak (Israel) and the head of the institutional review board. He is a professor of Neurology (Emeritus), at the Sackler Faculty of Medicine, Tel-Aviv University, Israel. He has obtained an MD degree from Hadassah Medical School, The Hebrew University, Jerusalem, in 1969. He has trained in Pediatric Neurology at the Johns Hopkins University Hospital in Baltimore USA (1972-1975). He is Israeli board certified in pediatric, adult and pediatric neurology and developmental pediatrics. He has served as the chairmen of the Israeli pediatric neurology society, the Israeli neurological society, and currently the chairman of the Israeli chapter of the European Federation of Clinical Neurophysiology. His scientific interests are in the areas of neurogenetics, clinical neurophysiology, the autonomic nervous system, neuromuscular disorders, sleep medicine and epilepsy in children and adults.

Ana Cristina Bohrer Gilbert is a psychotherapist and an independent researcher. Her academic background is in Psychology and Psychotherapy and she has been working at the intersection of Humanities, Social Sciences and Public Health since her graduation. She has a PhD in Women and Child's Health and her research interests include cultural studies, disability studies, disability, art and the body, cultural complex (in a Jungian perspective), and technologies of the self. She is the author of "*Vértice do impensável: um estudo de narrativas em síndrome de Down*" (2012, Editora Fiocruz).

Dafne D. G. Horovitz is a clinical geneticist and pediatrician at the National Institute of Women, Children and Adolescent Health Fernandes Figueira / Fiocruz, in Rio de Janeiro, Brazil. Her work involves diagnosis and management of birth defects and disabilities, prenatal diagnosis, genetic counseling, chromosomal abnormalities, new treatments for genetic diseases, and public health policies in genetics. She has a PhD in Public Health policies, having worked for the past 15 years in the inclusion of care for birth defects and genetic disorders in the agenda of the Ministry of Health and in the Brazilian Health System. Dr Horovitz has been in the board of directors of the Brazilian Society of Medical Genetics for several years and is a consulting member of the Brazilian Ministry of Health for the special policy on rare diseases. She has published and collaborated in research in medical genetics, lysosomal storage disorders, and in public health.

Isabell Koinig is a Postdoctoral Researcher at the Media and Communication at the University of Klagenfurt, Austria. In her PhD, she investigated how different pharmaceutical advertisement appeals are received in a cross-cultural context as well as, the degree at which these appeals facilitate consumer self-empowerment. Her research interests predominantly concern the areas of health communication (advertising, social media, mHealth, health for sustainable development, and wearables), intercultural advertising, organizational health, and media and convergence management.

Maria Angelica de F. D. de Lima is a medical geneticist, with specialization in neurology and oncogenetics. She works at the Gaffrée e Guinle University Hospital. Her work involves disability studies, public health policies in genetics and genetic counselling. She has a PhD in Women and Child's Health.

Michaela Liuccio is a Professor in Sociology at the Department of Communication and Social research, "La Sapienza" University of Rome (Italy). She has a degree in Humanities and Sociology and a Ph.D. in Sociology of culture and political processes, from "La Sapienza" University of Rome. She has been awarded with fellowships from the Centre d'Etude sur l'Actuel et le Quotidien, University René Descartes, La Sorbonne, Paris, the 'Institute of Communication and Health, University of Lugano-Switzerland, the School of Journalism and Communication and Tsinghua University of Beijing. Michaela is the president for the master's degree in Scientific Biomedical Communication at La Sapienza University of Rome, where she also lectures "Health and Society". Member of Editorial Board: Journal of Communication in Healthcare: Strategies, Media, and Engagement in Global Health Director publishing series "Communication and health", Aracne Editrice Project leader of the research observatory "Chiediloqui" http://www.coris.uniroma1.it/unit-di-ricerca/18291. Specialized in sociology, her research focuses on communication and health.

Catarina Pinheiro Mota is a Clinical Psychologist, Psychotherapist and Professor at the University of Trás-os-Montes and Alto Douro (UTAD, Portugal). She earned her PhD in Familiar and Clinical Psychology in 2008 from the University of Porto (Portugal). She is also a Researcher in the Center for Psychology from the University of Porto.

Cláudia Pernencar is working as an Independent consultant in digital healthcare industry. She holds a PhD in Digital Media (FCSH.UNL - University of Austin Portugal Co-Lab) where she studied how IBD Portuguese patients were able to track specific disease symptoms using mobile apps. Between 2017 and 2019 she was involved in a funded multidisciplinary project - the TeenPower –, as a collaborator researcher from LIDA - Design and Arts Research Lab from the Institute Polytechnic of Leiria. She worked in how gamification techniques could prevent obesity through strategic assignments implemented in a mobile app. Currently, as a researcher from the ICNova (NOVA School of Social Sciences and Humanities, University NOVA of Lisboa) she is working with DigiMedia - Aveiro University. In this collaboration project, she is studying how opinion leaders are using Instagram to promote eating behavior and how health challenges are being used by them, and what is the impact on behavior change in the general public. Her work relates to EMR UX, Digital Health, Healthy behavior promotion, Human Factors for Wellbeing, Health Service Design, User Experience Design, and Usability testing.

Inga Saboia is a teacher at the Federal University of Ceara, Brazil. Her main university subjects are User Interface Design, Human Computer Interaction, Web Design, and Visual Communication. She is also a PhD candidate in Information and Communication in Digital Platforms in a conjoint doctoral program from the Universities of Aveiro and of Porto. She is also a collaborating researcher at DigiMedia research center from The University of Aveiro. Her topics of interest are social media, opinion leaders and eating behavior. Her work has been focused in how gamification techniques can be developed into a mobile app for weight control, as well as how opinion leaders influence the eating behavior of their Instagram followers and how the online health challenges are promoted by Instagram leaders. Other interests include digital health, health communication, healthy behavior promotion and usability testing.

Beatriz Moreira Silva Santos has a master's degree in Clinical Psychology from the University of Trás-Os-Montes and Alto Douro (UTAD, Portugal). Currently, she is a research fellow under the CareME project: "Efficacy of an attachment-based intervention in residential care: A randomized controlled trial on the effects on the caregivers' relational skills and the adolescents' psychosocial adaptation".

Ana Isabel Veloso is an Assistant Professor with habilitation (*agregação*) and the Dean of the Department of Communication and Art of the University of Aveiro. Throughout years, Ana Veloso has been supervising many students of master's and doctoral degree levels. She has also been the coordinator of several research projects, such as SEDUCE 2.0, SEDUCE, EYES ON GAMES, IMP.cubed. She did her Ph.D. in Communication Sciences and Technologies at the University of Aveiro. Before her doctoral studies, in 2006, she obtained her MSc in Biomedical Engineering and bachelor's in Informatics Engineering from the University of Coimbra. Her research interests include video games, gerontechnology and other applications of information and communication in technological mediated contexts.

Paloma Lopez Villafranca is a lecturer at the Audiovisual Communication and Advertising Department at the University of Malaga (Spain) since 2009. She has been a visiting researcher at the University of Sheffield (UK), University of Minho (Braga, Portugal) and University of Sapienza (Rome, Italy). Her field of study includes communication on radio, narrative, health and strategic communication. She has participated in several international conferences and has authored several articles published in communication journals. She has worked in Prisa, Recoletos, RNE (Radio Nacional de Espana) and local communication groups.

Index

S

T

U

www.ingramcontent.com/pod-product-compliance
Lightning Source LLC
LaVergne TN
LVHW080909300926
849162LV00003B/619